Confronting Critical Health Issues
OF ASIAN AND PACIFIC ISLANDER AMERICANS

Confronting Critical Health Issues

OF ASIAN AND PACIFIC ISLANDER AMERICANS

edited by

Nolan W. S. Zane
David T. Takeuchi
Kathleen N. J. Young

Published under the auspices of the Asian
& Pacific Islander American Health Forum

SAGE Publications
International Educational and Professional Publisher
Thousand Oaks   London   New Delhi

For information address:

SAGE Publications, Inc.
2455 Teller Road
Thousand Oaks, California 91320

SAGE Publications Ltd.
6 Bonhill Street
London EC2A 4PU
United Kingdom

SAGE Publications India Pvt. Ltd.
M-32 Market
Greater Kailash I
New Delhi 110 048 India

Printed in the United States of America

Library of Congress Cataloging-in-Publication Data

Main entry under title:

Confronting critical health issues of Asian and Pacific Islander
   Americans / edited by Nolan Zane, David Takeuchi, Kathleen Young.
      p.   cm.
   Includes bibliographical references and index.
   ISBN 0-8039-5113-2 (cl)
      1. Asian Americans—Health and hygiene. 2. Pacific Islanders—
Health and hygiene. 3. Asian Americans—Medical care. 4. Pacific
Islanders—Medical care. 5. Asian Americans—Diseases. 6. Pacific
Islanders—Diseases. I. Zane, Nolan. II. Takeuchi, David.
III. Young, Kathleen.
RA448.5.A83C66 1994
362.1'089'95073—dc20   93-34623

94 95 96 97 98 10 9 8 7 6 5 4 3 2 1

Sage Production Editor: Diane S. Foster

Contents

Preface:
Beyond "Black, White, and Other"

Asian and Pacific Islander Americans make up the fastest-growing ethnic community in the United States today. While that growth affords us a tremendous opportunity to take a greater role in the life of this nation, it presents challenges as well. Building a responsive health care system must certainly rank among the greatest of those challenges.

The undeniable truth is that many Asian Pacific Americans must deal with critical health issues in a health care system that does not respond to their needs as individuals or as a community. For far too long, those problems have gone unrecognized by public health policy makers and political leaders. It is my hope that this is finally beginning to change, as we work to educate our fellow Americans about our histories, our cultures, and our communities.

More than anything else, the story of Asian Pacific American health is one of dealing with diversity. We have long understood that we cannot rely on systems of data collection and health research that combine all Asian Pacific populations into one illusory homogeneous whole. Perhaps more than any other group of Americans, we recognize that statistics are meaningless if the lives and hopes of individuals remain hidden within them.

The passage of the Disadvantaged Minority Health Improvement Act of 1990 was a hallmark achievement, finally signaling federal recognition that existing health data collection systems were inadequate for Asian Pacific Americans. Three years after its passage, the National Center for Health Statistics, the principal health data collection agency of the federal government, now collects and reports ethnically detailed vital statistics data on 75% of the Asian Pacific American population. Previously, it had not collected any such ethnicity-specific data. In addition, the funding of research studies to discover the health variations among these communities is producing findings that can only facilitate better health policy and enhanced services for these communities.

Clearly, much more needs to be done. Our national health data collection system must be expanded until all Asian Pacific Americans are included, not only in vital statistics registries but in disease surveillance by the Centers for Disease Control and in research at the National Institutes of Health. But ultimately, the success of the Disadvantaged Minority Health Improvement Act should be a source of hope. We have learned that our fellow Americans *can* be educated about the unique characteristics within our communities, and that positive results can be achieved.

The research reported in this volume is an important part of our efforts at the local, state, and national levels to finally break through the ironclad categories of "black, white, and other" into which health data have traditionally been divided. This book constitutes the first major critical appraisal of the health status of Asian Pacific Americans. Experts from a variety of scientific disciplines have been brought together to provide comprehensive analyses of what we know about Asian Pacific health and health care and, more important, what more we need to know. This volume also represents another major contribution by the Asian and Pacific Islander American Health Forum in moving our community forward. Our challenge is to build on this empirical work to establish a truly responsive health care system for all Asian Pacific American communities. It is a challenge that we will not ignore.

Congressman Norman Mineta
State of California

Introduction

NOLAN ZANE
DAVID T. TAKEUCHI

This book is a product of the Asian & Pacific Islander American Health Forum's visionary leadership for improving health services and research in Asian Pacific American communities. In 1988 the Forum sponsored a national conference to address some of the serious health problems among the Asian Pacific population. The conference convened leaders in policy, research, health care, and community issues to focus on confronting these problems. One concern was the lack of a strong empirical base to assess the health status and need for health services among Asian Pacific Americans. Policy makers and service providers have had to rely on outdated studies, anecdotal material, and research with serious methodological or conceptual flaws to make decisions about the health care needs of Asian Pacific Americans. In the past, the absence of a substantial research foundation often resulted in government policies that minimized their health needs and reduced the likelihood that important prevention and treatment programs would be established for high-risk groups in these communities. These problems were compounded because the Asian Pacific American population is increasing at a rapid rate, placing even greater demands on policy makers to respond to the growing health needs of the communities that make up this population.

Issues raised during the conference underscored the need to compile a publication that would examine the state of knowledge about Asian Pacific American health. Accordingly, this book follows the spirit and intent of the 1988 conference, and we are indebted to the participants for setting the agenda for much of what follows. The primary purpose of this volume is to review and critique the existing knowledge about Asian Pacific American health status. Our hope is that this evaluation and interpretation of what is known, as well as what is not known, about the health of Asian Pacific Americans will stimulate a reexamination of their health issues in a sensitive and comprehensive manner that moves beyond the common stereotypes associated with the "model minority" myth, namely, that most Asian Pacific Americans have good health and receive adequate health care. Given President Clinton's emphasis on reorganizing the U.S. health care system, the issues examined by the contributing authors are timely and salient; the chapters presented here should provide the bases for the establishment of better health priorities for the various Asian Pacific American populations. Equally important, the chapters articulate some critical strategies and directions for the next generation of empirical studies that address Asian Pacific American health concerns.

At this point, it is important that we address the terms that will be used to refer to Asian American and Pacific Islander populations. We use the term *Asian Pacific Americans* to refer to the collective set of Asian American and Pacific Islander American populations. However, although many Asian Pacific groups share certain value orientations, migration experiences, and so on, use of this term is in no way meant to imply that these populations or communities are homogeneous in nature. In fact, it will become apparent throughout this book that the heterogeneity of the Asian Pacific populations with respect to health problems and needs constitutes an important health issue that has often been neglected. Finally, we have adopted the convention of referring to people from the Philippines as *Filipinos*, rather than *Pilipinos*. The latter term was developed by community activists in the 1960s and 1970s to honor the old immigrants. In most languages and dialects spoken in the Philippines, there is no *f* sound, and the term *Pilipino* was developed as an alternative to Filipino, which was considered to be associated with the colonization of the Philippines by Western European nations. However, as Chan (1991) notes, "Today's highly educated immigrants consider it an insult to imply they cannot pronounce the *f* sound, so *Filipino* is now more acceptable."

This book is divided into three general sections that address the context, health status, and health service and policy issues concerning Asian Pacific Americans. Because empirical health research on this population has been neglected in the past, each chapter could have begun with a general critique about the lack of data and the problems inherent in conducting health research in these minority communities. Rather than reiterating these themes in each chapter, however, the two chapters in Part I highlight some common methodological and conceptual problems researchers often confront in conducting research on Asian Pacific American communities. Specific concerns unique to an area are discussed in the individual chapters. In the first chapter, David T. Takeuchi and Kathleen N. J. Young provide an overview of the Asian Pacific American populations. They describe the diversity of the ethnic groups that are categorized under the *Asian Pacific* or *Asian American* rubric and discuss some general conceptual issues that must be considered in understanding the social construction of health in minority communities. Whereas the overview presents some common problems in conducting health research in Asian Pacific American communities, in Chapter 2, Elena S. H. Yu and William T. Liu provide a comprehensive methodological essay on the nature of epidemiological studies. Yu and Liu draw upon their vast research experience to discuss the problems in previous national surveys on Asian Pacific American health status. In their conclusion, they establish an insightful agenda for future work in this area.

Part II, on health status, comprises eight chapters that address mortality, specific diseases, and health problems. Robert Gardner begins this section by reviewing the mortality data on Asian Pacific Americans. The chapter centers on three salient dimensions of Asian Pacific American mortality: levels and patterns of mortality, comparison of Asian Pacific mortality rates with those of the white population in the United States, and factors that explain the observed levels and patterns. To address these dimensions, Gardner conducts an extensive review of the literature, providing valuable commentary about the meanings and implications of the studies he discusses.

One in four Americans will develop some form of cancer. Despite the ubiquitous nature of this disease, very few epidemiologic data are available on cancer among Asian Pacific Americans. Christopher N. H. Jenkins and Marjorie Kagawa-Singer strip the disease of its mystery and critically evaluate the empirical investigations on cancer in this population. The authors enhance our understanding of cancer by commenting on specific types of cancers rather than using only the generic category. Their discussion of how the risks for different cancers vary among specific Asian Pacific ethnic groups is particularly revealing.

Hie-Won Lee Hann points out that more than 200 million persons in the world are chronically infected with the hepatitis B virus. In addition to having the disease, these people are also considered carriers of the virus. Carriers make up 5% of the world's population, but 75% of these carriers live in Asia. It has been estimated that about 5% to 20% of immigrants who come from Asia to the United States are hepatitis B carriers. Accordingly, with the large number of Asians who have immigrated to the United States over the past two decades, hepatitis B has emerged as one of the leading medical concerns in Asian Pacific American communities. Hann describes the medical nature of the disease and addresses the clinical treatment of the problem. She also articulates public health implications by listing the social correlates of the disease.

In Chapter 6, Douglas E. Crews provides a comprehensive summary of research on diabetes and obesity. Despite being a major health problem among Pacific Islander Americans, particularly Samoans and Native Hawaiians, the extent of obesity and diabetes in this population has not been adequately documented. Crews demonstrates his keen understanding of the problem by describing the nature of obesity and diabetes and then establishing the epidemiology and risk factors associated with these two problems. He also offers practical strategies for increasing Asian Pacific American participation in health promotion, disease prevention, and medical intervention.

As Ayala Tamir and Shirley Cachola indicate in Chapter 7, collectively, diseases of the heart continue to be a leading cause of death among Asian Pacific Americans. They examine each of the major risk factors for cardiovascular disease, namely, hypertension, smoking, hypercholesterolemia, high alcohol consumption, and lack of physical activity. Based on their review, they present specific recommendations for more responsive health research and better prevention and treatment interventions.

Terry S. Gock begins Chapter 8 by asserting that the mainstream media and Asian Pacific American communities have participated in a "conspiracy of silence" related to acquired immunodeficiency syndrome (AIDS) by maintaining the notion that AIDS is a disease contracted only by gay white men and drug users. Gock provides a compelling argument for dispelling myths surrounding AIDS in Asian Pacific American communities. He describes the disease in lay terms, then establishes the fact that incidence of AIDS in Asian Pacific American populations matches the rate found in other ethnic groups. He concludes his chapter by suggesting some creative avenues for research and intervention.

Like HIV/AIDS, mental health problems have not generally been seen as a critical concern in Asian Pacific American communities. In Chapter 9, Stanley Sue writes a critical review disputing this stereotyped notion. He provides extensive discussion of the epidemiological evidence that can be used to evaluate whether Asian Pacific Americans have equal, elevated, or reduced levels of psychopathology when compared with whites. The chapter provides an informative review of interventions that are meant to be culturally responsive to Asian Pacific Americans. The notion of culturally responsive services has wide application for the delivery of prevention and intervention health services.

Narratives on infectious diseases form the basis of the next two chapters. Richard S. Hann has written medically informed treatises on tuberculosis and parasitic infestations. Because immigrants and refugees constitute a substantial proportion of the Asian Pacific American population, a discussion of infectious diseases is extremely timely and valuable. These chapters establish a medical point of view of these diseases and provide an engaging contrast to other chapters in the book. The chapters conclude with some astute observations for providing clinical therapy in Asian Pacific American communities.

Substance use and abuse have emerged as significant health concerns for many Asian Pacific communities. In Chapter 12, Nolan Zane and Jeannie Huh Kim note the great variances in use and abuse rates among Asian Pacific American populations. They identify certain methodological problems that have impeded the accurate assessment of substance abuse issues in these communities and present empirical findings that dispute stereotypes about Asian Pacific drinking and other substance use habits. They show that, contrary to popular belief, certain Asian Pacific subgroups do drink heavily or are at high risk for drug use, that ethnicity-based physiological differences in metabolizing alcohol (e.g., the fast flushing response) do not "protect" Asian Pacific Americans from abusing alcohol, and that lower use rates do not necessarily imply less need for drug treatment and prevention services. Zane and Kim also discuss certain prevention strategies that may prove to be especially culturally appropriate for interventions in Asian Pacific American communities.

Laurin Mayeno and Sherry M. Hirota begin Part III, on health service and policy, by providing a critical commentary on the issues pertinent to the provision and receipt of quality health care. Unemployment, lack of health insurance, and lack of education and literacy are some of the common obstacles that often prevent Asian Pacific Americans from using health services in their communities. Mayeno and Hirota also address the obstacles that are common to various Asian Pacific groups. They conclude their review with recommendations for overcoming some of these barriers.

One possible barrier to the provision of health care for Asian Pacific Americans is a lack of health care professionals who come from these ethnic communities. In Chapter 14, Laura Uba tackles the issue of whether Asian Pacific Americans have reached parity with whites in numbers of health care professionals. She addresses the complexity of determining the numbers of health care providers of particular ethnicities and argues that the ways in which policy makers have defined this issue may be detrimental to Asian Pacific Americans.

The final chapter presents a framework that captures the formulation of health policy for Asian Pacific Americans. Ninez Ponce and Tessie Guillermo make use of their extensive experience on national health policy issues to assist readers in understanding the often complex maze of the national health care system. They conclude by offering a number of policy themes that have been used to advocate for the health care and research needs of Asian Pacific Americans. It is only fitting that this book conclude with a chapter on policy. The complexities and specific health needs of the various Asian Pacific populations in the United States have long gone unattended. Policy changes are necessary if we are to develop true "cultural responsiveness" in health care for Asian Pacific Americans.

In many ways, this book represents the beginning of a reexamination of the health statuses of populations that have often been relegated to the "other" category in previous health data collection efforts. If the issues highlighted in these chapters help bring about some recognition that the "other" designation is no longer tenable, then this beginning has been a successful one.

Reference

Chan, S. (1991). *Asian Americans: An interpretive history.* Boston: Twayne.

PART I

The Context

1

Overview of Asian
and Pacific Islander Americans

DAVID T. TAKEUCHI
KATHLEEN N. J. YOUNG

Asian Pacific American Ethnic Groups

It is only within the past 20 years that the term *Asian American* has been used to refer to a broad selection of ethnic groups. In the late 1960s and early 1970s, scholars engaged in ethnic studies sought a new label to sever ties with past stereotypes that created images of Asians as "exotic" or "inscrutable" Orientals (Takaki, 1987). However, as the Asian Pacific American population grew, the demand to extend analyses beyond a single label also increased.

In 1990 the population of Asian Pacific Americans exceeded 7.2 million, nearly doubling the 3.7 million figure in 1980. A little more than half of all Asian Pacific Americans live in the western United States, although the Asian and Pacific Islander population has also increased in other regions: by 139% in the South and Northeast, and by 97% and 95% in the Midwest and West, respectively. The majority of the Asian Pacific American population live in the states of California, New York, and Hawaii. There was a 127% increase in California's Asian Pacific American population between 1980 and 1990. The largest number of Asian Pacific Americans live in California

AUTHORS' NOTE: Research reported in this chapter was supported in part by National Institute of Mental Health Grants 44331 and 47526.

and, at 9.6% of California's population, they constitute the state's second largest minority group, after Latinos. In Hawaii, Asian Pacific Americans constitute 61.8% of the state population.

Overlooked in these figures is the fact that Asian Pacific Americans are often seen as a homogeneous ethnic category. The failure to make distinctions among specific ethnic groups can lead to faulty conclusions about important health needs among Asian Pacific Americans. The necessity of examining the health care issues of *specific* Asian Pacific American groups (e.g., Chinese, Filipino, Native Hawaiian, Samoan, Vietnamese) is a consistent theme in this book.

The emergence of Asian Pacific American communities demonstrates the diversity of the ethnic groups in the United States. Historical developments help shape the way ethnic groups relate to the dominant group and form the boundaries in which ethnic groups can express their cultural norms. A number of excellent resources are available that document the heterogeneity of the Asian Pacific American experience (see, for example, Chan, 1991; Takaki, 1987). Selected facets of some Asian Pacific American ethnic groups are presented below to illustrate the diversity within the group known as Asian Pacific Americans.

Chinese Americans

Although there are scattered reports of Asians inhabiting parts of the United States as early as 498 A.D., the migration of significant numbers of Asians, specifically the Chinese, began with the California Gold Rush of 1849 (Daniels, 1988). Between 1849 and 1882, more than 275,000 Chinese entered the United States. Of these, more than 90% were male. Initially, the Chinese immigrants worked primarily in mines, but they also labored on the western leg of the transcontinental Central Pacific Railroad, in agriculture, and in service trades. Some researchers have proposed that the Chinese, like other European ethnic groups who immigrated to the United States, were sojourners who intended only to work in the United States in order to make money and then return to their country of origin. However, unlike European immigrants, the Chinese became the first ethnic group to be barred legally from immigrating to the United States, by the Chinese Exclusion Act of 1882. The Chinese Exclusion Act represented, at a federal level, the culmination of anti-Chinese sentiment that had been present throughout many western states and localities. Because of the Chinese Exclusion Act, the early Chinese population, consisting primarily of unmarried males, declined until the 1920s.

The advent of World War II marked a change in U.S. policy toward the Chinese. The laws that had excluded Chinese immigration to the United States were repealed in 1943 by the Magnuson Act. The Magnuson Act also set a Chinese immigration quota of 105 per year and allowed those of Chinese descent to be eligible for naturalization. The McCarran-Walter Act of 1952 was a turning point in U.S. policy of discrimination along racial lines in citizenship eligibility. The McCarran-Walter Act allowed the Chinese, and all Asians, to become naturalized citizens of the United States. Because of changes in immigration and refugee policies, between 1960 and 1985 the Chinese American population quadrupled (Kitano & Daniels, 1988).

At the time of the 1990 U.S. Census, Chinese Americans, at more than 1.6 million, were found to be the largest Asian Pacific American group, making up 22.6% of the Asian Pacific American population. Between 1980 and 1990, the Chinese American population doubled, with most of the growth owing to immigration. Currently more than 63% of Chinese Americans are foreign-born (U.S. Commission on Civil Rights, 1992).

Japanese Americans

Early immigration from Japan to the United States and Hawaii commenced in large numbers around 1885 and peaked between 1900 and 1910. The National Origins Act barred Japanese Americans and other Asians from entering the United States after 1924. This immigration pattern created a unique layering of generations that is important to understand when conducting research within the Japanese American community (Fugita & O'Brien, 1991). The Issei, or first generation of Japanese Americans, for example, had a strong sense of nationalism, with a set of social boundaries that distinguished them and other peoples of the world. At the time of the Issei immigration, the Japanese had a single language without significant variations in dialect (Haglund, 1984; Nakane, 1970). In addition, Japan's Constitution and the Imperial Rescript of Education formally stated the uniqueness of its people (Ichioka, 1971). This is a significant point because, unlike many European and other Asian groups who came to the United States during the same period, the Japanese immigrants did not share problems associated with a national identity.

As with most groups, the sense of a national identity is most salient with the Issei and becomes less so with each succeeding generation (O'Brien & Fugita, 1991). However, it is an error to equate the changes in identity with the lack of a strong identification with the Japanese American community. Japanese Americans have shown the ability to acculturate on many dimensions while maintaining a viable ethnic community. Even if Japanese Americans appear similar to middle-class Caucasians in lifestyles and behaviors, most have not given up their identity and involvement with their ethnic community (Fugita & O'Brien, 1991).

Based on the 1990 U.S. Census, Japanese Americans are the third-largest Asian Pacific American group, with a population of 847,562. In contrast to many other Asian American groups, more than 70% of the Japanese American population were born in the United States. More than 80% of Japanese Americans currently live in the western United States (U.S. Commission on Civil Rights, 1992).

Filipino Americans

Initial Filipino immigration to the United States was markedly different from Chinese or Japanese immigration. Unlike earlier Asian immigrants, who were considered aliens, because of American imperialism in the Philippine Islands Filipinos were considered to be American nationals (Kitano & Daniels, 1988). Between 1903 and 1910, those in the first wave of Filipino immigrants, the *pensionados*, were sponsored by a U.S. government program to attend American educational institutions. In what is considered to be a second wave of immigration, after World War I, significant numbers of Filipinos began arriving in the United States and Hawaii to work in agriculture, a labor niche previously occupied by the Chinese and Japanese immigrants.

The third major wave of Filipino immigration began after the discontinuation of the quota system in 1965 and continues to this day. The Filipino American population increased by 81% from 1980 to 1990. Currently at 1.4 million, Filipino Americans make up the second-largest Asian Pacific American ethnic group. More than 64% of Filipino Americans are foreign-born (U.S. Commission on Civil Rights, 1992).

Korean Americans

There have been three waves of immigration of Koreans to the United States. The Tonghak Rebellion, the Sino-Japanese War, the Russo-Japanese War in the late 1800s and early 1900s, a cholera epidemic, a drought, a locust plague, and famine all created unstable conditions in Korea, which prompted displaced Koreans to migrate to Hawaii to work on plantations (Kitano & Daniels, 1988). Between 1951 and 1964, the second wave of Korean immigration consisted of the wives of Americans who had gone to Korea during the Korean War, Korean children orphaned by the Korean War who were adopted by American families, and students (Kitano, 1991). The largest wave of Korean immigration, which continues today, followed the 1965 Immigration and Naturalization Act.

According to the 1990 U.S. Census, the population of Korean Americans is 798,849, making up 11% of the Asian Pacific American population. More than 80% of Korean Americans are foreign-born, and between 1980 and 1990 the Korean population in the United States more than doubled. Koreans who are currently immigrating to the United States tend to come with their families, and the adults tend to be highly educated.

Pacific Islander Americans

Prior to the 1980 U.S. Census, the populations of the different Pacific Islander ethnic groups, such as the Native Hawaiians, Samoans, Tongans, Tahitians, Guamanians, Fijians, Northern Mariana Islanders, and Palauans, were not presented by ethnic group. However, in the 1980 U.S. Census, the populations of some of the different Pacific Islander groups were detailed. At 211,014 at the time of the 1990 U.S. Census, Native Hawaiians are the most numerous of the Pacific Islanders, followed by the Samoans (62,964), Guamanians (49,345), and Tongans (17,606). Because of the limited scope of this chapter, Native Hawaiians are the only Pacific Islander group we discuss in detail.

Native Hawaiians are the indigenous people of Hawaii, who settled that land more than 2,000 years ago. At the time of Captain Cook's arrival in Hawaii in 1778, the population of Native Hawaiians may have been as large as one million people (Stannard, 1989). With contact from Westerners, tuberculosis, measles, influenza, leprosy, and other infectious diseases decimated the Native Hawaiian population. From 1778 to 1883, the population was reduced to approximately 40,000 Native Hawaiians. Within this period, the number of foreigners outnumbered Native Hawaiians by more than 10,000 people. Although Native Hawaiians currently total more than 200,000 in Hawaii, there are only 8,000 full-blooded Native Hawaiians left (Ikeda, 1987).

Native Hawaiians evolved a web of cultural values that served as the basis for social relationships. These values imparted a deep concern for unity (*lokahi*) with a living, conscious, and communicating cosmos. The values emphasized harmony with self—*na'au* (feelings), *kino* (body), and *'uhane* (spirit). Equally important was harmony with kin (*'ohana*), elders (*kupuna*), and land (*'aina*). This worldview encouraged supportive interpersonal relationships and low reliance on personal responsibility (Howard, 1974).

The Hawaiian language played an important part in reinforcing this harmonic relationship between the person and the community, nature, and spiritual world. The language was an oral tradition until the missionaries arrived in 1820. An example of the power of this oral tradition came when unfamiliar chiefs met in Hawaii. Chief genealogy was proof of rank, which dictated protocol. When these chiefs met, their *kahuna* or priests would step out and repeat thousands or more lines of poetry related to genealogy. Only after these chants did the chiefs know who had the higher rank and was deferred to. A memory lapse, lengthy pause, or mispronunciation was sufficient for a kahuna to be put to death (E Ola Mau, 1985).

In the past two centuries, Hawaiian culture and traditional methods of resolving problems have been devalued through Westernization and capitalism. For example, as important as the Hawaiian language is, it is estimated that there are only 10,000 people who can carry on a conversation in Hawaiian; about 4,000 Native Hawaiians—many of whom are elderly—can speak it fluently. In recent years, Native Hawaiians have recognized the importance of the Hawaiian language in defining culture and community in Hawaii. Language preschools have been established on different islands as one method of making the Hawaiian language prosper once again.

Southeast Asian Americans

Prior to 1975, the number of Southeast Asians migrating to the United States was small. Immigration records show that Southeast

Asians totaled no more than 55 annually during the 1950s, increased from 100 to 1,000 during the 1960s, and ranged from 1,500 to 4,700 during the early 1970s. Vietnamese constituted about 97% of these admissions (Gordon, 1984). However, this migration pattern changed dramatically in the mid-1970s. Beginning in 1975, more than 1.5 million people left their homes in Cambodia, Laos, and Vietnam to escape war, internal political conflicts, and famine. By September 1988, about 900,000 Southeast Asians had relocated to the United States (Rumbaut, 1991). Vietnamese represented 60% of this refugee group and Cambodians and Laotians made up equal proportions (20%) of the remaining people (U.S. Committee for Refugees, 1988). Despite initial efforts by the federal government to settle Southeast Asians throughout the United States, a substantial proportion (40%) now live in California.

Southeast Asians came to the United States in two waves. The first occurred during April 1975 to December 1977, the period following the fall of Saigon. Vietnamese made up this first group of refugees, who were seen as sympathizers with the American and South Vietnamese governments. The second wave of refugees ensued between 1978 and 1980, as political turmoil escalated in Cambodia, Vietnam, and Laos. The Vietnamese escaped in small, overcrowded boats that were often stopped by Thai pirates. Many were tortured, raped, or killed. The people who survived the long journey were forced to remain in camps for months in Malaysia, Singapore, Indonesia, Hong Kong, or the Philippines before resettling in another country (Chung & Okazaki, 1992). Cambodians, Hmong, and Laotians overcame traumatic circumstances to escape their countries. Many of the Hmong and Laotians who eventually resettled in the United States were poor, illiterate, and unfamiliar with Western culture, which made their adjustment to life in the United States even more difficult.

By the 1990 U.S. Census, there were 614,547 Vietnamese, 147,411 Cambodians, 149,014 Laotians, and 90,082 Hmong in the United States. The rates of poverty among Southeast Asian American ethnic groups are high: In 1980 a third of Vietnamese immigrants and over half of Cambodian and Laotian immigrants lived in poverty (O'Hare & Felt, 1991). Given the tremendous increases in Southeast Asian American populations owing to immigration, it is likely that the poverty rates among these groups has also increased substantially.

The brief descriptions of ethnic groups offered above help to demonstrate the different paths Asian Pacific Americans have taken to establish communities in the United States. Next, we explore this diversity further by calling attention to selected demographic features of these communities.

Sociodemographic Characteristics

Sociodemographic factors can provide a general assessment of a community's well-being, because some variables are strongly linked to health status. In this section we explore some differences in demographic characteristics among Asian Pacific American groups.

One of the prevailing images of Asian Americans is their phenomenal level of economic success. This stereotype has led to unfortunate policies that attempt to exclude Asian Americans from minority programs (Laura Uba, in Chapter 14 of this volume, discusses this issue in more detail). Equally important, using data based on the U.S. Census, policy makers often conclude that Asian Americans are not at high risk for health problems. However, the image of economic success is not supported under closer scrutiny (Kim & Hurh, 1983; Suzuki, 1977). Educational attainment and income levels are often used to support the argument that Asian Americans are doing well. Most Asian American ethnic groups have relatively high levels of education and income compared with the national average, and it is usually assumed that high educational attainment leads to well-paying jobs, high status, and prestigious occupations. For Asian Americans, however, this is often not the case. A high level of education does not necessarily lead to more pay and status. Barringer, Takeuchi, and Xenos (1990) found that Asian Americans do not reap the same benefits of education that whites receive; only for Japanese Americans does the relationship between education and attainment come close to the association found for whites. This is an important finding, because Asian Americans use education as the primary path for social mobility (Sue & Okazaki, 1990).

A close examination of sociodemographic characteristics reveals that some Asian Pacific American ethnic groups may be more at risk for health problems than others. Immigrant status is related to a number of adjustment stressors that are linked to health. A recurring hypothesis regarding immigrants is that they experience more stressors than do native-born individuals. Fabrega (1969), for example, argues that migrants encounter stressors that originate from leaving the country of origin, the difficulties of passage, the adaptation process in the host society, and the expectations of social and economic attainment. More recently, investigations on Asian immigrants have documented that migrants are facing many stressors, including those created by the acculturation process, stressful life events, employment, and economic hardships (Kuo & Tsai, 1986; Lin, Masuda, & Tazuma, 1984). Chinese, Filipino, Asian Indian, Korean, and Vietnamese Americans are among the ethnic groups with large proportions who were born in another country.

A consistent finding in the social sciences is the inverse relationship between socioeconomic status and illness (Williams, 1990). Studies provide indirect evidence that economic factors can have pernicious consequences for the health of adults. Poverty status, per capita income, and employment status are often used as indicators of socioeconomic status. Of 17 Asian American groups, 14 have poverty levels above the U.S. average (9.6%). Laotians, Hmong, and Cambodians have poverty levels above 45%. Per capita income is a useful measure of socioeconomic status because it takes into consideration the number of people the household income is intended to support. In 1980 Asian Americans had an average household income of $6,900, compared with the U.S. average of $7,400. Only Indonesian, Chinese, and Japanese American groups had average per capita incomes at or above the U.S. average. In 1980, 7% of all Asian Pacific Americans were unemployed. Although the average unemployment rate for Asian Pacific Americans was below the U.S. average (5%), Hmong (20%), Laotians (15%), Cambodians (11%), and Samoans (10%) had unemployment rates in double figures.

Using a general Asian Pacific American category masks the diversity and heterogeneity of different ethnic groups. A global ethnic category can underestimate the health problems of specific ethnic groups or lead to erroneous conclusions about risk factors. Uehara, Bates, and Takeuchi (1993) specifically address the consequences of examining Asian Americans as a single category or as disaggregated ethnic groups. They conducted analyses examining the level of functioning drawing upon data from a large-scale study of adults with serious mental illness in King County, Washington. Because data on level of functioning are used as a basis for resource allocation to community mental health programs in King County, the analyses had important consequences for program planning.

Uehara et al. first compared Asian Americans as an ethnic category to whites. Asian Americans, on the average, had higher community functioning scores than whites. On the basis of these data, planners might reasonably conclude that fewer resources are required to meet the needs of Asian American consumers. Further analyses suggest, however, that such conclusions would have been premature. When analyses were conducted of specific Asian American groups (i.e., Chinese, Japanese, Filipino, Laotian, and Vietnamese), the results indicated that only the Chinese had higher scores than whites on level of functioning. Thus the investigators were able to demonstrate systematically the actual analytic and programmatic consequences for categorizing Asian and Pacific Islander ethnic groups.

Conceptual Considerations

A number of different paradigms are possible in organizing a book on health issues. One common way is to focus on the general issues of health and discuss specific subpopulations, such as the elderly and children. Another way, the one chosen for this book, is to examine specific illnesses and discuss their prevalence among the population of interest, in this case, Asian Pacific Americans. Because empirical health research on Asian Pacific Americans has been neglected in the past, each chapter could begin with a lament about the lack of data and the problems inherent in conducting health research in these minority communities. Rather than have the chapter authors spend time on these issues, however, we highlight in this chapter some common conceptual and methodological issues scientists confront in conducting research in Asian Pacific American communities. Specific concerns unique to particular areas are discussed in the individual chapters.

Because so little has been published about risk factors and special populations within Asian Pacific American communities, the Asian & Pacific Islander American Health Forum decided to emphasize the prevalence of diseases, with some attention to the issues of the health professions and access to care. One problem with this approach is the inadequate coverage given to theoretical issues that help to guide research. Although we cannot adequately address conceptual concerns in this overview, we can raise an issue that is missing from the chapters that follow.

Public health policy has begun to emphasize a "lifestyle" approach to the study of illnesses and diseases. Activities such as heavy alcohol consumption, inadequate diets, and smoking are often seen as precursors to poor health. However, the focus on lifestyle factors can overlook the importance of social structural factors that are linked to both lifestyle and health problems. It is important to recognize that macro social structures (e.g., an individual's position in the social structure) shape behavior and values that in turn partially explain health behavior. Asian Pacific American ethnic groups differ along a number of socioeconomic status (SES) indicators. As mentioned earlier, SES has a consistently strong inverse relationship with health status. SES position is also strongly related to the conditions of life that promote certain lifestyles (Berkman & Breslow, 1983; Schoenborn, 1986). Thus a focus on changing lifestyles at the expense of ignoring macro SES factors may do little to change the health status of a group (Williams, 1990).

Investigators seeking to establish linkages between social structural position and health status among Asian Americans can benefit from a more systematic research plan (Williams, 1990). First, there is a need to conceptualize and measure dimensions of SES that are most salient in predicting health status. Few studies have explored the social factors that are important in determining social positions and the conditions of life among Asian Pacific Americans. Although empirical investigations can enhance our understanding of the role conventional measures of SES—education, occupation, and income—play in Asian Pacific American communities, more research is required to examine alternative measures of social position that are unique to these communities. This has been a useful strategy in investigations in African American communities. Dressler (1991), for example, demonstrates that darker skin color as a measure of social position is related to hypertension among high-SES African Americans.

Second, social position factors affect individual health through smaller, intermediary structures. In health research, these structures include stress, social support, and attitudes toward health. Lifestyle behaviors such as smoking and alcohol consumption are also considered as part of the linkages between the macro levels and health status. Studies that measure these intermediate structures specify that their linkages with health status and use are critically needed. Stress, for example, is associated with health status, but few studies have examined what stressors are meaningful among

Asian Pacific Americans. Equally important, we do not know whether the stress-health model is a fruitful avenue of research for Asian Pacific Americans.

Finally, empirical investigations are needed to identify the social psychological processes through which people respond to the social structure. Significant others and the media are some common parties that transmit information to individuals (Hacker, Collins, & Jacobson, 1987). In addition to this relay function, significant others and the media often provide models of health behavior for people. To understand these processes, research on Asian Pacific Americans requires more substantive attention to the types of individuals and media that play significant relay functions among Asian Pacific Americans. For example, the Asian American Health Forum has effectively used health promotion campaigns targeted at ethnic newspapers and radio stations. We need to determine whether other sources of influence are salient in the Asian Pacific American communities. An assessment of the impact of different influences and an understanding of how these processes work in these communities are also needed.

The study of linkages between macro structures and health status and behavior provides a systematic understanding of the context of health and illness in Asian Pacific American communities. Investigations on these linkages provide an alternative to viewing disease as simply a medical problem. The attendance to social and psychological factors can have a significant impact on preventing illness and promoting health in Asian Pacific American communities. It is important to keep this point in mind as one reads through these chapters.

Methodological Considerations

One reason for the lack of empirical studies on Asian Pacific American health issues is that a number of methodological issues must be considered in the research designs, making the implementation of a project complex and costly. In fact, these methodological problems make health research in minority communities more difficult to conduct and administer than health research in predominantly white communities. In this section we provide short descriptions of some common methodological problems that must be considered in health research among Asian Pacific Americans.

Public Records

In public records, such as those of public health clinics, some problems call into question the quality of the data:

1. Diagnostic data from public records are limited by interviewer reliability. Often assessments are made by a number of interviewers. Different interviewers create biases, especially when interviewers must rate clients on a number of dimensions. Some clinicians may be more thorough in their assessments than others, and some patients may describe their problems more openly with some clinicians than with others.

2. Ethnic identification is often problematic from public records. When a client does not provide ethnic information, an interviewer may guess about ethnicity based on the client's last name or physical appearance.

3. Health indicators from public records provide a confounded variable of health status and service utilization. It is well documented that Asian Pacific Americans delay seeking professional care for their health problems; thus they may have more severe problems when they enter health facilities than do whites.

4. Missing data are a common problem in public records, especially data on income, occupational status, and education level. These three variables are important in determining whether differences in health status among groups can be attributed to ethnicity or socioeconomic status.

5. Some variables that are critical in understanding Asian Pacific American health status may not be recorded on health clinic forms, such as primary language, place of birth, and generation.

6. There is uncertainty about the meaning of some information found in public records. For example, suicides are recorded on death certificates by medical examiners or coroners across the country. Aside from the technical expertise of medical examiners or coroners to make this assessment, there are often cultural, political, economic, or religious pressures on a coroner not to label a death as suicide. Asian Pacific Americans may be reluctant to cooperate with a suicide investigation because such a determination would lead to a loss of face for the family of the deceased.

Secondary Analyses

Because Asian Pacific American health studies are difficult to conduct, researchers often rely on analyses of secondary data. In addition to problems associated with any secondary analysis, two related issues are involved in studies that include Asian Pacific Americans. Most large-scale studies include only small samples of Asian Pacific Americans. Large-scale studies usually weight the data to the population figures of the community or geographic region, or the nation as a whole. These weights may disguise the fact that the Asian Pacific American samples are actually quite small. Small samples do not have sufficient statistical power to detect significant health needs. In addition, complex multivariate analyses are not possible to identify high-risk subgroups. When a large sample of Asian Pacific Americans is collected, they are often collapsed into one category. As described earlier, because Asian Pacific Americans are quite heterogeneous, the use of a general category makes it difficult to assess their health care needs accurately.

Original Data Collection

Three issues are especially salient in the study of the health care needs in Asian Pacific American communities: measurement, sampling, and access in the community. It is well established that culture affects the perception of physical and emotional conditions (Kleinman, 1980; Mechanic, 1980; Zola, 1964). Medical technology can reliably detect physical disease, but cultural factors can constrain the ways individuals define and evaluate their health problems, present their problems to the physician, and seek help for their problems. Without adequate information from the patient, the physician may not be able to detect the disease.

The measurement of health status, especially that relying on survey techniques, has become increasingly sophisticated over the past decade with the development of standardized instruments. Too often, however, researchers have used standardized instruments without also assessing the reliability and validity of these instruments for specific ethnic and racial subpopulations, assuming that concepts and measurements of health and illness are uniform from one cultural group to another (Angel & Thoits, 1987). This assumption is unwarranted, because cultural groups vary in their definitions of normality and abnormality, and these variations affect models of health and illness (Higginbotham, 1984). Some of the factors affected by culture include types and parameters of stressors, coping mechanisms, personality patterns, language systems, and expression of illness (Marsella, 1982). Without proper consideration of these issues, errors are often made in diagnosis, assessment, and treatment.

Manson, Walker, and Kivlahan (1987) assert that some standardized self-rating scales and interview schedules can accurately assess health status among ethnic minorities if they are modified to reflect important aspects of the minority culture and history. In the past, researchers often took this to mean that standardized instruments should be translated into different languages for non-English-speaking minorities. The problems in this process are illustrated by the following anecdote. A major health study translated a standardized instrument from English into Spanish. Shortly after the study went into the field, the researchers noticed that Latinos were scoring very low on one particular question: "How often do you kiss your child?" The researchers were quite puzzled by this response pattern and did not know how to interpret this finding, given that it could be very controversial. After checking and double-checking the original questionnaire, someone thought to check the translation. Instead of asking Latinos "How often do you kiss your child," the translated question read, "How often do you kiss your puppy?"

Most translation problems are more subtle. To avoid these types of problems, instruments are translated back into English. However, translation procedures cannot correct for other measurement problems. Let us give another example. We conducted a meta-analysis of an evaluation study that was intended to improve the self-esteem of Hawaiian children. We examined an instrument that measured self-esteem and that was modified to incorporate the pidgin English that Hawaiian children often use. We reviewed the responses for a sample of children and observed their behavior. We were particularly struck by one girl who had scored poorly on the self-esteem instrument but whose other records showed that she had good grades, received excellent evaluations by teachers, and behaved in a manner that demonstrated a positive sense of self. We took her aside and talked with her. We asked her why she answered no on such items as "My friends like me," "My teacher likes me," and "I do good work." In her best pidgin English, she said, "Eh, I no like brag."

This anecdote leads us to other measurement issues. Besides translation considerations, researchers must be concerned with conceptual equivalence, scale equivalence, and norm equivalence. *Conceptual equivalence* refers to similarities in the meanings of concepts used in assessment. For example, do minorities and whites think of well-being, depression, or self-esteem in the same way? *Scale equivalence* refers to the use of standard formats in questionnaire items that are familiar to all groups. For example, among well-educated groups, most are familiar with answering survey questions using responses along a scale that includes "strongly agree," "agree," and so on, or with a true-false dichotomy. Recent immigrants or individuals who have not been educated in the Western system may not understand this format, however. *Norm equivalence* refers to the application of standard norms developed in one sample to another group. Because statistical norms are the basis upon which we judge "normal" and "abnormal" or "high functioning" and "low functioning," it is important to understand whether the normative sample is similar to the study group. For example, standards of weight and height developed among whites may not be suitable for Asian Pacific Americans.

Sampling

Sampling is another issue that must be considered in conducting research in Asian Pacific American communities. In selecting a sample, researchers are concerned about the representativeness of the people they choose to interview. Although many Asian Pacific Americans live in certain parts of given cities, substantial numbers do not. In Los Angeles County, for example, 22% of Chinese Americans live in census tracts with 500 or more Chinese Americans. The remaining 78% live in areas not populated by large numbers of Chinese Americans. Although it is easier to select a sample of Chinese Americans from geographic areas where large numbers reside, such a sample may not be representative of all Chinese Americans living in Los Angeles County.

The issue of sampling from small populations has been one of the reasons no large-scale health or psychiatric epidemiological study has been conducted for an Asian Pacific American group. Some researchers have resorted to the use of telephone or ethnic directories to obtain a universe of ethnic populations. However, such sampling frames have their own biases. Elena Yu and William Liu address this sampling issue in more detail and propose several solutions to this problem in Chapter 2 of this volume.

Access in the Community

In addition to enhancing their own careers, health researchers conduct studies in minority communities because they want their work to have an impact in resolving social problems, guiding policy, or serving as a basis for programs that will improve the quality of life in these communities. Researchers can provide minority communities with needed data that can be used to secure resources for new programs, assess interventions that may be useful, or identify high-risk groups. However, to conduct studies, investigators must rely on the community to provide access to minority samples as well as a laboratory in which to test innovative intervention strategies. Unfortunately, there is often an uneasy tension between researchers and the community. Community leaders often see researchers as exploiters whose studies are divorced from real issues and real-life problems. On the other hand, researchers often view community leaders as compromising the science of the research enterprise. This tension makes it difficult to initiate new research projects in minority communities. If this tension is unresolved, both researchers and the communities are unable to meet their objectives.

Concluding Note

Although this overview has focused on some conceptual and methodological issues in conducting health research, future generations of researchers will need to pay closer attention to theoretical issues. Epidemiological research designs must be incorporated with theory (Mechanic, 1980). This statement is especially appropriate to Asian Pacific American mental health research, where few studies are driven by theoretical issues (Sue & Morishima, 1982). An understanding of the biological, psychological, social, and cultural processes that lead to well-being and illness in Asian Pacific American communities will be accomplished only through a more established link between the theoretical and empirical levels.

References

Angel, R., & Thoits, P. (1987). The impact of culture on the cognitive structure of illness. *Culture, Medicine and Psychiatry, 11,* 465-494.

Barringer, H., Takeuchi, D., & Xenos, P. (1990). Education, occupational prestige, and income of Asian Americans: Evidence from the 1980 census. *Sociology of Education, 63,* 27-43.

Berkman, L., & Breslow, L. (1983). *Health and ways of living.* New York: Oxford University Press.

Chan, S. (1991). *Asian Americans: An interpretive history.* Boston: Twayne.

Chung, R. C., & Okazaki, S. (1992). Counseling Americans of Southeast Asian descent: The impact of the refugee experience. In C. C. Lee & B. L. Richardson (Eds.), *Multicultural issues in counseling: New approaches to diversity* (pp. 107-126). New York: American Association for Counseling and Development.

Daniels, R. (1988). *Asian America: Chinese and Japanese in the United States since 1850.* Seattle: University of Washington Press.

Dressler, W. (1991). Social class, skin color, and arterial blood pressure in two societies. *Ethnicity and Disease, 1,* 60-77.

E Ola Mau. (1985). *Native Hawaiian health study.* Honolulu: Alu Like.

Fabrega, H. (1969). Social psychiatric aspects of acculturation and migration: A general statement. *Comprehensive Psychiatry, 10,* 314-392.

Fugita, S., & O'Brien, D. (1991). *Japanese American ethnicity: The persistence of community.* Seattle: University of Washington Press.

Gordon, L. (1984). *Southeast Asian refugee migration to the United States.* Paper presented at the Conference on Asia-Pacific Immigration to the United States.

Hacker, G., Collins, R., & Jacobson, M. (1987). *Marketing booze to blacks.* Washington, DC: Center for Science in the Public Interest.

Haglund, E. (1984). Japan: Cultural considerations. *International Journal of Intercultural Relations, 8,* 61-76.

Higginbotham, N. (1984). *Third World challenge to psychiatry: Cultural accommodation and mental health care.* Honolulu: University Press of Hawaii.

Howard, A. (1974). *Ain't no big thing: Coping strategies in a Hawaiian-American community.* Honolulu: University of Hawaii Press.

Ichioka, Y. (1971). A buried past: Early Issei socialists and the Japanese community. *Amerasia, 1,* 25-37.

Ikeda, K. (1987). *Demographic profile of Native Hawaiians: 1980-1986.* Honolulu: University of Hawaii, Department of Sociology.

Kim, K. C., & Hurh, W. M. (1983). Korean Americans and the "success" image: A critique. *Amerasia, 10,* 3-21.

Kitano, H. H. L. (1991). *Race relations* (4th ed.). Englewood Cliffs, NJ: Prentice Hall.

Kitano, H. H. L., & Daniels, R. (1988). *Asian Americans: Emerging minorities.* Englewood Cliffs, NJ: Prentice Hall.

Kleinman, A. (1980). *Patients and healers in the context of culture.* Berkeley: University of California Press.

Kuo, W. H., & Tsai, Y. M. (1986). Social networking, hardiness, and immigrant's mental health. *Journal of Health and Social Behavior, 27,* 133-149.

Lin, K. M., Masuda, M., & Tazuma, L. (1984). Adaptational problems of Vietnamese refugees: Part IV. Three year comparison. *Psychiatric Journal of the University of Ottawa, 9,* 79-84.

Mechanic, D. (1980). The experience and reporting of common physical complaints. *Journal of Health and Social Behavior, 21,* 146-155.

Manson, S., Walker, R., & Kivlahan, D. (1987). Psychiatric assessment and treatment of American Indians and Alaska Natives. *Hospital and Community Psychiatry, 38,* 165-173.

Marsella, A. (1982). Culture and mental health: An overview. In A. Marsella & G. White (Eds.), *Cultural conceptions of mental health and therapy* (pp. 359-388). Boston: G. Reidel.

Nakane, C. (1970). *Japanese society.* Berkeley: University of California Press.

O'Brien, D., & Fugita, S. (1991). *The Japanese American experience.* Bloomington: Indiana University Press.

O'Hare , W. P., & Felt, J. C. (1991). *Asian Americans: America's fastest growing minority group.* Washington, DC: Population Reference Bureau.

Rumbaut, R. G. (1991). The agony of exile: A study of the migration and adaptation of Indochinese refugee adults and children. In F. L. Ahearn & J. L. Athey (Eds.), *Refugee children: Theory, research and practice.* Baltimore: Johns Hopkins University Press.

Schoenborn, C. (1986). Health habits of U.S. adults, 1985: The Alameda 7 revisited. *Public Health Reports, 101,* 571-580.

Stannard, D. E. (1989). *Before the horror: The population of Hawai'i on the eve of Western contact.* Honolulu: University of Hawaii Press.

Sue, S., & Morishima, J. (1982). *The mental health of Asian Americans.* San Francisco: Jossey-Bass.

Sue, S., & Okazaki, S. (1990). Asian American achievement: A phenomenon in search of an explanation. *American Psychologist, 45,* 913-920.

Suzuki, B. (1977). Education and socialization of Asian Americans: A revisionist analysis of the "model minority" thesis. *Amerasia, 4,* 23-51.

Takaki, R. (1987). *Strangers from a different shore.* Boston: Little, Brown.

Uehara, E., Bates, R., & Takeuchi, D. (1993). *The effects of combining disparate groups in the analysis of ethnic differences: Variations among Asian American mental health consumers in level of community functioning.* Unpublished manuscript.

U.S. Bureau of the Census. (1989). *We, the Asian Pacific Americans.* Washington, DC: Government Printing Office.

U.S. Commission on Civil Rights. (1992). *Civil rights issues facing Asian Americans in the 1990s.* Washington, DC: Government Printing Office.

U.S. Committee for Refugees. (1988). *Refugee reports.* Washington, DC: American Council for Nationalistic Services.

Williams, D. (1990). Socioeconomic differentials in health: A review and redirection. *Social Psychology Quarterly, 53,* 81-99.

Zola, I. (1964). Illness behavior of the working class: Implications and recommendations. In A. Shostak & W. Gomberg (Eds.), *Blue collar world: Studies of the American worker* (pp. 350-361). Englewood Cliffs, NJ: Prentice Hall.

2

Methodological Issues

ELENA S. H. YU

WILLIAM T. LIU

Between 1980 and 1990, the Asian Pacific American population in the United States—officially counted at 7.3 million—increased by at least 40% in all states except Hawaii. The slower growth rate in Hawaii (17%) is attributable to the fact that the Asian Pacific American population constitutes a majority in that state. The rising economic power of the Pacific Rim countries and the shift in U.S. funding policies toward support for more research on understudied populations, such as women and minorities, mean that the health and well-being of Asian Pacific Americans have finally become the new frontiers for research.

For the most part, our knowledge of the health risks and morbidity patterns of different Asian Pacific subgroups have been drawn primarily from the following general sources of data:

AUTHORS' NOTE: This chapter is an expanded version of a paper titled *Estimating the Health Status of Asian Americans,* which was presented at the annual meeting of the American Public Health Association, September 30 to October 4, 1990, in New York City. We are grateful to Ninez Ponce and other staff of the Asian and Pacific Islander American Health Forum for sharing with us their unpublished compilation of NCHS data collection programs, which facilitated our preparation of Table 2.1 in this chapter. We wish also to acknowledge the staff of the National Center for Health Statistics, particularly John E. Patterson, Ed Hunter, and Paul Placek, for their helpful suggestions. The comments of David Takeuchi, Nolan Zane, and Anthony Graham-White on an earlier version and the bibliographic assistance of Y. M. Kean are also appreciated.

- investigator-initiated epidemiological surveys conducted in Hawaii and on the West Coast (Curb et al., 1991; Kagan et al., 1974; Kato, Tillotson, Nichaman, Rhoads, & Hamilton, 1973; Reed & Yano, 1987; Rhoads & Feinleib, 1983; Robertson et al., 1977; Stavig, Igra, & Leonard, 1984; Stemmermann, Chyou, Kagan, Nomura, & Yano, 1991; Takeya et al., 1984; Tillotson et al., 1973; Yano & MacLean, 1989; Yano, Reed, Curb, Hankin, & Albers, 1986)
- Surveillance, Epidemiology and End Result (SEER) cancer registry data maintained in selected cities (Hinds, Kolonel, Lee, & Hirohata, 1980; Kolonel et al., 1981; Yu, 1986)
- descriptive clinic-based studies, such as the Kaiser Permanente prepaid health plan (Angel, Armstrong, & Klatsky, 1989; Klatsky & Armstrong, 1991)
- mortality statistics compiled by the National Center for Health Statistics (NCHS) (Haenszel & Kurihara, 1968; King, 1975; Kleinman, 1990; Li, Ni, Schwartz, & Daling, 1990; Liu & Yu, 1985; Lynberg & Muin, 1990; Yu, 1982)

Because of the lack of better information, findings from these seemingly abundant data may have unwittingly sustained the myth—begun in the 1960s—that Asian Pacific Americans are quite healthy compared with black or white Americans. As scientists have continued to use the prevailing morbidity risks of white and black Americans as the basis for research, scientific and public awareness of more troubling Asian Pacific American health risks (such as tuberculosis and hepatitis B) have for some time remained low, until the media's recent dissemination of the fact that these diseases are affecting mainstream populations at an alarming rate. In the absence of alternative data sources, continuing use of the data and implicit acceptance of their methodological approaches have had four negative consequences:

1. a slower rate of development of knowledge about the morbidity risks more commonly encountered in Asian Pacific American subgroups than in the majority white population
2. a general lack of rigorous study designs in ethnicity and health research, particularly on Asian Pacific Americans
3. inertia in the explorations of alternative sampling procedures that would take into account the ethnic diversity within, and the peculiar geographic distribution of, Asian Pacific Americans
4. a general lack of interest and delays in the development of culturally appropriate measures, in non-English languages, that would enable

researchers to have a precise understanding of the health status and
morbidity patterns of subgroups of Asian Pacific Americans

Issues concerning the unique morbidity risks of Asian Pacific
Americans, though very important, require a separate and independent discussion. The purpose of this chapter is to present, in lay
language, an overview of the major limitations of the existing data
sources insofar as Asian Pacific Americans are concerned, as well
as to discuss in detail the major methodological problems that we
must overcome during the 1990s if we are to conduct scientifically
sound, culturally appropriate, and policy-relevant surveys on the
health risks and morbidity patterns of Asian Pacific Americans.

Limitations of Existing Data Sources

Fascinating as they are, health and epidemiological studies on
Asian Pacific Americans are beset with many difficulties not often
encountered in studies of the mainstream population or other ethnic minorities. The best-known investigator-initiated studies of
Asian Americans conducted in Hawaii and California are "migrant
studies," which are by nature comparative. Typically, members of
a specific population—usually the Japanese—are sampled in three
locations (e.g., Japan, Hawaii, and California) and compared, or
they are studied in two locations (e.g., Japan and Hawaii or California) and then compared with a white American population.
Using similar study designs and questionnaires to the extent possible, inferences are drawn about the health status or morbidity
patterns of the Japanese as an example of Asian Pacific Americans.
Sampling the Japanese has often been viewed as a simple "statistical" exercise, because they are easily identifiable by their surnames,
belong to formal organizations, have telephones, and are prominent in Hawaii and California. Although seemingly logically sound,
this approach has the unintended consequence of using the most
established Asian Pacific American subgroup—which happens to
have an extremely large percentage of English speakers and also
the highest socioeconomic attainment of all Asian Pacific Americans—to represent *all* Asian Pacific Americans, an ethnic minority
characterized by a heavy representation of persons from low socioeconomic status who are nonnative English speakers. Thus it is easy
for both the media and policy makers to gloss over the issue of

ethnic diversity in health and morbidity. Furthermore, comparisons between the Japanese and white Americans have often led to the conclusion that the Japanese are in "better" health than white Americans. This may have inadvertently buoyed the myth of Asian Pacific Americans as a healthy minority, at the expense of rigorously controlling for social class or socioeconomic status—a key variable in any health study. In several epidemiological studies of Asian Pacific American subgroups, social class or socioeconomic status has often been poorly measured, even if it can be and has been properly "controlled for" statistically. Consequently, the general public or mainstream researchers are not always aware that other Asian Americans or Pacific Islanders are *unlike* the Japanese.

Routinely collected registry data in selected cities (such as the SEER cancer data) contain standardized information on specified subgroups of Asian Pacific Americans that, though useful, suffer from certain limitations. First, they are focused exclusively on specific types of diseases that are well defined in terms of pathological manifestations and clinical diagnoses. They cannot address a broader array of concepts such as "health status," "health utilization," or "health behaviors." Second, these data are almost always collected from selective locations and are therefore of limited use in providing a *national* picture of the health status of Asian Pacific Americans. Third, important concepts affecting the incidence, prevalence, and clinical course of disease—such as social class or socioeconomic status—remain poorly measured, if they are assessed at all.

The third type of data on Asian Pacific American health, based on clinic populations, may offer specific insights into the health problems of Asian Pacific Americans who use the services of the clinics under study but provide no information as to how representative that clinic population is of the Asian Pacific American community in any single region of the country, much less the entire United States. Although a concerted effort has been launched among a handful of clinics nationwide to coordinate data collection procedures, statistics on the socioeconomic status of persons utilizing these clinics are often lacking. Thus the impact of social class on the self-selection of clinic patients, and the patterns of diseases that may commonly afflict Asian Pacific Americans, cannot be determined with great precision.

Only the data maintained by The National Center for Health Statistics (NCHS) provide *national* estimates of health. Nevertheless, these data are not without their share of limitations. In what follows, we describe the major obstacles in analyzing and interpreting findings from existing national data routinely collected by NCHS. We also elaborate further on the major methodological obstacles confronting surveys by independent investigators during the 1990s.

Existing National Health Data

Established in 1959, NCHS has the mission is to collect, analyze, and disseminate national health statistics; administer the Cooperative Health Statistics System; conduct research in survey and statistical methodology; coordinate the efforts of various federal agencies in health statistics to the maximum extent feasible; cooperate in international health statistics activities; and serve as a focal point for health data (National Center for Health Statistics, 1979). Table 2.1 summarizes the major data collection programs maintained by NCHS, which are broadly divided into population-based surveys and record-based surveys. In anticipation of future health statistics needs, four of the center's record-based surveys will be merged by 1993 and expanded into one integrated survey of health care providers called the National Health Care Survey. These four surveys are the National Hospital Discharge Survey, the National Ambulatory Medical Care Survey, the National Nursing Home Survey, and the National Master Facility Inventory. The last of these is now called the National Health Provider Inventory.

NCHS's variegated and highly integrated research programs are probably the most sophisticated taxpayer-supported national health data collection systems in the world. They provide the best estimates of the health characteristics of Americans from several vantage points, both subjective and objective. To illustrate, the National Health Interview Survey (NHIS), conducted annually using a probability sample of 50,000 households in the continental United States, yields estimates of health characteristics based on the sampled respondents' self-reports; the National Health and Nutrition Examination Survey (NHANES) and HANES Epidemiologic Followup Study obtain estimates of health characteristics through physical examinations conducted by qualified physicians or medical practitioners in mobile units that travel across the country.

Both the NHIS and NHANES programs, based on face-to-face contacts with a probability sample of individual Americans, are complemented

text continued on page 32

Table 2.1 Summary of Surveys and Data Systems: National Center for Health Statistics

Programs and Surveys	Data Sources/Methods	Health Estimates	Year Started	Data Years	Ethnicity Identifiers
Record-Based Programs					
Vital Statistics Cooperative Program	state-operated vital registration records submitted to NCHS according to NCHS's specification	births, deaths, and fetal deaths, sample of marriages and divorces, termination of pregnancy for selected reporting	1973	annual	9 race codes[a]
National Maternal and Infant Health Survey	follow-back of state vital records, based on questionnaires administered to mothers, physicians, hospitals, and other medical care providers; medical records of approximately 10,000 live births, 4,000 fetal deaths, 6,000 infant deaths	factors associated with poor pregnancy outcomes, barriers to and facilitators of prenatal care, effects of maternal risk factors on pregnancy outcomes, use and evaluation of public programs for Medicaid mothers and children	1988	natality, 1963, 1964-66, 1968-69, 1972, 1980, 1988; fetal mortality, 1980; infant mortality, 1964-66; birth, fetal death, and infant death survey in 1988	9 race codes[a]
National Mortality Followback Survey	follow-back of state death records by mailed questionnaires, telephone, and/or personal interviews with persons providing information on death certificates on the 1986 sample is approximately 1% of U.S. deaths of persons age 25 and over	mortality by socioeconomic factors, premature death, use of and payment for health care and cost of health care during the last year of life, disability prior to death; mortality associated with suspected risk factors, such as smoking	1961	annually from 1961 through 1968; 1986	9 race codes[a]

(continued)

Table 2.1 Continued

Programs and Surveys	Data Sources/Methods	Health Estimates	Year Started	Data Years	Ethnicity Identifiers
National Death Index	central computerized index of death record information from state registration; death certificates for all deaths	facilitates epidemiological follow-up studies; verification of death for individuals under study	1979	annual	9 race codes[a]
Linked Birth/Infant Death Records	all birth and death certificates and infant deaths	infant mortality rates by birth cohort, infant mortality rates by birth weight, mother's age, prenatal care, linked to information on death certificate	1983	annual	9 race codes[a]
Population-Based Surveys					
National Health Interview Survey	face-to-face interviews in approximately 50,000 households	CORE questions: health, illness, and disability; utilization of health care and other topics; supplement on AIDS knowledge and attitudes, cancer risk factors and smoking, health insurance, child health, and aging	1957	annual	Asian Pacific Islanders
National Health and Nutrition Examination Survey	direct physical examination, clinical and laboratory testing, and nutritional assessment	total prevalence of disease or conditions, unrecognized or undetected disease or conditions, heart disease, diabetes, osteoporosis, iron deficiency anemia, and other nutritional disorders	1959	1959, 1970, 1988, 1982-1984 = Hispanic HANES ($N = 12,000$)	Asian Pacific Islanders

NHANES I Epidemiologic Followup Study	longitudinal follow-up of NHANES I cohort of 14,407 persons aged 25-74 years by personal and telephone interviews, use of medical records, hospitals and nursing homes, death certificates	chronic disease and functional impairment, mortality and morbidity associated with suspected risk factors, hospital and nursing home utilization	1982	Wave 1, 1982-84 household interviews of 14,407 age 25-74; Wave 2, 1986 follow-up 5,677 elderly age 55-74; Wave 3, 1987 follow-up full cohort, 11,750 age 25-74	Asian Pacific Islanders
National Survey of Family Growth	face-to-face interviews with approximately 10,000 ever-married women 15-44 years of age	contraception and sterilization, teenage sexual activity and pregnancy, family planning, adoption, breast-feeding	1973	1973, 1976, 1982, 1988	Asian Pacific Islanders

Targeted Population Studies

Longitudinal Study of Aging, Supplement to NHIS	personal interviews with telephone and mail follow-ups, Medicare records, National Death Index, death certificates	changes in functional status and living arrangements, use of hospitals and nursing homes over time, migration, economic status, death rates by social, economic, family, and health characteristics of 7,000 persons age 70 and older in 1984	1984	1984, 1986, 1988, 1990	Asian Pacific Islanders
Teenage Attitudes and Practices Survey	telephone interviews and mailed questionnaires on 12,000 adolescents 12-18 years of age	prevalence of tobacco use among teenagers, determinants of tobacco use among teenagers	1988	1988	Asian Pacific Islanders

(continued)

29

Table 2.1 Continued

Programs and Surveys	Data Sources/Methods	Health Estimates	Year Started	Data Years	Ethnicity Identifiers
National Health Care Surveys					
National Hospital Discharge Survey	hospital records and computerized data sources abstracted from a sample of 500,000 from 542 hospitals	inpatient utilization of hospitals, expected source of payment, and length of stay, hospital patterns of use of care, and patient characteristics	1965	annual	Asian Pacific Islanders
National Ambulatory Medical Care Survey	mailed questionnaires to 2,500 probability sample of physicians in office-based practices	characteristics of patients' visits to physicians, services provided, diagnostic procedures, patient management and planned future treatment	1974	annual until 1981, 1985, 1989; annual after 1989	Asian Pacific Islanders
National Nursing Home Survey	self-administered questionnaires and interviews with administrators and staff in a sample of about 1,200 facilities	information on LTC facilities: size, ownership, Medicare/Medicaid certification, occupancy rate, days of care provided, and expenses; for patients, data on demographic characteristics, health status, and services received	1973	1973-1974, 1977, 1985	Asian Pacific Islanders

National Master Facility Survey (now part of NHPI)	mailed questionnaires to facilities or data collected by other federal agencies, national associations, and state programs	listing of inpatient health facilities including hospitals, nursing homes, and other facilities such as those for the mentally retarded or physically disabled	1967	1967, 1969, 1971, 1973, 1976, 1978, 1980, 1982	Asian Pacific Islanders
National Health Provider Inventory	health care facilities, state licensing agencies, professional associations, all licensed facilities in covered categories	characteristics of hospitals, nursing and related care homes, characteristics of board and care homes and hospices	1991	1991	Asian Pacific Islanders
National Nursing Home Survey, Follow-up on 11,181 persons at 1985 baseline survey	proxy or next-of-kin CATI interviews, nursing homes, Medicare records	nursing home utilization patterns, estimates of length of stay, changes in payment sources, survival time	1985 baseline	continuous follow-up 1987, 1988, 1990	Asian Pacific Islanders

NOTE: a. White (includes Mexican, Puerto Rican, and other Caucasian), Black, Indian (American, Alaskan, Canadian, Mexican Indian, Eskimo, and Aleut), Chinese, Japanese, Hawaiian (includes part Hawaiian), Filipino, other Asian Pacific Islander, and other races.
SOURCE: National Center for Health Statistics, unpublished table, modified by the author.

by information collected from various components of the U.S. health care delivery systems. For example, the National Ambulatory Medical Care Survey collects data through self-administered questionnaires sent to a probability sample of office-based physicians throughout the country, whereas the National Hospital Discharge Survey investigates the flow and characteristics of patients discharged from the nation's hospitals. To provide information on facility and resident characteristics, a new survey called the National Health Provider Inventory was initiated in 1991 that collects data from questionnaires mailed out to all (approximately 80,000) nursing homes, board and care homes, home health agencies, and hospices in the United States.

In addition to the aforementioned surveys, there are other types of programmatic research targeted toward specific populations. Some surveys have been established for quite some time; others have started only recently. The National Survey of Family Growth (NSFG), conducted in 1973, 1976, 1982, and 1988, has focused on a variety of topics, including contraceptive use and family planning, teenage sexual activity and pregnancy, adoption, and breast-feeding. NSFG has a national sample of approximately 10,000 households in which only one woman 15 to 44 years old is interviewed. During the decade of the 1980s, two new data collection programs were added: the Longitudinal Study of Aging, a special survey of some 7,000 persons who were 70 years and older in 1984; and the Teenage Attitudes and Practices Survey, which examines tobacco use and HIV infection in a sample of 12,000 adolescents 12 to 18 years of age.

Finally, NCHS also has several data maintenance programs based on the vital statistics routinely maintained by each of 50 states: the Vital Statistics Cooperative Program, which serves as a network of communication for state vital registration offices and facilitates the standardization of a set of minimum information collected from vital records; the National Linked Birth-and-Death Files program, established in 1983, which provides precise estimates of the true infant mortality rates experienced by different groups in the country; the National Death Index, which makes possible the verification of death nationwide for epidemiological studies; the National Maternal and Infant Health Survey, which examines factors associated with low birth weight and infant death, prenatal care, and maternal risk factors; and the National Mortality Followback Survey, which traces state death records for useful information on factors associated with premature or infant deaths, use of health care resources in the last year of life, disability prior to death, and mortality associated with suspected risk factors.

Through these complex data collection systems, NCHS supplies Congress with useful annual statistics on the health of the nation that are necessary for legislative planning. However, in the 30 years since its establishment, none of the programmatic *surveys* has provided useful, valid, and reliable information on Asian Pacific American subgroups. Most of the programs have, by now, provided data for Asian Pacific Americans as a broad category (see the last column of Table 2.1), which are not useful. A couple contain information on specific Asian Pacific American subgroups (see Table 2.1), which is of limited use. Methodological problems in concepts and measurements abound in all of NCHS's *survey* programs, insofar as the extrapolation of Asian Pacific American health data is concerned. These are discussed below.

Accuracy of the Numerator

Through vital statistics records routinely maintained by state departments of health, NCHS collects and publishes data on births, deaths, marriages, and divorces in the United States. Fetal deaths are classified and tabulated separately from other deaths. However, ethnicity identifiers for Asian Americans have been rather limited. The recognition of Japanese, Chinese, and Filipinos as separate groups of Asians—begun in the late 1960s—is an improvement over earlier practices in which Asians were classified as "other" together with Native Americans and other nonwhites. However, not coded in the vital statistics are the fastest growing and more recent Asian immigrants and refugees (e.g., Koreans, East Indians, Vietnamese, Cambodians, Laotians, Hmongs, Thais, Burmese, Malaysians, and Indonesians). Changes are underway beginning with 1992 data.

Because the natality and mortality data files at present distinguish only Japanese, Chinese, Filipinos, Hawaiians, Guamanians, Samoans, and "other Pacific Islanders," we have no national estimates of the mortality rates for Koreans, East Indians, and Vietnamese, much less other emerging Asian subgroups such as Malaysians, Thais, Indonesians, Cambodians, Laotians, and Hmongs. What is perhaps most bothersome about NCHS's vital statistics system is the lack of accurate information—until very recently—on the extent of race/ethnic classification errors that may exist in both mortality and natality files for small ethnic groups. The establishment of the

National Linked Birth-and-Death Files since 1983 have finally enabled NCHS to determine the direction and magnitude of recording errors for Asian Pacific Americans in the U.S. infant mortality data. One investigator has determined that "for whites and blacks, the race coding on the birth certificate differed from that on the corresponding death certificate in < 2% of the linked files; however, 25% to 40% of the infant deaths among births coded as American Indian/Alaska Native or Asian on the birth certificate were coded to a different race on the death certificate" (Kleinman, 1990). Another study revealed that although inconsistency in the coding of race for white infants is low (1.2%), it is quite high for nonwhite, nonblack groups, especially Asian Americans—33.3% for Chinese, 48.8% for Japanese, and 78.7% for Filipinos (Hahn, Mulinare, & Teutsch, 1992).

These reports present an alarming message on the futility of continued reliance on unlinked mortality files to determine the infant—and, by extension, adult—death rates for Asian Pacific Americans prior to 1983, even though we still have very little information with which to assess the quality of adult mortality data for Asian Pacific Americans. With the benefit of hindsight, we are now convinced that previous reports of low infant mortality rates for certain Asian Pacific subgroups may have been, in part, an artifact of racial or ethnic classification, even though we cannot ascertain the magnitude of this error for the period prior to the time when national birth and death data were linked. Especially for the top 10 states (California, New York, Hawaii, Texas, Illinois, New Jersey, Washington, Virginia, Florida, and Massachusetts) where 79% of the Asian Pacific American population resides and for the 15 selected standard metropolitan statistical areas (Los Angeles-Long Beach, New York, Honolulu, San Francisco, Oakland, San Jose, Anaheim-Santa Ana, Chicago, San Diego, Seattle, Houston, Sacramento, Philadelphia, Riverside-San Bernardino, and Boston) with the largest Asian or Pacific Islander population in 1990, it would be productive and informative to conduct research to determine if the direction and magnitude of misclassification errors on existing vital records is greater for some groups of Asians compared with others, and whether the misclassification has significantly altered the different measures of infant health from the neonatal to the postneonatal period. Such an effort was undertaken for Washington State at a time when Asians were still small in numbers (Frost & Shy, 1980). During the late 1960s, this issue had also emerged in relation to the California data files. However, Norris and Shipley (1971) noted that although the misclassification significantly altered the measures of infant health for Japanese relative to those for white Americans, it did not change the relative position of Chinese Americans compared with whites. More recent presentations of the 1983 to 1985 national birth cohorts indicate that Chinese, Japanese, and Filipinos all have lower infant mortality rates than do white Americans (Feinleib, 1991; Hahn et al., 1992), even after one corrects for inconsistencies in racial coding between the birth and death certificates. These findings provide strong evidence for the need to identify subgroups of Asian Pacific Americans whose infant mortality rates may be higher than those reported for the white American, Chinese, Japanese, and Filipino groups.

It is important to emphasize that the residual category labeled "other Asian or Pacific Islanders" is now the largest Asian Pacific American group in NCHS's coding system for the natality data, and the one with the highest infant mortality rate (Hahn et al., 1992; Kleinman, 1990). Just what does "other Asian or Pacific Islanders" refer to? According to Taffel (1984), the term includes Asian Indian, Burmese, Cambodian, Ceylonese, Chamorro, Dutch East Indian, Fijian, Gilbertese, Guamanian, Javanese, Korean, Laotian, Malaysian, Maori, Marshallese, Pakistani, Ponapean, Samoan, Siamese, Thai, and Vietnamese. We are unable to decompose the category of "other Asian Pacific Americans" in order to determine which specific subgroup may warrant special attention. A population that may be at risk thus remains unidentified and unserved as we attempt to reach the nation's health objectives for the year 2000.

The Denominator Problem

The denominator for calculating the *national* mortality and morbidity rates of Asian Americans can be obtained only from the U.S. Census. Two serious limitations exist with the data: population undercount and lack of intercensal estimates.

Population undercount. It was reported originally that the 1990 census missed 4.7 million people, compared with 2.9 million left out in 1980 ("Cities Press Campaign," 1991). A later news report, however, put the undercount figure at 8.3 million, including up to 1.5 million Californians (Fulwood, 1991). The U.S. General Accounting Office is reported to have estimated that "the census may have missed counting as many as 9.7 million people" ("Sawyer Trying," 1991). One source stated that "Los Angeles was the most severely undercounted city in the nation" and "California was the most dramatically undercounted of any state in the nation," representing one fifth of the total census undercount nationwide (Waugh, 1991). In the absence of systematic studies on undercount of minority populations, it is difficult to evaluate the accuracy of these news reports, but they do point up the fact that the undercount problem may be worse for some cities than others.

Table 2.2 shows the 1990 census undercount, as officially acknowledged in the *Congressional Quarterly Weekly Report* (Elving, 1991a). The report puts the nationwide undercount at 5.27 million, or about 2.1%. States with a large influx of immigrants in recent years (California, Arizona, New Mexico, and Texas) also had the worst undercount problem. Given that Asian Pacific Islanders are largely immigrants, one can expect this group to be seriously undercounted. It is interesting to note that Commerce Secretary Robert A. Mosbacher reported only that "blacks were undercounted by 4.8%, American Indians by 5%, and Hispanics by 5.2%." His selective omission of the extent of undercount among Asian Americans is noteworthy (Elving, 1991b).

Needless to say, census data have enormous political implications because they are used for reapportioning the 435 seats in the U.S. House of Representatives and state legislatures, and they form the basis for allocating federal revenues to state and local governments, which ultimately affect research, training, and health and human services programs for underserved populations. It comes as no surprise that more than 20 cities, counties, states, and civil rights organizations have reportedly filed lawsuits to demand census adjustment of population figures.

Lack of intercensal estimates. Updated statistics on Americans in general are obtainable through the application of demographic methods by the U.S. Bureau of the Census and independent investigators. Inasmuch as the magnitude of errors in natality and mortality for Asian Pacific Americans have not been critically assessed, there is great difficulty in obtaining valid estimates of the annual growth in terms of the excess of births over deaths. Furthermore, although immigration figures are available, there are no emigration statistics for Asian Pacific Americans. Hence it is not possible to obtain intercensal estimates for this ethnic group.

Questions have been raised as to whether the Current Population Surveys (CPS) that are conducted annually around special topics

Table 2.2 1990 Census Undercount

	Official 1990 Census	1991 Survey Data Projection	Estimated Undercount %
U.S. total	248,709,873	253,978,000	2.1
Alabama	4,040,587	4,146,000	2.5
Alaska	550,043	561,000	2.0
Arizona	3,665,228	3,790,000	3.3
Arkansas	2,350,725	2,403,000	2.2
California	29,760,021	30,888,000	3.7
Colorado	3,294,394	3,376,000	2.4
Connecticut	3,287,116	3,306,000	0.6
Delaware	666,168	687,000	3.0
District of Columbia	606,900	639,000	5.0
Florida	12,937,926	13,278,000	2.6
Georgia	6,478,216	6,633,000	2.3
Hawaii	1,108,229	1,136,000	2.4
Idaho	1,006,749	1,035,000	2.7
Illinois	11,430,602	11,592,000	1.4
Indiana	5,544,159	5,586,000	0.7
Iowa	2,776,755	2,807,000	1.1
Kansas	2,477,574	2,506,000	1.1
Kentucky	3,685,296	3,768,000	2.2
Louisiana	4,219,973	4,332,000	2.6
Maine	1,227,928	1,240,000	1.0
Maryland	4,718,468	4,869,000	1.8
Massachusetts	6,016,425	6,039,000	0.4
Michigan	9,295,297	9,404,000	1.2
Minnesota	4,375,099	4,419,000	1.0
Mississippi	2,573,216	2,632,000	2.2
Missouri	5,117,073	5,184,000	1.3
Montana	799,065	822,000	2.8
Nebraska	1,578,385	1,595,000	1.0
Nevada	1,201,833	1,232,000	2.4
New Hampshire	1,109,252	1,116,000	0.6
New Jersey	7,730,188	7,836,000	1.4
New Mexico	1,515,069	1,586,000	4.5
New York	17,990,455	18,304,000	1.7
North Carolina	6,628,637	6,815,000	2.7
North Dakota	638,800	648,000	1.4
Ohio	10,847,115	10,933,000	0.8
Oklahoma	3,145,585	3,214,000	2.1
Oregon	2,842,321	2,898,000	1.9
Pennsylvania	11,881,643	11,957,000	0.6
Rhode Island	1,003,464	1,006,000	0.3
South Carolina	3,486,703	3,590,000	2.9
South Dakota	696,004	707,000	1.6

(continued)

Table 2.2 Continued

	Official 1990 Census	1991 Survey Data Projection	Estimated Undercount %
Tennessee	4,877,185	5,012,000	2.7
Texas	16,986,510	17,551,000	3.2
Utah	1,722,850	1,757,000	1.9
Vermont	562,758	571,000	1.4
Virginia	6,187,358	6,353,000	2.6
Washington	4,866,692	4,987,000	2.4
West Virginia	1,793,477	1,842,000	2.6
Wisconsin	4,891,769	4,924,000	0.7
Wyoming	453,588	466,000	2.7

SOURCE: Elving (1991a).

can be redirected to provide some estimates of the births and deaths of Asian Pacific Islanders. But, because of current practice of sampling in proportion to population size, it is not possible to have a sufficient number of Asian Pacific American subgroups in any given year of the CPS to warrant separate analysis, even if it were to focus its data collection activities on obtaining estimates of births and deaths. This means that annual data from the Current Population Surveys are not of much use for epidemiological studies on Asian Pacific American subpopulations. Thus the denominators required to calculate national mortality and morbidity rates for Asian Pacific American subgroups between census years are simply nonexistent.

An alternative sampling strategy better suited for studying Asian Pacific Americans needs to be developed. In a slow-growth economy with a shortage of federal funds, special sample surveys in the top 10 states and 15 SMSAs with the largest Asian Pacific American populations could be a cost-effective way of obtaining intercensal population estimates for specific regions of the country. However, such a strategy would require the collaboration of federal, state, and local governments, working in conjunction with Asian Pacific American scientists and community advocates.

Difficulty in Assessing Risks

As a result of the lack of national health data on Asian Pacific Americans, the mortality files at NCHS are often used to provide an indirect estimate of Asian Pacific American health risks. However, the absence of denominator data between census years means that, in assessing the mortality risks of Asian Pacific Americans from specific causes of death, researchers can measure risks only in a very rudimentary manner. The simple task of age adjustment, used in making comparisons of risks across populations, requires extreme caution in interpretation. More often than not, the researcher can use only the indirect, instead of the direct, method of adjustment. With the indirect method, an expected number of deaths for the Asian Pacific subgroup of interest is obtained by using the age-specific rates of another group, usually either the U.S. total or the white population in a given year. A standard mortality ratio (SMR) is calculated by dividing the observed number of deaths for the Asian Pacific population of interest by the expected number of deaths, which is then expressed as a percentage. Such an exercise, however, provides only limited information as to whether a certain subgroup of Asian Americans is experiencing more or fewer deaths than expected *if the U.S. total or white population's age-specific rates were to prevail in the Asian subpopulation.* It does *not* allow the researcher to make comparisons across subgroups of Asian Pacific Americans, or between Asian Pacific Americans and other minorities. Cross-group comparisons are often desirable to provide evidence of higher risk for a particular disease in one Asian Pacific subgroup compared to another, or to justify the need for special services targeted toward a special subpopulation, or to document *differences within* the category of people labeled "Asian Pacific Americans." Computations based on SMRs do not lend themselves to such comparisons and are thus of limited use.

Because of the absence of intercensal estimates for Asian Pacific Americans, researchers have often used the intercensal numerator data to obtain an approximate measure of mortality "risk" in an extremely limited way by calculating the proportional mortality ratio (PMR). The magnitude of the PMR, however, is influenced by other competing causes of death, which makes comparisons among groups a limited exercise. If intercensal surveys can be conducted in selected states or cities with the largest numbers of Asian Pacific Americans, we will be making a positive step toward solving at least the denominator problem for these states or cities. At the same time, we will be in a better position to assess the morbidity and mortality risks of Asian Pacific Americans outside of Hawaii.

Feasibility of Pooling Data

In all of NCHS's data collection systems except for the National Vital Statistics System, the category "Asian Pacific Islanders" is the only ethnicity identifier for the diverse groups of people who originate from the Pacific Rim countries and surrounding territories, and it is not possible to disaggregate this group further to distinguish Japanese from Chinese, Filipinos, Koreans, Vietnamese, Asian Indians, and others. In some data sets prior to the mid-1980s, Asian Pacific Americans were often combined with American Indians and Alaska Natives as "other" in the data tabulation stage. Pooling information from different years of these surveys, though often recommended as a strategy to increase the precision of estimates, actually becomes problematic for two reasons: The number of Asian Pacific Americans remains small because of the practice of sampling in proportion to population size, and interpretation is difficult because it is not always clear what the "mix" of ethnic subgroups is from year to year (Yu, Drury, & Liu, 1981).

Obstacles in Studies by Independent Investigators

Funded projects and community surveys conducted by individual investigators are an alternative source of health data on Asian Pacific Americans. However, with the exception of the Ni-Hon-San study and other studies of Japanese Americans patterned after it, the data collection procedures and question contents of most health surveys on Asian Pacific Americans have not been standardized across studies to facilitate comparison of specific health measures with either the national U.S. data or other major health surveys. Each piece of research is simply not designed to shed light on the national or cross-national health profile of major Asian Pacific American subgroups. Despite several past attempts to encourage different investigators in certain major cities to conduct collaborative and coordinated studies on the health of Asian Pacific Americans, where each site replicates the work of the other sites in anticipation of subsequently pooling data for analysis, we have yet to see such a plan come to fruition. Problems seem to exist at various levels. First, a unique mix of linguistic, cultural, methodological, and substantive expertise is required to conduct any large-scale epidemiological study of specific Asian or Pacific Islander subgroups in a single site, not to mention multisite studies of different groups. Even in cities where Asians are highly concentrated it is not easy to assemble such a team of competent investigators with complementary skills. Second, a complex set of issues confronts any team of researchers interested in conducting epidemiological studies. The elements in this set of issues are described below.

Defining the Study Population

The term *Asian Pacific Americans* covers myriad cultures and at least 45 linguistic groups whose ancestries can be traced to places that include Mongolia to the north, the islands near Australia to the south, India-Pakistan to the west, and Hawaii to the east. In their native habitats, some are nomads living on horseback; others ride the "bullet trains" to work in modern high-rise buildings, and still others go to work in chauffeur-driven Rolls Royces. In terms of indigenous diet, some are vegetarians, others shun pork, and still others do not eat beef. Suffice to say that they differ immensely in terms of racial origin, religion, lifestyle, diet, and health. As a consequence of the U.S. "open-door" immigration policy begun in 1965, we find varying numbers of Asians and Pacific Islanders across the vast expanse of the United States. How does one scientifically define this special population in any piece of epidemiological research without inadvertently excluding some groups—and thereby risking political fallout? Yet this was precisely what had happened in the past when funding became available for research on Asian Pacific Americans. Some members of the National Institutes of Health's IRBs are not always aware that the inclusion of each Asian Pacific American ethnic group would double the cost of research if the added group speaks only one non-English native language. The cost increases each time a different language group is included, even within the same ethnic population. At some point, the epidemiological concept of sampling by selective respondent characteristics must be used and defended to ensure adequate sample size for meaningful interpretation of health data.

Identification and Sampling Issues

It is difficult in epidemiological studies of Asian Americans and Pacific Islanders to defend the selection of respondents for health surveys using less than scientifically rigorous sampling methods (e.g., snowball sampling, quota sampling, purposive sampling, or other nonprobability sampling procedures) and still obtain the critical approval of sampling statisticians who are accustomed to using conventional sampling schemes in their own research (e.g., simple random sampling or multistage probability sampling procedures) but have had no previous working experiences with Asian Pacific Americans. Recently, some investigators have used sampling lists from telephone directories or a combination of different directories created by survey or marketing firms. But the accuracy of these lists for Asian Pacific Americans has so far never been tested. The differential biases expected from identifying Asian Pacific Americans inherent in the use of these phone directories or other merged records have, therefore, not been addressed. A concerted effort to tackle this issue is essential if we are to conduct health surveys of Asian Pacific Americans that will be credible to the mainstream scientific community.

Several issues need to be examined with regard to sampling lists obtained from marketing firms: How accurate are they in representing the surnames of persons from particular ethnic backgrounds? For example, does the list of surnames for, say, Chinese households in fact contain large proportions of non-Chinese names mistakenly identified as Chinese? Are there specific Chinese names that are fairly common but that have been systematically omitted by the surname identification procedure used by the marketing firms? Part of the problem is that not all Asian American investigators are able to read and write fluently in native Asian languages and so are unable to ascertain the adequacy of their purchased sampling lists. But even if this problem were solved by the inclusion of foreign-educated Asian American researchers as research colleagues or assistants, the scrutiny and analysis of surnames will increase accurate identification of groups only within certain limits. First, the results will be more accurate for groups with low rates of interracial marriages than for those with high rates. Second, the "yield" will be greater when the Asian group of interest is highly concentrated within a defined geographic boundary than when it is not. Third, although the method of surname identification may be practical for surveys on the health of Chinese, Japanese, Koreans, and Vietnamese, it is doubtful that it would work for Filipinos—many of whom have Spanish surnames—or Hawaiians—many of whom have an assortment of Asian, Polynesian, and other last names not always distinguishable from those found among mainstream Americans.

A second major problem with sampling lists purchased from marketing firms is the timeliness of the household addresses and telephone numbers found for a given list of surnames. Because intercensal counts or estimates are nonexistent, marketing firms' data sources for their lists of ethnic surnames ultimately come from matching a list of surnames-by-ethnicity obtained from the census to available records in the public domain that contain names, addresses, and telephone numbers (e.g., telephone and street directories, driver's license registrations, and motor vehicle registrations). For those Asian subgroups with large immigrant populations that are constantly in a state of flux, few investigators—Asian Americans included—are aware that the census-generated surnames are accurate only in those cases where there has been *no* new influx of a different group of immigrants. To illustrate, in April 1980, when the census was taken, the United States had established diplomatic relationships with the People's Republic of China for only three months. Extremely few Chinese from Mainland China were able to immigrate directly to the United States then. In the ensuing years, however, the United States has experienced a rapid influx of this new group of immigrants. It is important to note that these Chinese have surnames (in English) that are spelled using the Pinyin romanization system developed and standardized throughout Communist China (e.g., Zhang instead of Chang; Xia instead of Hsia; Qu instead of Ju). Thus marketing firms whose source of Chinese surnames was initially derived by matching 1980 census-generated surnames to existing lists of, say, telephone directories or driver's license registration files will miss all Chinese from Mainland China whose last names are spelled differently under the Pinyin system from the way they would have been spelled under any other romanization system (e.g., the Yale or Wade-Giles systems) commonly used previously. Health and epidemiological surveys conducted throughout the 1980s using samples of Chinese surnames generated in the manner described above will have *systematically missed* a segment of the Chinese American population whose sociodemographic characteristics (such as age, income, education, and ability to speak English), health behaviors (such as smoking, drinking, physical exercise, and health care coverage), and outcome measures (such as depression and anxiety) are distinctly different from those of other Chinese Americans.

To date, there have been no studies to determine the accuracy and timeliness of sampling lists purchased from marketing firms for purposes of doing surveys on Asian Pacific Americans. How many of the occupants in any surname list have in fact changed residences by the time the marketing firms generated their sampling lists and the researchers contacted the addressees? What distortions are introduced when investigators capture only those whose residences remain stable? Questions on accuracy and timeliness have been ignored for too long in community surveys of Asian Pacific Americans. There has been concern in some circles that to investigate this matter would be to open a can of worms, to bring on professional doubts about the external validity of findings obtained from such research, and to make health surveys on Asian Pacific Americans even more difficult to get funded in the future than they are now.

Language and Culture

In studying Japanese, Koreans, or Vietnamese, only one foreign-language version of the instrument is required besides an English version. But in studying Chinese, or segments of the Filipino or Indian populations, who do not speak English, one faces unique translation problems because of the existence of diverse languages or dialects—of which some are sufficiently different as to be considered distinct languages in and of themselves. The cost of research increases as one expands a study to include different language or dialect groups in order to increase sample size and to improve generalizability. In conducting surveys on certain Asian Pacific American subgroups, such as Chinese Americans, there is the added difficulty that respondents may not be able to read a dialect (e.g., Cantonese) even though they may speak it well. And as one expands the translation to include *major linguistic groups*, the ominous task begins of ensuring that the different dialect versions are the same as the native-language version and the original English version. Endless pretests are required to establish equivalence between different dialect and language versions of an instrument, a task for which the investigators themselves may be totally unprepared.

Response Rates

With the exception of surveys conducted in Hawaii, few health surveys on Asian Pacific Americans in the continental United States have explicitly reported response rates. Obtaining a high response rate in studies of populations overrepresented by immigrants and refugees is not an easy task for a number of reasons: First, these groups are often geographically mobile; second, their members frequently have more than one job and are thus difficult to reach, making it nearly impossible at times for interviewers to reach them at home; and third, they may not always have telephones. Rather than detracting from the scientific value of the research efforts, researchers' candid reporting of response rates and frank discussion of methodological problems in epidemiological surveys of Asian Pacific Americans will improve our ability to do better research in the future. At the very least, it will enable both funding agencies and researchers to have a more realistic comprehension of the difficulties involved in conducting minority research.

Obtaining Informed Consent

For majority Americans, who have experienced more than 40 years of surveys, giving informed consent to interviewers is less of a problem than it is for Asian Pacific Americans. Recently arrived immigrants and refugees from politically controlled areas in Asia understandably associate surveys with police interrogations or punitive political actions. Even without such suspicions, some immigrants refuse to give consent because they are unable to write their own names; others simply cannot understand why they must sign their names in order to answer a series of harmless questions. Does the signature not violate the promise of anonymity and confidentiality? How much freedom should review boards give investigators to obtain verbal consent when written informed consent is viewed with fear or anxiety by respondents? Few authors of published studies on Asian Pacific Americans have admitted their difficulties in obtaining written informed consent. Investigators are often caught between the rules concerning the use of human subjects and field conditions that are generally not widely known to non-Asian Pacific American researchers.

Discussion and Conclusions

Over the past 30 years, our knowledge of the health status, characteristics, and behaviors of different Asian Pacific American subgroups have been based on a few epidemiological surveys conducted in Hawaii and on the West Coast as well as on inferences drawn

from available data compiled by the NCHS, even though they are
not designed to focus on the health of special minority populations.
Through the routinely collected vital statistics records and the
National Linked Birth-and-Death Files, we have counts of death for
some of the major and "older" Asian Pacific American groups, but
not of the new immigrants and refugees whose numbers are increasing at an astounding rate. Thus we have only the most rudimentary estimates on the status and determinants of Asian Pacific
Americans' health, in spite of more than 30 years of continuing
programmatic support from the U.S. Congress for NCHS to conduct
periodic nationwide surveys on the health of Americans.

With the exception of Hawaii, where the importance of maintaining health data by ethnic groups has long been appreciated, health
surveys on Asian Pacific American groups must confront numerous
methodological problems in defining the study population, sampling of rare elements, developing instruments that may need to be
translated into several languages and/or dialects, determining actual response rates, and obtaining written informed consent. The
National Center for Health Statistics was established primarily to
collect health and epidemiological data on the *general population*—a
mission that does not easily justify expenditures on minority populations that appear to be insignificant in terms of size or political power,
unless these are specifically funded by the U.S. Congress in the form
of "special projects." The sampling procedures NCHS has used in its
surveys over the past 30 years have not been designed to study small
groups of ethnic minority populations unevenly distributed across the
nation, of which Asian Pacific Americans are one example. Thus, even
if funding were available today for NCHS to do special surveys on
Asian Pacific Americans, the methodology for conducting such studies in a scientifically acceptable manner remains to be discussed,
debated, and deliberated. Moreover, the National Center for Health
Statistics, as it is currently organized, is not equipped to deal with the
complex linguistic and cultural issues of instrument development
beyond English and Spanish.

At the level of the individual investigator, lack of communication
between qualified mainstream and Asian Pacific American health
investigators, and intense competition among trained Asian Pacific
American researchers for limited resources, as well as the classic
"town-and-gown" conflict between "community advocates" and
"academics" on the objectives of research (immediate services and jobs
for minorities versus generating basic data and building theories)

constitute the major obstacles to studies on the health of Asian Pacific Americans.

In the 1990s there is renewed opportunity for Asian Pacific American community advocates and scientific researchers to work cooperatively toward a common goal. A more favorable climate now exists for research on Asian Pacific American health, including mental health, than has ever existed in the past 100 years of Asian Pacific Islander presence in the United States. The U.S. Congress has been much more receptive to the idea of appropriating special allocations for understudied populations, such as women and minorities. An example is the passage of the Disadvantaged Minority Health Improvement Act of 1990 (P.L. 101-527); another is the 1991 Cooperative Agreement issued by the Centers for Disease Control to the Asian and Pacific Islander American Health Forum and the National Coalition of Hispanic Health and Human Services Organizations to advance the understanding of the health of racial and ethnic populations or subpopulations, authorized under Section 306 (42G U.S.C. 242K) of the Public Health Service Act. This agreement provides an unprecedented opportunity for researchers to analyze previously collected health data and improve existing research methodologies or test innovative methodological techniques used in gathering information on special populations.

We believe that the time has finally come also to confront the methodological problems in studying the health of Asian Pacific Americans and to design methodological studies that will explore important issues in sampling Asian Pacific Americans outside of Hawaii. In addition, in future years of the National Health Interview Survey, a special supplement to study selected Asian Pacific American subgroups by means of oversampling, augmented sampling, or other selective regional sampling schemes should be discussed seriously. Given the fact that the sampling procedures for the next several years of the NHIS program are based on census data collected in 1990, the time to plan for an NHIS Asian Pacific supplement for the year 2000 is now. On several occasions, and in a recent editorial (Yu, 1991), we have recommended that until the NHIS Asian survey becomes a reality, a good place to begin is the improvement of at least one question in the current NHIS program: the ethnicity identifier. We are pleased that, beginning with the 1992 data year, NCHS began a new code structure for natality, mortality, fetal deaths, and induced termination of pregnancy data in order to distinguish the six major Asian American subgroups (Filipinos,

Chinese, Japanese, Vietnamese, Asian Indians, and Koreans) and
gain a better understanding of their respective health risks through
pooled analysis of consecutive years of data. If, as we suspect will
be the case, those data remain unusable because of extremely small
numbers even after they are pooled over several years, NCHS will
have a firmer basis for rethinking the current sampling design used
in its surveys, as the inadequacy of that design for studying the
health risks of Asian Americans will have been demonstrated.
There is a need to lobby for the expansion of NCHS's new "race"
coding structure to all of NCHS's survey programs as well as to
other data collection systems maintained by other federal agencies,
such as the Alcohol, Drug Abuse, and Mental Health Administration, the Health Care Financing Administration, and the Agency for
Health Care Policy Research. In a separate paper, we plan to make
a set of recommendations to the National Center for Health Statistics to help improve the quality of national health data to be collected on subgroups of Asian Pacific Americans in future years of
its vital statistics system and survey programs.

References

Angel, A., Armstrong, M. A., & Klatsky, A. L. (1989). Blood pressure among Asian-
Americans living in Northern California. *American Journal of Cardiology, 64,* 237-240.
Cities press campaign to fix census undercount. (1991, April 2). *Los Angeles Times,*
p. B1.
Curb, J. D., Aluli, N. E., Kautz, J. A., Petrovitch, H., Knutsen, S. F., Knutsen, R.,
O'Conner, H. K., & O'Conner, W. E. (1991). Cardiovascular risk factor levels in
ethnic Hawaiians. *American Journal of Public Health, 81,* 164-167.
Elving, R. D. (1991a, June 15). Bureau releases new estimates, remains wary of
adjustment. *Congressional Quarterly Weekly Report, 49.*
Elving, R. D. (1991b, July 20). Refusal to adjust undercount spurs protest, renews suit.
Congressional Quarterly Weekly Report, 49.
Feinleib, M. (1991, December 4-6). *Overview of federal data systems and issues.* Paper
presented at the conference, Setting a Research Agenda: Challenges for Minority
Health Grants Program, Bethesda, MD.
Frost, F., & Shy, K. K. (1980). Racial differences between linked birth and infant death
records in Washington State. *American Journal of Public Health, 70,* 974-976.
Fulwood, S., III. (1991, April 19). Census may have skipped 8.3 million, studies show.
Los Angeles Times, p. A1.
Haenszel, W., & Kurihara, M. (1968). Studies of Japanese migrants: I. Mortality from
cancer and other diseases among Japanese in the United States. *Journal of the
National Cancer Institute, 40,* 43-68.

Hahn, R. A., Mulinare, J., & Teutsch, S. M. (1992). Inconsistencies in coding of race and ethnicity between birth and death in U.S. infants. *Journal of the American Medical Association, 267,* 259-263.

Hinds, M. W., Kolonel, L. N., Lee, J., & Hirohata, T. (1980). Associations between cancer incidence and alcohol/cigarette consumption among five ethnic groups in Hawaii. *British Journal of Cancer, 41,* 929-940.

Kagan, A., Harris, B. R., Winkelstein, W., Johnson, K. G., Kato, H., Syme, S. L., Rhoads, G. G., Gay, M. L., Nichaman, M. Z., Hamilton, H. B., & Tillotson, J. (1974). Epidemiologic studies of coronary heart disease and stroke in Japanese men living in Japan, Hawaii and California: Demographic, physical, dietary and biochemical characteristics. *Journal of Chronic Disease, 27,* 345-364.

Kato, H., Tillotson, J., Nichaman, M. Z., Rhoads, G. G., & Hamilton, H. B. (1973). Epidemiologic studies of coronary heart disease and stroke in Japanese men living in Japan, Hawaii, and California: Serum lipids and diet. *American Journal of Epidemiology, 97,* 372-385.

King, H. (1975). Selected epidemiologic aspects of major disease and causes of death among Chinese in the United States and Asia. In A. Kleinman, P. Kunstadter, E. R. Alexander, & J. L. Gale (Eds.), *Medicine in Chinese cultures: Comparative analysis of health Care in Chinese and other societies* (Publication No. NHI 75-653, pp. 487-550). Washington, DC: Government Printing Office.

Klatsky, A. L., & Armstrong, M. A. (1991). Cardiovascular risk factors among Asian Americans living in Northern California. *American Journal of Public Health, 81,* 1423-1427.

Kleinman, J. C. (1990). Infant mortality among racial/ethnic minority groups, 1983-1984. *Morbidity and Mortality Weekly Report, 39*(SS-3), 31-39.

Kolonel, L. N., Hankin, J. H., Lee, J., Chu, S. Y., Nomura, A. M. Y., & Hinds, M. W. (1981). Nutrient intakes in relation to cancer incidence in Hawaii. *British Journal of Cancer, 44,* 332-339.

Li, D. K., Ni, H., Schwartz, S. M., & Daling, J. R. (1990). Secular change in birthweight among Southeast Asian immigrants to the United States. *American Journal of Public Health, 80,* 685-688.

Liu, W. T., & Yu, E. S. H. (1985). Asian Pacific American elderly: Mortality differentials, health status, and use of health services. *Journal of Applied Gerontology, 4,* 35-64.

Lynberg, M., & Muin, J. K. (1990). Contribution of birth defects to infant mortality among racial/ethnic groups, United States, 1983. *Morbidity and Mortality Weekly Reports, 39*(SS-3), 1-11.

National Center for Health Statistics. (1979). *NCHS fact sheet* (Publication No. 861-384). Washington, DC: Government Printing Office.

Norris, F. D., & Shipley, P. W. (1971). A closer look at race differentials in California's infant mortality, 1965-67. *HSMHA Health Reports, 86,* 810-814.

Reed, D., & Yano, K. (1987). Epidemiological studies of hypertension among elderly Japanese and Japanese Americans. *Asia-Pacific Journal of Public Health, 1,* 49-56.

Rhoads, G. G., & Feinleib, M. (1983). Serum triglyceride and risk of coronary heart disease, stroke, and total mortality in Japanese-American men. *Arteriosclerosis, 3,* 316-322.

Robertson, T. L., Kato, H., Rhoads, G. G., Kagan, A., Marmot, M., Syme, S. L., Gordon, T., Worth, R. M., Belsky, J. L., Dock, D. S., Miyanish, M., & Kawamoto, S. (1977). Epidemiologic studies of coronary heart disease and stroke in Japanese men living in Japan, Hawaii, and California. *American Journal of Cardiology, 39,* 239-243.

Sawyer trying to free data for use in redistricting. (1991, September 14). *Congressional Quarterly Weekly Report, 49.*

Stavig, G. R., Igra, A., & Leonard, A. R. (1984). Hypertension among Asians and Pacific Islanders in California. *American Journal of Epidemiology, 119,* 677-691.

Stemmermann, G. N., Chyou, P. H., Kagan, A., Nomura, A. M. Y., & Yano, K. (1991). Serum cholesterol and mortality among Japanese-American men. *Archives of Internal Medicine, 151,* 969-972.

Taffel, S. (1984). Characteristics of Asian births: United States, 1980. *Monthly Vital Statistics Report, 32*(Suppl. 10).

Takeya, Y., Popper, J. S., Shimizu, Y., Kato, H., Rhoads, G. G., & Kagan, A. (1984). Epidemiologic studies of coronary heart disease and stroke in Japanese men living in Japan, Hawaii, and California: Incidence of stroke in Japan and Hawaii. *Stroke, 15,* 15-23.

Tillotson, J. L., Kato, H., Nichaman, M. Z., Miller, D. C., Gay, M. L., Johnson, K. G., & Rhoads, G. G. (1973). Epidemiology of coronary heart disease and stroke in Japanese men living in Japan, Hawaii, and California: Methodology for comparison of diet. *American Journal of Clinical Nutrition, 26,* 177-184.

Waugh, D., (1991, June 14). Dramatic census revision. *San Francisco Examiner,* p. C4.

Yano, K., & MacLean, C. J. (1989). The incidence and prognosis of unrecognized myocardial infarction in the Honolulu, Hawaii, Heart Program. *Archives of Internal Medicine, 149,* 1528-1532.

Yano, K., Reed, D. M., Curb, J. D., Hankin, H. H., & Albers, J. J. (1986). Biological and dietary correlates of plasma lipids and lipoproteins among elderly Japanese men in Hawaii. *Arteriosclerosis, 6,* 422-433.

Yu, E. S. H. (1982). The low mortality rates of Chinese infants: Some plausible explanatory factors. *Social Science and Medicine, 16,* 253-265.

Yu, E. S. H. (1986). Health of the Chinese elderly in America. *Research on Aging, 8,* 84-109.

Yu, E. S. H. (1991). The health risks of Asian Americans. *American Journal of Public Health, 81,* 1391-1393.

Yu, E. S. H., Drury, T. P., & Liu, W. T. (1981). *Using National Health Interview Survey data in secondary analysis of health characteristics of Asian Pacific Americans: Problems and prospects.* Paper presented at the annual meeting of the American Statistical Association, Detroit.

PART II

Health Status

3

Mortality

ROBERT GARDNER

In this chapter I hope to answer the following questions:

1. What are the levels and patterns of mortality among Asian Americans?
2. How does Asian American mortality compare with mortality of the white population?
3. What factors explain the observed levels and patterns?

Before attempting to answer these questions, I must first present the data available for the study of Asian American mortality. Following this, I will devote some discussion to the factors that affect mortality; this discussion will set the stage for the remainder of the chapter.

Before going any further, it should be noted that "Asian Pacific Americans" do not constitute a homogeneous group. The six largest groups are Chinese, Filipinos, Indians, Japanese, Koreans, and Vietnamese; there are numerous smaller groups as well.[1] These groups are not homogeneous either, but vary internally along a number of dimensions. Regardless of the size of the group being dealt with here (e.g., all Asian Americans or a specific group such as Japanese Americans) and regardless of its heterogeneity, I will not be discussing individuals but *averages* and rates for the *group,* for instance, the death rate for all Asian Americans.

It should also be noted that, although this chapter is about mortality, there will be inevitable overlap with morbidity, the incidence and prevalence of disease. *Incidence rate* refers to the number of new cases of a disease divided by the size of the population at risk; *prevalence rate* refers to the number of cases "on hand" at a point in time divided by the size of the population at risk (see Polednak, 1989). Morbidity levels and rankings never correlate 100% with mortality, but the relationship, especially for certain causes of death, is close, and in the absence of data dealing directly with mortality, morbidity data can be used to make useful inferences about mortality. Furthermore, for certain causes of death, such as cancer of the prostate, survival rates are quite high, and data on incidence may be especially enlightening in such cases (Kolonel, Hinds, & Hankin, 1980).

Finally, it should be noted that there is little separate consideration of the sexes in the discussion or data presented here. Separate data are not always available, but even when they are, there is simply not the space available to cover two groups (or three: total, male, and female).

Problems of Data

Any discussion of the mortality of Asian Americans should begin with some consideration of both the availability and the quality of data. Because Asian Americans are numerically still a rather small group in the total U.S. population, they do not appear in statistically significant numbers in sample surveys that might otherwise shed light on their mortality levels. Even when complete data are collected at the national level, they may not be reported; until 1966 the National Center for Health Statistics published data only on whites and nonwhites in its annual *Vital Statistics* volumes.

Apart from availability, there are problems of quality of data. For several reasons, data on the mortality of Asian Americans are simply not as good as those for whites. The most important reason has to do with difficulties of "matching." Mortality rates, like other demographic rates, are composed of two parts: a numerator and a denominator. The crude death rate (CDR), for example, has deaths in the numerator and "population at risk" in the denominator. If deaths are recorded completely and the population is counted accurately, the resulting CDR should be accurate. If, however, deaths are not recorded completely or the population is not counted accurately, then the CDR will not be correct.

For the total population of the United States, there is little question about the accuracy of the CDR. For Asian Americans, however, the situation is problematic, because of the difficulty of determining and assigning race consistently for different individuals. By *consistently*, I mean that if an individual appears in U.S. census counts as a Filipino, then when that person dies, he or she should be listed on the death certificate as Filipino. On the U.S. Census form, a person's ethnicity (or "race," in Census Bureau terms; I shall use the terms interchangeably here) is decided by that person; that is, ethnicity is self-identified (or determined by the household member filling out the form). If a person born of German parents wants to declare herself an Asian American, she can, simply by checking the appropriate box on the census form. An individual may change his or her ethnic self-identification from one census to the next. In addition, the census form makes no allowance for people who are of mixed race: a Chinese-Filipino must choose either Chinese or Filipino; if he writes in "Chinese-Filipino," the Census Bureau will assign him a category.[2] This eliminates the possibility of having to contend with an almost infinite number of combinations, but it does violence to the real complexity of the situation.[3] Of course, if everyone were of one ethnicity or another, things would be a lot easier; it is with mixed-ethnicity individuals that most problems occur.

The difficulty of collecting information on ethnicity, and the volatile nature of the topic, was underscored during the years preceding the 1990 census, when the U.S. Bureau of the Census, after much thought and pretesting of alternatives, sought to change its question on race and was met with a tremendous outcry from, among others, the Asian American community, which felt that the new approach would result in an undercount of Asian Americans. The bureau returned to a format similar to that used in 1980.

Although the individual (or a household member) records his or her own race on a census form, on a death certificate it is always someone else who records that person's race. Generally, the funeral director is responsible for completion of personal information on the deceased. The section of the certificate that includes the race question is answered on the basis of information obtained by the funeral director from an informant, usually a family member or friend of the decedent. The result of this situation is that, for example, a Chinese-white person who was listed as Chinese in the census may be listed on her death certificate as white. This would result in a downward bias in the death rate for Chinese Americans and an upward bias in the death rate for whites.

If all persons were assigned their "census races" on their death certificates, this problem would not arise. However, there is no easy way such a thing can be accomplished. As we shall see below, only one major research effort on adult mortality has been able to get past this problem of mismatch between numerator and denominator (Kitagawa & Hauser, 1973). There have been more studies looking at matching of birth and infant mortality records; these are reviewed below.

> A study by the National Center for Health Statistics on the comparability of racial data on death certificates and matching census records found that although agreement was very high for whites (99 percent) and blacks (98.2 percent), it was quite poor for Filipinos (72.6 percent) and Native Americans (79.2 percent), and less than satisfactory for Chinese (90.3 percent). The study concluded that *"observed death rates for the Indians, Chinese and Filipinos were much lower than death rates would have been if only census information had been used."* (Lin-Fu, 1988, p. 23, citing National Center for Health Statistics, 1969; emphasis added)

The reader should keep this in mind throughout the discussion that follows.

Determinants of Mortality

As we shall see below, Asian American mortality levels are not the same as those of whites. They are not the same because Asian Americans are not the same as whites. How are Asian Americans different from whites? In trying to answer this question, we could begin by listing all sorts of possible candidates: income, diet, and more. Although there are a variety of ways one could try to answer this question (e.g., Polednak, 1989), it will profit us here to use a simple framework of factors that distinguish Asian Americans from whites and that may affect mortality.

Genetic Considerations

One factor is genetics. Although there is a large literature on the genetic basis of disease, relatively little of it refers to Asians or

Asian Americans. Young (1990) discusses the topic, noting the well-known examples of "sickle-cell disease in Afro-Caribbeans, Tay-Sachs disease in Ashkenaze Jews, cystic fibrosis in western European Caucasians, and thalassaemia in Greek Cypriots" (p. 193). Looking at (mainly South) Asians in Great Britain, Young finds relatively high levels of thalassemia (impairment of hemoglobin synthesis) and neural tube defects (NTDs), both traceable to high levels in the origin populations. (NTD incidence in Great Britain among Asians, however, "is probably lower than their country of origin, but higher than for the indigenous British population. This is in keeping with the observation that ethnic differences for NTDs are influenced considerably by migration, pointing to a major environmental aetiological contribution"; p. 205.)

With regard to Asian Americans, there are only a few clear examples of genetic sources of mortality differentials. There is more information on several nonlethal disorders. Lin-Fu (1988) notes that many health workers "are not aware of the high prevalence of alpha and beta thalassemia and hemoglobin E carrier state [HbE] in Asian Pacific Americans" (p. 23) and goes on to discuss other genetic disorders, such as lactose intolerance, which may be more prevalent among Asian Americans than in the host white population. Polednak (1989) lists single-gene disorders that are relatively frequent and relatively infrequent in several ethnic groups, including Japanese and Koreans, Chinese, and Thais. High-frequency single-gene disorders for Japanese and Koreans are acatalasia, cyschromatosis universalis hereditaria, Oguchi's disease, and G6PD deficiency; low frequencies are found for alpha thalassemia and phenylketonuria. For Chinese, high-frequency disorders include alpha thalassemia, G6PD deficiency (Chinese type), and beta thalassemia (southern China); low frequency is found for HbE, except in Yunnan province. For Thais, high-frequency disorders include HbE (abnormal hemoglobin), alpha and beta thalassemia, combined HbE-thalassemia syndromes, and G6PD deficiency. HbE is also found in high frequency among Asian refugees in the United States, especially Khmers (Polednak, 1989, p. 78).

The "persistence of low breast-cancer rates among the second-generation Nisei (Japanese) suggests a role for genetic factors," according to Haenszel and Kurihara (1968, p. 57). The extremely high levels of nasopharyngeal cancer observed among Chinese, especially those from certain high-risk areas of China, have been attributed to genetic causes (Hu & White, 1979; King & Haenszel,

1973). However, recent observation of dramatic differences in the incidence of the disease among Chinese in China, China-born immigrants to the United States, and U.S.-born Chinese indicates that other factors are also at work (Dickson, 1981). One study found that in Hong Kong "90 percent of cancers may be attributable to childhood consumption of salted fish" (Polednak, 1989, p. 212, citing results from Yu, Ho, Lang, & Henderson, 1986).

Even if genetic factors are the source of some Asian American mortality, they are not necessarily of much relative importance. Kolonel (1988) states that "available evidence suggests that purely genetic factors probably account for less than 2% of cancer incidence overall" (p. 133). The evidence "has failed to suggest that differences in mortality and health care are due to genetic (racial) differences, as Asians have achieved both high and low mortality rates relative to the U.S. general population" (Liu, 1986, p. 164).

Selection

Asian Americans are composed of both immigrants and U.S.-born individuals. The immigrants may have been "selected" in their country of origin—that is, people leaving the home country may have been in better overall health (or worse overall health) than the average citizen of that country. Indeed, they also may have had better or worse health than the average citizen of their new country, the United States. Any discussion of the health and mortality of Asian Americans must consider that the immigrants among them may have arrived with levels of health different from those of the origin and the host populations. Kuo and Tsai (1986) found that, with regard to immigrant *mental* health, "a migratory selection factor does exist" (p. 147). Selection is thus not a way in which Asian American immigrants and whites differ, but a possible source of those differences in various factors.

A number of studies have found that immigrant mortality levels are often intermediate between those of the origin population and those of the host population. "This 'shifting' phenomenon does not necessarily constitute an assimilation of mortality patterns" (Trovato, 1990, p. 96), but may be caused by the fact that immigrants were positively (or negatively) selected. That is, "migrants may reflect a select group which in turn exemplify a superior mortality experience [or] there may be an assimilative phenomenon which operates upwardly or downwardly in aligning life expectation of immigrants with [that of] the indigenous host population" (p. 97). "The overall evidence suggests that migration is a selective process with respect to mortality" (p. 106).

Characteristics

Another way in which Asian Pacific Americans differ from whites has to do with socioeconomic and demographic characteristics, such as age, sex, and marital structures, average income, occupational distribution, and average educational attainment. One might argue that if two groups have the same characteristics, they would have the same mortality. This perspective would predict that, as Asian Americans become more "assimilated"—that is, as their characteristics become more and more like those of whites—their mortality levels would become more and more like those of whites (Evans, 1987).

"Racial and ethnic differences in certain diseases may be due largely or entirely to differences in socioeconomic status (SES) and environmental factors associated with SES" (Polednak, 1989, p. 6). Polednak emphasizes "the overwhelming importance of socioeconomic status . . . factors in explaining racial/ethnic differences in incidence and mortality rates for many diseases . . . both infectious and chronic." "The effects of poverty go beyond variables of personal risk factors or medical-care services, and suggest the influence of a broad range of environmental factors including differential exposure to crowding, psychosocial stress, and noxious environmental agents" (p. 280).

The study of differential mortality mentioned earlier focused on characteristics. Kitagawa and Hauser (1973) looked at productivity, standards of living, environmental sanitation, personal hygiene, public health measures, and modern medicine. The ethnic mortality levels they observed were inversely related to group incomes. Yu, Chang, Liu, and Kan (1984) note, "The evidence suggests the presence—on an aggregate level—of an inverse relationship between socioeconomic status and mortality which may account for some of the observed inter-ethnic mortality differentials" (p. 19).

According to Polednak (1989), "The predominant role of socioeconomic status in explaining racial/ethnic differences in disease patterns actually operates through environmental influences associated with SES. These factors include crowding, poor nutrition and sanitation, and social stresses as well as inadequate medical care"

(p. 23). At least for cancer, "socioeconomic status is not a risk factor for cancer per se, but a proxy for other real environmental exposures or genetic predispositions that are more prevalent in particular groups in our society" (Goodman, 1989, p. 42).

Culture

"Filipinos and Hawaiians, both of lower socioeconomic status in Hawaii, have widely divergent rates for many types of cancer. Ethnicity or race may therefore exert a significant effect on the incidence of cancer that is independent of education, income, or other socioeconomic indicators" (Goodman, 1989, p. 42). A cultural perspective on mortality seeks to find sources of differentials in differences in "cultural" (racial or ethnic) factors. Of course, "culture alone is . . . not a sufficient explanation for the types of lives that people lead" (Helman, 1990, p. 23), or their mortality levels.[4]

For immigrants, and for later generations, the very process of acculturation may affect health and mortality. "Acculturative stress" can lead to "a reduction in the health status of individuals, and may include physical, psychological, and social aspects," according to Berry, Kim, Minde, and Mok (1987, p. 493). "Population or racial/ethnic differences in some cancers and cardiovascular diseases are apparently related largely to differences in intake of specific dietary constituents such as total fats or specific types of fats, vitamins, fiber, and sodium. Other habits of importance include smoking and alcohol" (Polednak, 1989, p. 282).

Diet may vary between two groups that are virtually indistinguishable in terms of their census "characteristics." Because diet affects mortality, levels of mortality might well be different between the two groups in spite of their similar characteristics. Studies of diet among different ethnic groups in Hawaii showed considerable variation in the consumption of various items (Kolonel, 1988; Kolonel, Hankin, & Nomura, 1986; Kolonel, Hankin, Nomura, & Chu, 1981; Kolonel et al., 1980, 1983; Kolonel, Nomura, Hirohata, Hankin, & Hinds, 1981). The items listed by Kolonel (1988) include rice (Filipinos ate the most, followed by Japanese, Chinese, Hawaiians, and Caucasians), beef (Caucasians, Hawaiians, Chinese, Japanese, and Filipinos), broccoli (Caucasians, Chinese, Hawaiians, Japanese, and Filipinos), fat (Caucasians, Hawaiians, Chinese, Japanese, and Filipinos), protein (Caucasians, Hawaiians, Japanese, Chinese, and Filipinos), and vitamin C (Caucasians, Japanese, Hawaiians, Chinese, and Filipinos). Kolonel (1988) states that "environmental, especially dietary, influences are major determinants of risk for cancers of such sites as the breast, prostate, stomach, colon and lung" (p. 133).

Diet may well change after immigration. A decrease in the sodium content of their diet may be partially responsible for the drop in levels of stroke for Japanese Americans compared with the levels found in Japan. Hankin, Kolonel, Yano, Heilbrun, and Nomura (1983) found differences in diet between Japanese migrants (Issei) and second-generation Japanese (Nisei) in Hawaii, with "greater intakes of total fat, total and animal protein and total carbohydrate in Nisei as compared to Issei, whereas Issei consumed more total cholesterol than Nisei. . . . Moreover, there was consistency among the cohorts in the consumption of more traditional food items by Issei and more western foods by Nisei" (p. 22). A study of Southeast Asian refugees found that they "maintained strong ties to their native foods and traditional diets . . . [but], although most adults prefer eating their native foods, their children prefer both American and native foods" (Story & Harris, 1989, p. 800).

Diet is only one of many cultural factors that may affect mortality. A second set has to do with smoking and drinking. Apparent low Asian American levels of smoking and alcohol consumption may lie behind low Asian American perinatal and adult death rates for certain causes of death for which tobacco and alcohol have been shown to be major risk factors (Yu, 1982; Yu et al., 1984). However, levels of smoking among Asian Americans are not necessarily low. Muto (1991) notes, "Studies indicate that in California, 71 percent of Cambodian men, 72 percent of Laotian men and 60 percent of Vietnamese men smoke. In contrast, 33 percent [of] the general population in California smokes. . . . Asian and Pacific Islander immigrants have the highest prevalence of smoking among young males in the U.S." (p. 25).

Other cultural factors are less tangible. Many researchers have found a steep gradient in coronary heart disease (CHD) mortality rates, from low in Japan through intermediate for Japanese in Hawaii to high for Japanese in California (Gordon, 1957, 1967; Kagan et al., 1974; Marmot et al., 1975). Marmot and Syme (1976) looked at factors such as use of language, ethnicity of associates, and religion in causing CHD among Japanese American males in eight San Francisco Bay Area counties. Their study showed that traditional Japanese males in the Bay Area tended to have low levels of CHD, whereas nontraditional Japanese males had high levels. The most traditional group had a prevalence rate for CHD only one fifth the rate of the group most acculturated to the United States. Nontraditional, U.S.-acculturated Japanese males tended to be characterized by relative lack of stability and accent on the individual rather than the group. Possible confounding factors such as diet, age, smoking, high blood pressure, serum triglycerides, weight, and levels of serum cholesterol were controlled for (but only one at a time, not in a multivariate approach).

The importance of culture is also emphasized by Liu (1986): "The changes of mortality rates over time can only be explained by changes of life styles, environment, and the way people take care—or fail to take care—of their health. Social class [characteristics] differences have not lent themselves as convincing explanation" (p. 164). Trovato (1990) notes, "There is now some convincing evidence, based on controlled follow-up studies of immigrants, that factors such as acculturation to the new society (e.g., diet, lifestyle), degree of traditionalism (maintenance of ethnic traditions), and the extent of social support systems in the immigrant community have a significant bearing on the incidence and prevalence of diseases such as elevated blood pressure and coronary heart disease" (p. 107).

Rumbaut and Weeks (1989) also place emphasis on the importance of culture, finding that groups with poor economic status nevertheless can achieve quite low infant mortality rates. They suggest that "the low rate of infant mortality within this seemingly high-risk population is at least partly due to such sociocultural factors as a generally nutritious diet in socially supportive familial and coethnic contexts, combined with virtual nonuse of drugs, alcohol and tobacco by Indochinese women" (p. 191). A similar perspective on infant mortality is provided by Fung, Wong, and Lau (1989), who found that low infant mortality among Chinese (in China, Singapore, and Hong Kong) might be explained by "favourable ethnic determinants": a low incidence of very low birth weight (VLBW) babies resulting from "optimal age at conception as well as rarity of teenage pregnancy, diabetes mellitus, and of mothers who smoke and drink alcohol" (p. 130). They conclude that "studying the lifestyle, nutrition and the sociocultural patterns of the Chinese may offer strategies to developed countries to shift the distribution of VLBW infants which could have considerable impact on perinatal mortality" (p. 130). Genetic factors may also be at work, given that the populations studied had relatively low rates of lethal congenital anomalies.

Also important, if not consciously health related in the minds of individuals, may be the existence of a personal support system (Berkman & Syme, 1979). The important factor may not be something specific to a particular culture's support system, but simply the existence of a support system. Berkman and Syme (1979) note that "the association between social ties and mortality was found to be independent of self-reported physical health status at the time of the 1965 survey, year of death, socioeconomic status, and health practices such as smoking, alcoholic beverage consumption, obesity, physical activity, and utilization of preventive health services as well as a cumulative index of health practices" (p. 186). Berry et al. (1987) state that "social support variables are found to mediate the acculturation and stress relationships among Koreans" (p. 507).

With regard to immigrants, who make up a majority of most Asian American groups, Helman (1990) notes, "The process of being an immigrant is a stressful one, and the individual may only be protected from this by his or her social support networks: religious organizations, community groups, extended family, circle of friends, and traditional healers" (p. 25). Kuo and Tsai (1986) found that, at least regarding immigrant mental health, "as long as the individual has a sufficient number of close ties—preferably with a high degree of interrelationship among them—he/she enjoys a better mental health status" (p. 147). Regardless of the great importance culture is seen to play by many researchers, however, "one should avoid the dangers of 'culturalism'—reducing all aspects of a group's life down to its 'culture,' while ignoring such important factors as its members' social class or economic status" (Helman, 1990, p. 21).

Discussion

One should not expect any simple answers when dealing with questions about the determinants of mortality. When looking at Asian American mortality levels and patterns, for example, and how they differ from white levels and patterns, we cannot say that all of the differences are caused by differences in income, education, and so on, nor can we say that all of the differences are caused by differences in culturally prescribed behaviors, or by selection, or by genetic factors. All of these factors are probably important, and most researchers acknowledge this, even if they are not able to include them all in individual studies.

A word that has commonly been used to describe the Asian American mortality experience (and many other kinds of experience as well) is *adaptation*. As a group adapts to a new place, it seems reasonable to assume that the group's characteristics, its "culture," and even its genetic makeup will change (owing to outmarriage) toward those of the host population. If Asian Americans ever became "exactly like whites," then the mortality levels and patterns of the two groups would become indistinguishable.

When we look at immigrant studies, we often find that, as has been found for England and Wales as well as for the United States, "immigrants appear to be in an intermediate position (relative to countries of origin and destination), but they also demonstrate a general tendency to adopt the cause-of-death patterns and levels of the receiving population" (Trovato, 1990, p. 106). However, the situation is not quite so simple. An important set of factors that interact with those listed above has to do with place of birth and, for immigrants, age at arrival and length of residence in the United States. These factors affect the possibility and potential for adaptation along both characteristics and cultural behavioral dimensions. If they are not taken into consideration, it is difficult to say how important adaptation is.

For example, if Chinese had extremely low mortality and if we knew they had all immigrated very recently, then we would know that not much adaptation could have occurred. Chinese mortality could have been low because Chinese were positively selected for health at the origin *and/or* had come to the United States with exceptionally good characteristics *and/or* were genetically superior. However, if immigrant Chinese had arrived young and were all longtime U.S. residents, then adaptation could be playing a bigger role: movement toward the national averages in terms of income, perhaps, and probably in terms of cultural behavior. Genetic factors would remain important and the effect of initial selection would probably diminish. A third case might be if Chinese were all second generation or higher, that is, born in this country. Adaptation along both characteristics and cultural dimensions would be very important and selection not very important at all, and genetic factors would depend on outmarriage.

The factors of place of birth, age at arrival, and length of residence interact with selection, genetics, characteristics, and culture. To the extent that I cannot take all of these factors into account in this discussion of Asian American adaptation and mortality, the discussion cannot be precise.

Table 3.1 Crude Death Rates, 1940 to 1980, and Age-Standardized Death Rates, 1970 to 1980, by Race, United States

	Crude Death Rates					Age-Standardized Death Rates	
	1940	1950	1960	1970	1980	1970	1980
Total	10.8	9.6	9.5	9.5	8.8	7.1	5.9
White	10.4	9.5	9.5	9.5	9.1	6.8	5.6
Black	13.9	11.3	10.4	10.0	8.6	10.0	8.6
Chinese	15.3	9.0	6.8	4.7	3.7	4.9	3.5
Japanese	6.7	6.1	5.1	4.2	4.0	3.3	2.9
Filipino	—	—	—	—	2.4	—	2.5

SOURCE: For 1940 to 1960, National Center for Health Statistics (1963); for 1970 and 1980, Yu et al. (1984), reprinted with permission.
NOTE: Table presents deaths per 1,000 population. Standardized on the 1940 U.S. age distribution.

Levels, Patterns, and Differentials

Death Rates and Life Expectancy

A basic measure of the mortality of a population is the crude death rate, which is the number of deaths in a given year divided by the midyear population of the group. As with all crude death rates, crude death rates for Asian Americans are affected by the age compositions of the populations: a "young" population will have a lower CDR, all else equal, than an "old" population. In addition, published CDRs suffer from the data problems mentioned above.

Keeping this in mind, see Table 3.1, which presents the CDRs for U.S. whites, blacks, Chinese, Japanese, and Filipinos for each census year since 1940. These data suggest that Asian American mortality levels, at least for the groups listed, are substantially below those for the country as a whole and even those of the majority white population. The comparisons for the past two census years are more valid because of the calculation of age-adjusted death rates, which removes the effects of the differing age structures on the rates. However, these low rates may not be entirely accurate because of possible mismatch between numerator and denominator death data. Although there is no standard, simple way to correct for this problem, the authors of the study discussed next went to some effort to deal with it.

Kitagawa and Hauser's (1973) classic work on differential mortality was the best early national study of mortality that included data on Asian Americans. The researchers matched records for some 340,000 deaths that occurred from May through August 1960 to 1960 annual census records in order to obtain information about the decedents that is not ordinarily available (such as income, which does not appear on death certificates). The matching process also enabled adjustment of ethnic death rates by examination of discrepant reporting of race between the death certificates and the census. The resulting adjustments revealed that uncorrected data for whites, blacks, and Japanese were reasonably accurate, but that data on Chinese were affected by mismatch problems.

The most notable finding from this study was the low mortality of the Japanese. Mortality indexes for Japanese for infants, children under 5, and individuals over 5 were all about one third below the rates for whites. For Chinese males, the adjusted mortality index for ages 5 and over was 10% above that for whites, but for females it was about 9% lower.

In addition, Kitagawa and Hauser calculated life expectancies from uncorrected age-specific death rates for whites, blacks, and Japanese. The life expectancy for Japanese males was estimated to be 74.4 years, and for Japanese females 80.4 years. Comparable figures for whites were 67.6 and 74.7 years, respectively. These figures were similar to those from a California study by Hechter and Borhani (1965) for the same time period (Table 3.2).

A study of 1979 data by the National Center for Health Statistics (1985) replicates the earlier findings of relatively low levels of Japanese American and Chinese American mortality. Japanese and Chinese Americans were found to have age-specific death rates lower than those for whites, with Japanese rates lower than Chinese at most ages. Because the earlier study by Kitagawa and Hauser found that adjustment *increased* nonwhite-white differentials, the National Center for Health Statistics authors note that although "observed rates . . . may contain a large error component," their findings "may be assumed to understate true race differentials in mortality" (p. 33).

In a study of data on the health and mortality of minority groups, the National Institutes of Health Task Force on Black and Minority Health calculated the life expectancy of different minority groups. Life tables prepared for this effort (uncorrected for definitional discrepancies) show the values for life expectancy for 1979 to 1981 (Table 3.2). As in previous research, Asian and Pacific Islander Americans show lower mortality and higher life expectancy than whites or blacks.

Table 3.2 Estimated Life Expectancy at Birth, Combined Sexes, by
Ethnic Group, Hawaii, 1920 to 1980, and California and United
States, 1960 and 1979 to 1981

Year	White	Chinese	Japanese	Filipino	Hawaiian, Part Hawaiian	Total
Hawaii						
1920	56.5	53.8	50.5	28.1	33.6	45.7
1930	61.9	60.1	60.1	46.1	41.9	54.0
1940	64.0	65.3	66.3	56.9	51.8	62.0
1950	69.2	69.7	72.6	69.1	62.5	69.5
1960	72.8	74.1	75.7	71.5	64.6	72.4
1970	73.2	76.1	77.4	72.6	67.6	74.1
1980	76.4	80.2	79.7	78.8	74.0	78.0
California						
1960[a]	71.8	72.9	77.9	—	—	—
1979-1981	74.9	82.5[b]		—	—	74.8
United States[a]						
1960	71.2	—	77.4	—	—	—
1979-1981	74.5		81.9[c]			73.9

SOURCES: For Hawaii, Gardner (1984); for California 1960, Hechter and Borhani (1965); for
California 1979 to 1981, California Center for Health Statistics (1983); for the United States 1960,
Kitagawa and Hauser (1973); for the United States 1979 to 1981, Asian and Pacific Islanders,
Duke University Demographic Studies Center (1984); for the United States 1979 to 1981, white
and total, National Center for Health Statistics (1985).
NOTES: a. Simple average of male and female life expectancies.
b. Combined Chinese and Japanese.
c. Asian and Pacific Islander.

Another study undertaken as part of the work of the Task Force
on Black and Minority Health represented a major effort to summarize the recent mortality experience of Asian Americans (Yu et al.,
1984). Unpublished data from the National Center for Health Statistics were used to calculate measures of Asian American health
and comparable figures for the U.S. white population for 1980. The
data were restricted to Chinese, Japanese, and Filipinos. In the
absence of any linked birth-and-death files since Kitagawa and
Hauser (1973) until the mid-1980s, it was not possible to examine
what Kitagawa and Hauser term "discrepancies in the reporting of
race on death certificates and census records" (p. 101).

Yu et al. found that Asian Americans (Chinese, Japanese, and
Filipinos) had lower mortality than whites, with Filipino rates the
lowest. This was true for both 1970 and 1980, and the rankings did

Table 3.3 Age-Specific Death Rates by Ethnicity, United States, 1988
(deaths per 100,000 population)

Age Group	White	Black	American Indian	Asian Pacific Islander
1-14	30	49	44	24
15-24	95	145	162	57
25-44	149	367	271	77
45-64	790	1,380	856	402
65+	5,106	5,650	3,292	2,430

SOURCE: National Center for Health Statistics (1991, data for Figures 6-10).

not change when the data were adjusted for age-structural differences. (Filipino rates were not available for 1970.)

The most recent national data I have found for mortality by ethnicity come from the annual volume *Health, United States* (National Center for Health Statistics, 1991). In the edition for 1990, data from 1988 are presented for Asian Pacific Islanders as well as for Hispanics, Native Americans, blacks, and whites. The data are presented for different age groups, thus minimizing the effects of differing age structures. Denominators were calculated by the National Center for Health Statistics, and no matching was done.

In all 5 age groups, Asian Pacific Islanders had the lowest death rates (Table 3.3). In second place most often were whites; blacks and Native Americans had the highest mortality.

Data at the local level come from Los Angeles County, which contains substantial numbers of Asian Americans. Using 1980 data, Frerichs, Chapman, and Maes (1984) found substantially lower age-adjusted death rates for Japanese, Filipinos, Koreans, and Chinese than for whites, blacks, or Hispanics (Table 3.4). Ratios of Asian death rates to total county rates ranged from 0.17 for Filipinos to 0.59 for Japanese; the white ratio was 1.06. The authors make little attempt to explain such a spectacular advantage for the Asians, except to note that the Japanese, who are longer established, are probably benefiting less from the "healthy migrant" effect. Other factors mentioned are "the unique aspects of [Asian] medical care system, family structure, diet, and lifestyle" (p. 295).

Table 3.4 Population and Deaths Due to All Causes, by Ethnicity, Los Angeles County, 1980

Ethnic Group	Population 1980	Number of Deaths	Adjusted Rate per 100,000	Ratio to Total County
Total County	7,477,503	61,329	820	1.00
White	5,073,617	52,401	870	1.06
Black	943,968	7,413	1,038	1.27
Hispanic	575,829	3,588	815	0.99
Japanese	116,543	555	483	0.59
Filipino	99,043	103	137	0.17
Chinese	93,747	244	363	0.44
Korean	60,618	129	422	0.51

SOURCE: Frerichs et al. (1984, Table 1). Reprinted by permission of Oxford University Press.
NOTE: Standard is total county age and sex structure. Hispanic data are from census tracts in which 75% or more of the population is Hispanic.

Infant Mortality and Health

Infant Mortality Rates

The study of infant mortality and especially of ethnic differentials in infant mortality differs from the study of mortality at other ages in that the data for both the numerator and denominator come from vital statistics records, not, as in the case of the denominator for death rates at other ages, from census sources. This poses different problems of definition and interpretation and special opportunities as well.[5]

Rumbaut and Weeks (1989) note that "children of mixed-Asian origin seem especially likely to be classified as non-Asian on the death certificate, but Asian on the birth certificate" (p. 145). In recent decades a number of researchers have tried to adjust for classification problems by matching numerator and denominator data, that is, by physically matching death certificates to birth certificates and assigning consistent ethnic categories. In a study in Washington State, Frost and Shy (1980) found that babies of mixed ethnicity tended to be classified more often as white at death than at birth, which would bias white infant mortality rates upward and other infant mortality rates downward.

After adjusting for classification error, Norris and Shipley (1971) estimated that 1965 to 1967 California Japanese infant mortality rates (at 22.0 deaths per 1,000 births) were 62% higher than before adjustment and were actually higher than those for white Americans in California (19.3 per 1,000). On the other hand, Chinese infant mortality rates, which were 13.6 infant deaths per 1,000 births before adjustment, were 25% higher after adjustment but still the lowest for any racial group.

Yu (1982), in a study of infant mortality among Chinese infants, looked at matched birth and death records for 1973 to 1977 in California. She found that "the best available data suggest that the *true* infant mortality rate for Chinese Americans *may* be lower than that found for white Americans" (p. 263). In seeking explanations for the extremely low reported levels of Chinese infant mortality, Yu reports that she was

> tempted to posit that perhaps the Chinese American women . . . being 86% foreign-born (non-U.S. residents excluded)—compared to about 8% foreign-born in the white population—may have retained a traditional set of sociocultural health habits or lifestyles which contribute to their advantage in fetal survival . . . [lower levels of] smoking, drinking, substance abuse, . . . [use of] herbal medicine and dietary preferences. (p. 263)

A recent matching study in San Diego County, California, during 1978 to 1985 focused on Indochinese refugees but collected data on other ethnic groups as well (Rumbaut & Weeks, 1989). Data from this study (Table 3.5) clearly show that Asian American levels of infant mortality are substantially below those of other major ethnic groups. The data also indicate that there are differences among the separate Asian American groups. Although most of the predominantly refugee groups compare favorably with non-Asian groups, some refugee groups, in particular the Hmong, have infant mortality rates that are relatively high (although only marginally higher than the rate for white non-Hispanics and substantially lower than that for blacks).

The San Diego data on Vietnamese and other Indochinese groups are among the few pieces of information we have so far on the mortality of Asian American groups other than Japanese, Chinese, and Filipinos. According to Rumbaut and Weeks (1989), the low rates are especially significant:

> (1) because they reflect a very rapid reduction in infant death levels from those of their sending environments and their own prior experi-

Table 3.5 Infant Mortality Rates by Ethnic Group, San Diego County, 1978 to 1985

Ethnic Group	Infant Mortality Rate
All Indochinese	6.6
Hmong	9.1
Laotians	7.2
Vietnamese	5.5
Khmer	5.8
Filipino	7.2
Chinese	6.9
Japanese	6.2
Black	16.3
White (non-Hispanic)	8.0
Hispanic	7.3
Total	8.5

SOURCE: Rumbaut and Weeks (1989, Table 2). Reprinted by permission of Oxford University Press.
NOTE: Calculated from linked records.

ences, and thus a positive adjustment to the receiving environment in the United States; (2) because their currently observable patterns of infant mortality, especially among the Hmong and Lao, involve greater than average proportions of post-early neonatal deaths which may in principle be preventable, thus leaving open the likelihood that their IMRs [Infant Mortality Rate] can be reduced further still; and (3) because this major epidemiological transition has taken place in the context of their extraordinarily stressful migration and resettlement experiences, and *despite* the fact that these refugees generally . . . reflect high-risk socioeconomic profiles overall. (p. 189)

Recent national data on infant mortality rates, *unadjusted* for any definitional and matching problems, show levels that are very low for Asian Americans (National Center for Health Statistics, 1991). Compared with the white level of 8.6 deaths per 1,000 births, the national level of 10.1, and 17.9 for blacks, the infant mortality rate for Chinese in 1987 was 5.0 infant deaths per 1,000 births; for Japanese, the rate was 4.6, and for Filipinos it was 4.4. Data on infant mortality rates as early as 1966 indicate that similar differentials have existed for several decades (Table 3.6).

The National Center for Health Statistics has recently made available computer tapes of matched birth and death certificates. These tapes provide researchers with the opportunity, for the first time,

Table 3.6 Infant Mortality Rates by Race, 1966 to 1987

Year	All Races	White	Black	Chinese	Japanese	Filipino
1966 total	23.7	20.6	40.1	9.9	10.6	—
male	26.6	23.5	44.0	10.5	12.2	—
female	20.6	17.7	36.2	9.3	8.9	—
1967 total	22.4	19.7	37.5	9.5	10.7	—
male	25.2	22.4	—	—	—	—
female	19.6	16.9	—	—	—	—
1968 total	21.8	19.2	36.2	8.9	10.3	—
male	24.5	21.9	39.6	11.8	11.6	—
female	18.9	16.4	32.7	5.9	9.0	—
1969 total	20.9	18.4	34.7	6.9	9.4	—
male	23.4	20.9	38.3	7.3	10.5	—
female	18.1	15.8	31.1	6.4	8.3	—
1970 total	20.0	17.8	32.6	8.5	10.5	—
male	22.4	20.0	36.2	9.8	13.0	—
female	17.5	15.4	29.0	7.1	8.0	—
1971 total	19.1	17.1	30.3	7.8	7.9	—
male	21.4	19.3	33.3	8.0	10.9	—
female	16.7	14.7	27.3	7.6	4.8	—
1972 total	18.5	16.4	29.6	5.5	9.7	—
male	20.8	18.6	32.4	7.1	10.2	—
female	16.0	14.0	26.8	3.8	9.1	—
1973 total	17.7	15.8	28.1	5.2	9.6	—
male	19.9	17.9	30.9	6.5	11.5	—
female	15.4	13.6	25.2	3.9	7.6	—
1974 total	16.7	14.8	26.8	6.0	9.3	—
male	18.7	16.8	29.4	6.0	10.0	—
female	14.6	12.8	24.1	6.0	8.5	—
1975 total	16.1	14.2	26.2	4.4	6.9	—
male	17.9	15.9	28.3	4.7	6.7	—
female	14.2	12.3	24.0	4.1	7.0	—
1976 total	15.2	13.3	25.5	5.8	4.6	—
male	16.8	14.8	27.8	5.3	4.0	—
female	13.8	11.7	23.2	6.2	5.2	—
1977 total	14.1	12.3	23.6	5.9	6.7	—
male	15.8	13.9	25.9	6.4	5.7	—
female	12.4	10.7	21.3	5.3	7.6	—
1978 total	13.8	12.0	23.1	6.4	6.5	—
male	15.3	13.4	25.4	6.8	7.4	—
female	12.2	10.6	20.8	5.9	5.6	—
1979 total	13.1	11.4	21.8	5.9	4.6	3.8
male	14.5	12.8	23.7	6.5	5.8	4.1
female	11.6	9.9	19.8	5.2	3.2	3.4

(continued)

Table 3.6 Continued

Year	All Races	White	Black	Chinese	Japanese	Filipino
1980 total	12.6	11.0	21.4	5.3	4.5	5.0
male	13.9	12.3	23.3	4.7	4.9	5.1
female	11.2	9.6	19.4	6.0	4.0	4.9
1981 total	11.9	10.5	20.0	5.2	5.2	4.8
male	13.1	11.7	21.7	4.7	5.8	4.2
female	10.7	9.2	18.3	4.6	4.6	5.5
1982 total	11.5	10.1	19.6	6.1	4.6	5.8
male	12.8	11.2	21.5	7.6	5.8	6.1
female	10.2	8.9	17.7	4.6	3.3	5.4
1983 total	11.2	9.7	19.2	6.5	4.3	4.0
male	12.3	10.8	21.1	6.8	4.3	5.1
female	10.0	8.6	17.2	6.1	4.2	2.7
1984 total	10.8	9.4	18.4	5.3	4.3	4.4
male	11.9	10.5	19.8	6.2	3.6	4.9
female	9.6	8.3	16.9	4.4	5.0	3.9
1985 total	10.6	9.3	18.2	5.3	4.4	5.5
male	11.9	10.6	19.9	5.5	4.5	6.1
female	9.3	8.0	16.5	5.1	4.2	5.0
1983-1985 total	NA	9.0	18.7	7.4	6.0	8.2
1986 total	10.4	8.9	18.0	4.7	4.0	4.3
male	11.5	10.0	20.0	4.7	5.0	4.9
female	9.1	7.8	16.0	4.7	3.0	3.7
1987 total	10.1	8.6	17.9	5.0	4.6	4.4
male	11.2	9.6	19.6	5.1	6.2	4.7
female	8.9	7.6	16.0	4.9	2.9	4.1

SOURCE: National Center for Health Statistics, *Vital Statistics of the United States*, annual publication, except 1983 to 1985, which are from matched data found in National Center for Health Statistics (1991).
NOTE: Except for "all races," figures for total are generally simple unweighted averages of figures for male and female. NA = not available.

of examining infant mortality at the national level without having to take matching problems into account. The ethnicity used in such studies is that of the mother, regardless of who the father is and how the child's ethnicity might be classified.

Two recent publications utilize the first data from these tapes. Kleinman (1990) presents information on infant mortality for 1983 to 1984. He notes that "for whites and blacks, the race coding on the birth certificate differed from that on the corresponding death certificate in <2 of the linked files; however, 25% to 40% of infant deaths among births coded as American Indian, Alaskan Native or

Table 3.7   Infant Mortality Rates by Ethnicity, United States, 1983 to 1984
and 1983 to 1985

	(1) 1983-1984	(2) 1983-1985	(3) 1983-1985
All races	10.7	NA	10.9
White	9.1	9.0	9.5
Black	18.7	18.7	18.6
Asian	8.6	NA	NA
Chinese	8.3	7.4	5.7
Filipino	8.5	8.2	4.6
Japanese	6.0	6.0	4.3
Other Asian	9.0	NA	6.9

SOURCES: Column 1, Kleinman (1990), matched data; column 2, National Center for Health
Statistics (1991), matched data; column 3, National Center for Health Statistics, *Vital Statistics of
the United States*, annual publication, unweighted average of yearly unmatched data.
NOTE: "Other Asian" figure for 1983-1985 includes Pacific Islanders. NA = not available.

Asian on the birth certificate were coded to a different race on the
death certificate" (p. 32). The infant mortality rates from Kleinman's
study are found in Table 3.7 (column 1). Asian infant mortality was
below that of whites; within Asian groups, Japanese rates were
lowest, followed by Chinese, Filipino, and "other Asian." Low birth
weight, which is a major factor contributing to infant mortality, was
not less prevalent among Asians, but Asian infant mortality was nevertheless lower than that of whites, blacks, and American Indians
regardless of birth weight.[6]

The publication *Health, United States, 1990* contains some information on infant mortality for the period 1983 to 1985, again using
the linked data (Table 3.7, column 2) (National Center for Health
Statistics, 1991). Japanese, Chinese, and Filipino infant mortality
rates, in that order, were below those of whites and other groups
studied (with the exception that Cubans had a rate slightly lower
than Filipinos, and the Central and South American rate was the
same as the Filipino rate).

At the state level, matched Hawaiian data for 10 ethnic groupings
for a longer period, 1979 to 1988, showed Chinese had the lowest
infant mortality rates, followed in order by Japanese, Samoans,
Caucasians, Hispanics, Filipinos, Koreans, others, Hawaiians and part
Hawaiians, and blacks (Table 3.8) (Park, 1991).[7] "Demographic"
factors were partially at work. For example, although black infant

Table 3.8 Infant Mortality Rates by Maternal Ethnicity, Hawaii, 1979 to 1988

Ethnic Group	Neonatal	Mortality Rate per 1,000 Births Postneonatal	Total
Black	7.14	4.36	11.50
Caucasian	4.83	2.03	6.87
Chinese	4.05	2.02	6.07
Filipino	5.81	2.18	8.00
Hawaiian	6.28	3.52	9.80
Hispanic	4.93	2.90	7.82
Japanese	4.25	2.24	6.50
Korean	7.02	1.30	8.32
Samoan	4.38	2.29	6.67
Others	6.85	1.93	8.78

SOURCE: Park and Horiuchi (1991, Table 1). Reprinted by permission of the authors.
NOTE: Hawaiian includes part Hawaiian. Hispanic means Puerto Rican and Portuguese. Neonatal = during the first four weeks after birth; postneonatal = during the remainder of the first year after birth.

mortality rates were highest, they were *not* highest for any birth weight group (Table 3.9).[8] (Rumbaut & Weeks, 1989, found a similar result for San Diego County.) Standardizing by birth weight therefore resulted in some rearrangement: Japanese levels were lowest, followed in order by Chinese and Filipinos, Koreans, Hispanics, blacks, Caucasians, Hawaiians and part Hawaiians, and Samoans.[9] "Ethnic differences in postneonatal mortality were larger than those in neonatal mortality" (Park & Horiuchi, 1991, p. 11). Given that early infant deaths (neonatal, or in the first month) are more likely to be caused by genetic or intrauterine causes and later infant deaths (postneonatal, or in the remainder of the first year) are more likely to be caused by external or environmental factors, this finding is evidence against strong genetic ethnic differences in the factors that cause infant mortality.

Birth Records

Another perspective on infant mortality and survival is provided from birth records. When birth records are employed there is no problem of mismatch because only the race of the mother is used. Weight at birth is known to be significantly associated with infant survival; a birth weight of less than 2,500 grams is considered low; however, the optimum birth weight is not the same for all ethnic

Table 3.9 Infant Mortality Rates by Maternal Ethnicity and Birth Weight, Hawaii, 1979 to 1988

Ethnic Group	<1,501	1,501-2,500	2,501-3,000	3,001-4,000	4,001+	Total
		Mortality Rate per 1000 Births				
		Birth Weight (grams)				
Black	402.0	17.6	2.4	4.1	0.0	11.5
Caucasian	376.3	26.5	6.2	2.5	2.6	6.8
Chinese	265.7	16.8	4.6	3.0	2.8	5.6
Filipino	334.5	20.3	4.2	2.6	2.6	7.7
Hawaiian	394.9	26.1	6.0	3.9	2.9	9.5
Hispanic	(333.3)	16.7	5.5	4.0	0.0	7.5
Japanese	309.4	21.5	5.0	2.2	0.9	6.1
Korean	(408.2)	18.9	3.0	2.6	0.0	8.3
Samoan	(470.6)	36.7	6.9	4.2	1.1	6.3

SOURCE: Park (1991, Table 1A). Reprinted by permission of the authors.
NOTE: Hawaiian includes part Hawaiian. Hispanic means Puerto Rican and Portuguese. Figures in parentheses are based on fewer than 100 births.

groups (Mi, 1971). In the United States in 1988, 6.9% of all births were below 2,500 grams in weight (Table 3.10). The percentages for some Asian American groups, however, were lower: 4.7% for Chinese and 6.2% for Japanese. The Japanese percentage of low birth weight infants was slightly above that for whites (5.6%) but below that for the other Asian American group tabulated, Filipinos, whose figure was 7.1%. (These figures vary a bit from year to year, but the rankings remain about the same.)

A major factor involved with low birth weights is the educational status of the mother (Taffel, 1984). Asian American women tend to be relatively well educated, but when this factor is statistically controlled it does not account for all of the observed differences in birth weights. Taffel (1984) suggests that other factors, such as the low percentage of out-of-wedlock and teenage Asian American births, may account for some of the observed ethnic differences in the percentages of low birth weights.

A more detailed study found that, after a number of factors hypothesized to be related to birth weight are taken into account, Asian birth weights tend to be slightly lighter (by 210 grams) than white births (Shiono, Klebanoff, Graubard, Berendes, & Rhoads, 1986).[10] The researchers were unable to identify what factors might be involved in the relatively low birth weight for Asian babies. One

Table 3.10 Percentage of Births of Low Weight, by Ethnicity, 1970 to 1988

Group	1970	1975	1980	1981	1982	1983	1984	1985	1986	1987	1988
Total											
United States	7.9	7.4	6.8	6.8	6.8	6.8	6.7	6.8	6.8	6.9	6.9
White	6.8	6.3	5.7	5.7	5.6	5.7	5.6	5.6	5.6	5.7	5.6
Black	13.8	13.1	12.5	12.5	12.4	12.6	12.4	12.4	12.5	12.7	13.0
Asian and											
Pacific Islander	8.4	7.0	6.6	6.6	6.6	6.5	6.5	6.1	6.4	6.4	6.3
Chinese	6.8	5.3	4.9	5.6	5.3	5.0	5.1	5.0	4.9	5.0	4.7
Japanese	8.6	7.2	6.2	6.1	6.2	5.8	6.1	5.9	5.6	6.3	6.2
Filipino	9.4	8.0	7.4	7.3	6.9	7.3	7.7	6.9	7.3	7.3	7.1

SOURCE: National Center for Health Statistics (1991, Table 7).
NOTE: Percentage of births with weight less than 2,500 grams (5 pounds, 8 ounces). For comparison, 1980 figures for California are, from top to bottom, 6.0, 5.3, 11.7, —, 4.7, 6.3, and 7.3 (California Center for Health Statistics, 1983).

might conjecture, however, that relatively high percentages of low birth weight Asian babies may not carry the same negative implications for survival that the same figures might for whites. That is, maybe Asian babies are just slightly smaller, and low birth weight is not as dangerous for them; Rumbaut and Weeks (1989) argue in this vein. Whether this is true or not, birth weight seems to rise with longer maternal residence in the United States, at least for the babies of Southeast Asian refugees (Li, Ni, Schwartz, & Daling, 1990).

Another approach to infant health is the Apgar score, a measure of the physical condition of the infant at 1 minute and 5 minutes after birth: a score of less than 7 is cause for concern about the infant's health and survival chances. The 5-minute score is considered a better predictor of the long-term health and survival chances of the infant than the one-minute score (Taffel, 1984). The percentage of 5-minute Apgar scores less than 7 for all infants in the reporting states in 1982 was 2.1. For whites the figure was 1.8; for Chinese, 1.2; for Japanese, 1.1; and for Filipinos, 1.3.

The two previously discussed approaches to measuring infant health and potential survival both suggest that Chinese infants have the best chance for survival, followed by Japanese and then Filipinos. These rankings are in agreement with the data on infant mortality rates presented above and also with the overall mortality data from Hawaii. An earlier review of minority health by the

National Center for Health Statistics (1985) showed essentially the same results.

Causes of Death

Data for 1979 to 1981 from a U.S. Department of Health and Human Services (1985) study on several major causes of death by broad ethnic group are depicted in Table 3.11. Asian American death rates were lowest in comparison with white rates for accidents, pulmonary disease, liver diseases, and atherosclerosis; Asian American rates were relatively high (but still below white rates) for cancer, cerebrovascular disease, pneumonia and influenza, and diabetes (Figure 3.1).

Also of interest are the rankings of diseases by importance within a specific ethnic group. Such rankings are not seriously affected by matching problems, because only numerator data are necessary. Regarding 1980 data, Yu et al. (1984) note, "Insofar as the first 4 leading causes of death are concerned, all four groups have identical rankings" (p. 21). That is, heart disease, cancer, cerebrovascular disease, and accidents are the most important causes of death for Asian Americans and for whites as well (Table 3.12). Together, these account for just over 70% of the deaths in each of these groups. Data from 1988 show a similar pattern.

Data for 1988 from the National Center for Health Statistics (1991) give death rates (uncorrected for matching problems) for ethnic groups (Asians and Pacific Islanders are grouped as one) for the major causes of death and separate age groups as well (Table 3.13). As the text of the publication notes, "Asian persons in the United States have the lowest death rates across each age group and for nearly all of the causes of death compared" (p. 13). In the few cases where another group had lower death rates, Asians ranked second. As in Yu's study, heart disease, cancer, cerebrovascular disease, and accidents were the most important causes of death for Asian Americans, accounting for more than 67% of all deaths.

The National Cancer Institute (1986) produced age-adjusted site-specific cancer incidence and death rates (*not* adjusted for possible ethnic classification discrepancies) for three Asian American groups—Chinese, Japanese, and Filipinos—as well as whites, Hawaiians, and Native Americans. Results showed that Asian American cancer incidence and mortality rates for the period 1978 to 1981 were well below those of whites, Hawaiians, or Native Americans (Table 3.14).

Table 3.11 Age-Adjusted Death Rates and Death Rates From Specific Causes, 1979 to 1981

| | Rate per 100,000 | | | | | |
| | White | | Black | | Asian | |
Cause of Death	Male	Female	Male	Female	Male	Female
All causes	736.0	405.0	1084.6	611.7	449.8	244.4
Cancer	159.2	106.9	227.9	127.3	106.0	67.1
Heart disease	274.4	131.9	319.4	194.4	146.2	62.2
Stroke	41.2	34.7	76.0	60.2	34.4	26.7
Liver disease/ cirrhosis	15.4	6.9	29.4	13.5	6.9	2.6
Homicide	10.9	3.2	73.4	14.4	8.0	3.3

SOURCE: U.S. Department of Health and Human Services (1985, pp. 65, 90, 108, 111, 158).

Table 3.12 Leading Causes of Death by Ethnicity, United States, 1980 and 1988 (in percentages of total deaths)

| | 1980 | | | | 1988 Males | Asian | 1988 Females | Asian |
Cause of Death	White	Chinese	Japanese	Filipino	White	American	White	American
Heart disease	39.3	31.8	30.4	33.5	35.4	28.9	37.0	26.4
Cancer	21.3	27.8	25.4	20.5	23.3	23.7	22.0	27.1
Cerebrovascular disease	8.6	8.6	11.2	10.1	5.3	7.1	8.7	10.1
Accidents	5.2	4.2	5.4	6.7	5.6	7.7	2.9	5.5
Chronic obstruction/ pulmonary distress	3.0	2.4	2.0	2.0	4.6	3.2	3.5	2.2
Pneumonia and influenza	2.6	3.0	3.5	2.8	3.3	3.4	4.1	3.1
Diabetes mellitus	1.7	2.1	2.0	1.8	1.5	1.8	2.0	2.4
Chronic liver disease/ cirrhosis	1.4	1.2	1.2	1.2	1.5	1.3	0.8	1.0
Atherosclerosis	1.5	0.9	1.0	0.6	—	—	—	—
Suicide	1.5	2.2	2.3	1.5	2.3	2.3	0.6	1.4
Homicide	—	—	—	—	0.8	2.0	0.3	1.4
Human immuno- deficiency disease	—	—	—	—	1.1	0.9	0.1	0.1

SOURCE: For 1980, Yu et al. (1984, Table 13); for 1988, National Center for Health Statistics (1991, Table 25).
NOTE: Data for 1980 are age standardized; 1988 data are unstandardized.

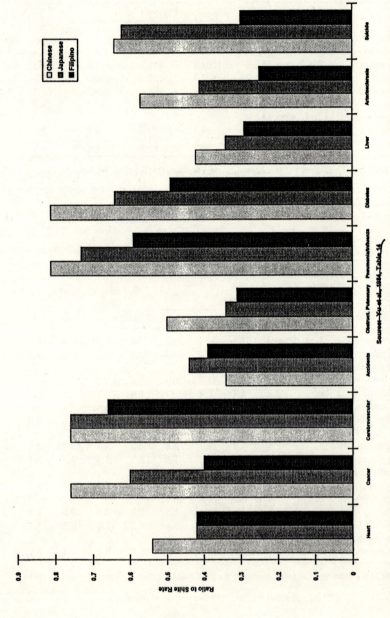

Figure 3.1. Ratios of Age-Standardized Cause-Specific Death Rates of Asian Americans to Those of Whites, 1980
SOURCE: Data from Yu et al. (1984, Table 14).

Table 3.13 Death Rates by Age, Cause, and Ethnicity, United States, 1988

Age Group and Cause	Deaths per 100,000 Population			
	White	Black	American Indian	Asian Americans
1-14				
injuries	13	20	24	10
homicide	1	5	2[a]	1[a]
cancer	3	3	2[a]	3
other	13	21	16	10
15-24				
injuries	52	37	89	29
homicide	8	59	22	7
suicide	14	8	26	6
other	21	41	24	15
25-44				
injuries	34	49	97	15
homicide	8	56	25	7
heart disease	17	44	20	7
HIV infection	12	43	4[a]	3
other	77	175	125	43
45-64				
injuries	31	52	77	18
heart disease	244	426	224	99
cancer	289	401	183	159
cerebrovascular disease	29	86	31	29
other	198	415	341	97
65+				
heart disease	2,079	2,181	1,128	870
cancer	1,062	1,241	606	549
cerebrovascular disease	425	526	248	260
other	1,540	1,702	1,309	752

SOURCE: National Center for Health Statistics (1991, data for Figures 6-10).
NOTE: a. Based on fewer than 50 deaths.

For all sites combined, the cancer death rate for Hawaiians was 200.5 per 100,000; for whites it was 163.6 per 100,000. Chinese rates were 131.5 per 100,000, Japanese were 104.2 per 100,000, and Filipino rates were lowest at 69.7 per 100,000.

For specific sites, there were a few instances where an Asian American rate was higher than that of whites. The most prominent example was for cancer of the stomach, where the Japanese rate (17.5 per 100,000) was more than three times the white rate.

Table 3.14 Average Annual Age-Adjusted Cancer Mortality Rates per
100,000 by Primary Site and Ethnicity, United States, 1978 to
1981

Primary Site	Whites	Japanese	Chinese	Filipinos
All sites	163.6	104.2	131.5	69.7
Bladder	3.9	1.8	1.7	1.5
Breast, female	26.6	9.9	13.0	8.0
Ages <40	1.6	1.1	0.8	0.9
Ages 40+	70.2	25.2	34.6	20.6
Cervix uteri	3.2	2.7	2.9	1.6
Colon and rectum	21.6	17.2	19.3	8.1
Colon	18.1	13.6	15.5	5.8
Rectum	3.5	3.6	3.8	2.3
Corpus uteri	3.9	3.9	4.3	2.0
Esophagus	2.6	1.9	3.3	1.9
Larynx	1.3	0.2	0.7	0.4
Lung, male	69.3	32.7	48.2	20.0
Lung, female	20.2	8.6	21.2	6.8
Multiple myeloma	2.4	1.2	1.2	1.2
Ovary	8.1	4.3	4.2	2.8
Pancreas	8.4	7.0	7.4	3.3
Prostate	21.0	8.8	7.5	8.2
Stomach	5.3	17.5	7.8	3.3

SOURCE: National Cancer Institute (1986, Table III-1).

Age-standardized cancer incidence (*not* death) rates for specific
sites from the National Center for Health Statistics (1991) for 1977-
1983 show that Asian rates were almost always lower than those of
whites (see also Table 3.15). Five-year survival rates, on the other
hand, showed relatively small differentials and in no particular
direction (see Table 3.16).

Data from Los Angeles County for 1980 (numerators and denominators not matched) indicate a large advantage for Asian Americans with regard to cardiovascular diseases, which accounted for
approximately half of all deaths in the county in that year. Compared to the total county, Asian death rates ranged from 0.21 for
Filipinos to 0.62 for Japanese (Table 3.17). For diseases of the heart,
a similar pattern was found; for cerebrovascular diseases, however,
all ratios were slightly higher, and the Japanese ratio was 1.07.

Table 3.15   Average Annual Age-Adjusted Cancer Incidence Rates per 100,000 by Primary Site and Ethnicity, SEER Program, 1978 to 1981

Primary Site	Whites	Japanese	Chinese	Filipinos
All sites	335.0	247.8	252.9	222.4
Bladder	15.4	7.7	7.7	5.1
Breast, female	86.5	53.1	54.0	43.4
Ages <40	8.2	8.6	7.4	7.1
Ages 40+	221.1	146.5	141.0	117.0
Cervix uteri	8.8	7.6	11.2	8.8
Colon and rectum	49.6	50.4	40.8	30.1
Colon	34.6	34.0	27.7	17.7
Rectum	15.0	16.4	13.1	12.4
Corpus uteri	25.1	18.6	17.6	11.7
Esophagus	3.0	2.4	3.4	3.6
Larynx	4.6	2.6	1.9	1.8
Lung, male	81.0	45.1	62.6	38.1
Lung, female	28.2	14.1	31.2	18.4
Multiple myeloma	3.4	1.2	1.6	4.1
Ovary	13.6	8.7	9.1	9.4
Pancreas	8.9	7.4	9.3	6.7
Prostate	75.1	44.2	26.1	48.9
Stomach	8.0	27.9	9.0	7.0

SOURCE: National Cancer Institute (1986, Table II-1).
NOTE: The SEER (Surveillance, Epidemiology, and End Results) Program collects data from 11 cancer registries. It currently includes six entire states (Connecticut, Hawaii, Iowa, New Mexico, New Jersey, and Utah), four large metropolitan areas (Atlanta, San Francisco, Detroit, and Seattle), and Puerto Rico.

Studies of Immigrant Groups: Evidence on Determinants

A study of a single ethnic group avoids criticisms that have been directed at the practice of looking at Asian Americans as if they represent a homogeneous group. As with socioeconomic status and culture, Asian Americans are a very heterogeneous group with respect to health status and mortality. A number of studies have been conducted to investigate the causes of disease and death for individual Asian American groups.

The two major diseases studied within Asian American groups have been cancer and heart disease, and the two ethnic groups most studied have been the Japanese and the Chinese. The studies of Japanese are especially interesting, because they have looked at the mortality of Japanese in Japan, of Japanese immigrants in the United

Table 3.16 Five-Year Relative Survival Rates for Cancer by Primary Site and Ethnicity, SEER Program, 1973 to 1981

Primary Site	Anglos	Japanese	Chinese	Filipinos
All sites	50	51	44	45
Bladder	74	72	74	49
Breast, female	75	85	78	72
Cervix uteri	68	72	72	72
Colon and rectum	51	59	50	41
Colon	52	61	53	38
Rectum	49	55	44	45
Corpus uteri	88	86	87	78
Esophagus	5	—	11	—
Larynx	67	75	67	57
Lung and bronchus	12	14	15	12
Multiple myeloma	24	30	24	29
Ovary	37	41	42	52
Pancreas	3	3	3	2
Prostate	69	76	76	73
Stomach	14	28	16	16

SOURCE: National Cancer Institute (1986, Table IV-1).
NOTE: Anglos are whites not of Hispanic origin or surname. Relative survival rates adjust for the possibility of dying from some other cause. For information on the SEER Program, see note to Table 3.15.

States, and of U.S.-born Japanese Americans. A theme running through many such studies is whether or not there is a "gradient" for the death rates of the various groups. The existence of such a gradient might suggest that environmental factors are implicated: as the environment changes from the home country to the new country, so too will death rates. A gradient might also imply that behaviors and characteristics change as individuals move from one country to another and as succeeding generations appear—that is, as adaptation occurs. Selection might also be a factor.

"Both in their native land and abroad the Japanese reveal an unusual pattern of cancer mortality" (Buell & Dunn, 1965, p. 656). Death rates from stomach cancer are unusually high, and death rates from female breast cancer and male prostate cancer are unusually low. For all causes of death, the Japanese American death rate in the period 1959 to 1962 was some 30% lower than that of whites.

Haenszel and Kurihara (1968) assert that there is no single pattern relating disease levels for origin and destination Japanese

Table 3.17 Population and Deaths Due to Cardiovascular Diseases, by
Ethnicity, Los Angeles County, 1980

Ethnic Group	Number of Deaths	Adjusted Rate per 100,000	Ratio to Total County
Major cardiovascular diseases			
total county	30,621	409	1.00
white	26,934	430	1.05
black	3,015	472	1.15
Hispanic	1,602	391	0.95
Japanese	286	255	0.62
Filipino	58	84	0.21
Chinese	97	157	0.38
Korean	32	144	0.35
Diseases of the heart			
total county	23,444	314	1.00
white	20,707	331	1.06
black	2,291	353	1.13
Hispanic	1,261	308	0.98
Japanese	182	162	0.52
Filipino	42	58	0.18
Chinese	59	99	0.32
Korean	19	82	0.26
Cerebrovascular diseases			
total county	5,559	74	1.00
white	4,798	76	1.02
black	571	94	1.27
Hispanic	261	64	0.85
Japanese	89	80	1.07
Filipino	13	20	0.27
Chinese	31	49	0.66
Korean	11	48	0.65

SOURCE: Frerichs et al. (1984, Tables 2-4). Reprinted by permission of Oxford University Press.
NOTE: Standard is total county age and sex structure. Hispanic data are from census tracts in
which 75% or more of the population is Hispanic.

populations, and Adelstein and Marmot (1989) note that "the relative
effect of the old and the new countries varies with different diseases" (p. 39). Cancers of different body sites show different patterns. Breast cancer among Japanese in the United States remains at
the relatively low levels characteristic of several "Mongolian" groups
(King & Haenszel, 1973, p. 641), "suggesting a genetic interpretation" (Kasl & Berkman, 1983, p. 77). Stomach cancer for Japanese
immigrants shows an "incomplete transition" from high death
rates in Japan to the relatively low rates characteristic of U.S.

whites. Haenszel and Kurihara (1968) expected further changes to take place among second-generation Japanese, because "stomach cancer mortality (among immigrants generally) relates more to country of origin than to country of destination" (p. 522); this indicates the possible importance of early exposure (Kasl & Berkman, 1983). For colon cancer, on the other hand, a "rather complete transition had occurred from the low risks in Japan to the characteristic high risks of U.S. whites. For colon, migrants (typically) gravitate to the experience of the host population" (Haenszel & Kurihara, 1968, p. 53).

Studies of cancer in Japanese in Japan and Hawaii show similar results:

> Cancers of the esophagus, stomach, bile duct, and uterine cervix have decreased relative to the native Japanese experience; while cancers of the colon, rectum, breast, endometrium, ovary, urinary bladder, and reticuloendothelial system have increased. The incidence of some tumors in Hawaii Japanese is intermediate between U.S. white and native Japanese rates, while the incidence of others now exceeds U.S. white rates (colon, rectum, leukemia). (Stemmermann, Nomura, & Kolonel, 1987, p. 99)

King and Haenszel (1973) and Locke and King (1980) looked at cancer among Chinese Americans in much the same way. Overall cancer mortality levels for Chinese males were close to those of U.S. whites, whereas levels for Chinese females were lower than those for white females. The researchers found relatively high risks for cancer of the nasopharynx, liver, and esophagus for males and for cancer of the nasopharynx, stomach, and liver for females. There were relatively low risks for cancer of the prostate and of the female breast. Patterns for breast and colon cancer generally paralleled those for Japanese (Kasl & Berkman, 1983). Other patterns more or less followed the general pattern for Chinese in Asia; King and Haenszel conclude that migration to the United States may have diluted risks for these sites but caused no fundamental change (p. 643). Locke and King speculate that perhaps a longer time had to elapse before a more substantial displacement toward U.S. white rates would appear.

Colon cancer *did* show a rise to the level of U.S. whites, "a likely environmental effect . . . consistent with the experience observed among migrants from Japan and from those European countries where a low risk of cancer at this site has prevailed" (King & Locke, 1980, p. 1147). As noted above, the hypothesis of a genetic basis for nasopharyngeal cancer seems "to have been confounded by our observations of a continuing decline since 1960 in this cancer among Erdai [second-generation Chinese] males" (p. 1147).

King and Locke (1987) note there has been "a downward transition for cancers with high risk among Asian Chinese and an upward displacement for those sites of low risk for Foshan and Hong Kong" (traditional origin areas of U.S. Chinese) (p. 566; see also King, Locke, Li, Pollack, & Tu, 1985). They state that the Chinese experience is "compatible with the transition experience noted for the U.S. Japanese migrant population" (p. 571). They suggest that, "in view of the fact that perhaps 85 percent of cancer is related to environmental and dietary factors . . . it seems advisable to look into . . . the degree of acculturation among different segments of Chinese population to Western dietary habits in reference to such cancer sites as esophagus, stomach, colon-rectum, liver, pancreas, gallbladder, lung, urinary bladder, kidneys, breast, endometrium, ovary and cervix" (p. 571; see also "Lung Cancer," 1989).

Colorectal cancer was the topic of a recent study by Chinese and American researchers (Whittemore, 1989; Whittemore et al., 1990). Comparing Chinese Americans in western North America with Chinese in the People's Republic of China, the study found that colorectal cancer was significantly associated with saturated fat consumption (the only dietary energy association) and with sedentary occupations. Among immigrants, the risk of colorectal cancer increased with the number of years lived in North America. Thus both dietary and lifestyle factors seem to influence this particular cancer. The levels of colorectal cancer among Chinese American men are comparable to those of white American men, whereas the rates among Chinese American women are intermediate between those of Chinese women in China and white American women. The different levels for males and females can be explained by longer average residence by males in North America and thus longer exposure to Western lifestyles.

Data on cancer among Filipinos is mainly limited to studies in Hawaii and California. According to Polednak (1989), Filipinos "have remarkably low incidence rates for total cancers and for most major specific sites" (p. 174). Kolonel (1980) found that

the results of the comparison between Manila and Hawaii agree with the general observation that cancer risks in migrants show a progressive shift from the rates of the parent country to those in the host country. . . . Thus increases are substantial between Manila and Hawaii in the incidence [*not* death] rates for colon, rectum, lung (in women), prostate, bladder, and corpus uteri cancers, all of which have relatively high rates in the U.S. compared with less developed or westernized countries like the Philippines. . . . However, some exceptions occur. For example, the rate of lung cancer in [Filipino] men in Hawaii is not higher than that in Manila. Equally dramatic are the decreases from Manila to Hawaii in the risk for sites with lower rates in the U.S. generally, such as liver, cervix, and stomach. (p. 96)

Turning from cancer to cerebrovascular accidents (CVA) or stroke, Haenszel and Kurihara (1968) found that death rates in Japan were much higher than those for whites in the United States; Japanese Americans (native and immigrant combined) showed rates close to the U.S. white levels, a relatively "complete transition."

For coronary heart disease (CHD), by way of contrast, U.S. white levels have been found to be much higher than rates in Japan; Japanese American rates are intermediate (Haenszel & Kurihara, 1968; on prevalence rates, see also Marmot & Syme, 1976; Marmot et al., 1975). Among Japanese Americans, immigrants have shown a rise from the low levels in Japan, and more change in an upward direction has been expected among second-generation Japanese (Haenszel & Kurihara, 1968). Filipino immigrants also showed an "upward displacement" in a Hawaii study (Hackenberg, Gerber, & Hackenberg, n.d.). Death rates for heart disease "generally reveal values for migrants that are intermediate between those for the country of origin and the host country; a longer period of residence tends to bring the rates closer and closer to the rates of the host country" (Kasl & Berkman, 1983, p. 77).

Haenszel and Kurihara (1968) conclude that "much of this [overall Japanese] advantage can be ascribed to the carry-over from Japan of the low risks of heart disease, coupled with a sharp reduction in mortality from vascular lesions of the central nervous system" (p. 46). Polednak (1989) concludes that "the low rates of IHD [CHD] death found in Japan could be approached by Japanese in Hawaii, and possibly by other racial/ethnic groups, if risk factor levels could be positively influenced" (p. 155).

King and Locke (1987) looked at levels of ischemic heart disease among Chinese immigrants, Chinese in major origin areas (Foshan and Hong Kong), and U.S. whites. They found that immigrant mortality far exceeded that of origin Chinese, but "remained significantly below that of the host white population" (p. 567).

An interesting recent study of older Chinese immigrants by Choi et al. (1990) sheds some light on cause-of-death patterns. These researchers found that "in 1976 the mortalities for stroke and myocardial infarction in urban mainland China were 138.7 and 29.6 per 100,000 population, respectively, while in the United States the respective rates were 87.9 and 301.0" (p. 413). A group of Chinese immigrants over 60 years of age in the Boston area "sought to preserve their traditional culture, including life-style, dietary habits, and usage of herbs . . . [and] their . . . physiochemical characteristics were found to be similar to those of the urban population of mainland China" (p. 417). That is, immigrants living in a style more like that of their origin had cardiovascular risk profiles closer to those in their country of origin than to those of their current area of residence: "conducive to stroke while protective against coronary atherosclerosis" (p. 417).

Similar results are noted by Marmot and Syme (1976), who found that the "most traditional group of Japanese-Americans had a CHD prevalence as low as that observed in Japan. The group that was most acculturated to Western culture had a three- to five-fold excess in CHD prevalence. *This difference in CHD rate between most and least acculturated groups could not be accounted for by differences in the major coronary risk factors*" (p. 225; emphasis added). Marmot and Syme suggest that "a stable society whose members enjoy the support of their fellows in closely knit groups may protect against the forms of social stress that may lead to CHD" (p. 245).[11] Yano, Reed, and Kagan (1985) note that "migrant Japanese men have a higher risk of CHD and a lower risk of stroke than indigenous Japanese men because of Westernization of their lifestyles and environmental changes through migration" (p. 297).

A study in Hawaii found less definite relationships of measures of acculturation to CHD, especially with regard to incidence (as contrasted with prevalence) (Reed et al., 1982).[12] Yano et al. (1985) summarize findings of studies of Japanese in Japan and Hawaii with the statement, "There was no evidence to support the hypothesis that social networks are especially protective among persons in the highest levels of stressful processes in terms of mobility and incongruity [which would include migrants]" (p. 312).

In a study on Filipinos in Hawaii, Gerber (1980) found that Filipino immigrants in Hawaii had rates of mortality from CHD that were intermediate, that is, higher than in the Philippines but lower than those of Hawaii whites. The findings about Filipinos, Gerber notes, "correspond to Gordon's [1957, 1967] reports that Japanese-American men have CHD mortality rates that are intermediate between the low levels in Japan and the high levels of Caucasian Americans" (p. 276).

Regarding infectious diseases, Polednak (1989) notes that "most of the burden of infectious disease, and the paramount importance of these diseases as contributors to mortality, is related to a combination of ecologic factors and low socioeconomic status. . . . Poor nutrition contributes to susceptibility to infection and infectious diseases . . . and thus to poor growth and development and increased mortality in a vicious cycle of interrelated effects" (p. 112).

Typically, countries and populations go through "transitions" from high mortality levels characterized by a dominance of infectious and parasitic diseases to low mortality levels characterized by dominance of chronic diseases. The disease and mortality patterns of Asian Americans, living in a developed country with advanced levels of public health and medicine, are of the low-mortality high-chronic-disease type. Nevertheless, high proportions of Asian American populations are composed of recent immigrants from countries that in general are not as developed economically as the United States and not as far along in the epidemiological transition. Immigrants are exposed to conditions and situations before they leave their home countries that are not duplicated in the United States, and this may result in health and mortality profiles after arrival that are different from those of U.S.-born Asian Americans and whites. In addition, insofar as some of the immigrant groups, notably the refugees, are composed of people who are not able to earn adequate incomes in the United States immediately, the factor of socioeconomic status and resources will affect disease and mortality patterns, even as it does for indigenous disadvantaged groups in this country.

In 1985, the rate of reported tuberculosis cases (incidence, not mortality) for Asian Pacific Americans was 49.6 per 100,000, 8.7 times higher than the rate of 5.7 per 100,000 for the white population. These cases were concentrated almost exclusively (93.6%) among the foreign-born. Almost half of the cases had developed within the first 2 years of arrival ("Tuberculosis," 1987).

Polednak (1989) notes that "racial/ethnic differences in infectious diseases are clearly due largely to factors subject to modification. These factors include nutritional deficiencies and poor host immune status, as well as poor sanitation and certain cultural practices" (p. 285).

There are only limited data on nondisease causes of death, but these reflect the same patterns of low Asian American mortality. Death rates from unintentional injury, suicide, and homicide among Asian Americans for the period 1977 to 1979 were below those reported for whites, blacks, and Native Americans (Baker, O'Neill, & Karpf, 1984; cited in U.S. Office of Disease Prevention and Health Promotion, 1987, p. 18-12).

In general, it appears that for some diseases and causes of death, and for some ethnic groups, there does seem to exist a gradient in level of death rate from the origin country to the United States, with first-generation (i.e., immigrant) groups showing intermediate rates and U.S.-born members showing mortality levels closer to those of the U.S. white population. The exceptions to this pattern are many, however, and Haenszel and Kurihara (1968) warn that, for cancers, not all types "present an orderly, uninterrupted sequence from home-to-host populations" (p. 56). Furthermore, with regard to cancer at least, convergence may be occurring, but it is not yet even close to complete (National Cancer Institute, 1986; U.S. Department of Health and Human Services, 1985).

Age Patterns

The age patterns of mortality for whites, Chinese, Japanese, and Filipinos for 1980, based on data uncorrected for any mismatch problems, are portrayed in Figure 3.2. All of the curves follow the familiar J pattern, with high rates at the very young and old ages (the curves would be higher for the youngest ages if age 0 were distinguished from ages 1 to 4). The curve for whites is higher at every age than the curves for any of the Asian American groups. At all ages except the oldest, Chinese rates are next highest, followed by Japanese and then Filipinos. Filipinos thus show the lowest mortality of any of the groups shown, a finding necessarily in agreement with the ranking of age-adjusted death rates from the same study.

Sex Patterns

As is generally true today no matter what population is being examined, the death rates for Asian American males are higher than

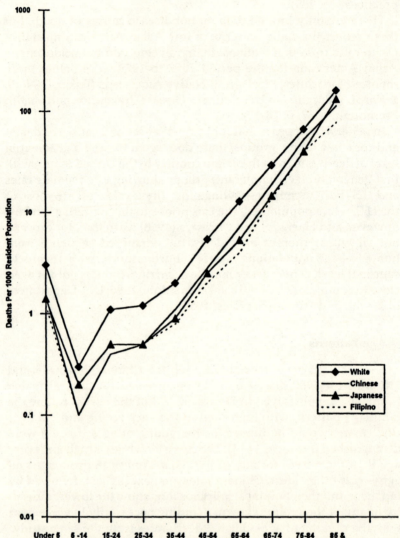

Figure 3.2. Age-Specific Death Rates for Whites and Asian Americans, 1980
SOURCE: Data from Yu et al. (1984, Table 11).

those for Asian American females at almost every age (the only exception, noted in Yu et al., 1984, Table 15, is for Chinese ages 5 to 14 years). A similar situation is observable for death rates for the major causes of death: Males die at higher rates almost without exception. These specific differences between males and females are summarized in the life-table values (for all Asian Pacific Americans) mentioned above, where the female value for e_0 is 8.5 years higher than that for males.

Place-of-Birth Differentials

The study of immigrant mortality provides an opportunity to explore a number of facets of mortality and its determinants. Genetic predisposition, environment, and self-selection are theoretically open to examination. In practice, however, "the data themselves do not allow for a direct determination of the influence of conditions in the host environment as opposed to 'origin' effects, selection and life stresses associated with migration itself" (Trovato, 1990, pp. 105-106). Nevertheless, immigrant studies have provided interesting results, some of which have been discussed above, in the section on determinants.

In 1980, both crude and age-adjusted mortality rates for Asians born abroad were found to be higher than the comparable rates for native-born Asian Americans (Yu et al., 1984): "For every one of the 10 leading causes of death, the mortality rates for foreign-born exceeded the native-born—on average—by a ratio of at least 2.0, if not larger" (p. 31).

Comments

Recent publications state that "the health status of Asian Americans as a group is remarkably good" (U.S. Office of Disease Prevention and Health Promotion, 1987, p. 18-1) and that "the Asian/ Pacific Island minority, in aggregate, is healthier than all [other] racial/ethnic groups in the United States" (U.S. Department of Health and Human Services, 1985, p. 81). Such results echo earlier studies, such as that by Breslow and Klein (1971), that find a consistent superiority of the Japanese "over a wide range of health measures . . . and over several defined California populations" (p. 772) and a strong showing by Chinese in comparison with whites and blacks.

Breslow and Klein found it "difficult to conceive of some artifact" that would explain the consistent rankings they found for a number of indexes of health and mortality (p. 773). Nevertheless, because of the data problems discussed above, it is difficult to come to any firm conclusions about the precise current levels of mortality of Asian Americans in general or of specific Asian American groups in particular.

The findings of many of the studies that have been conducted should be interpreted with caution, because, as noted earlier, many are based on vital statistics data unadjusted for comparability with census data and may contain discrepancies. Mortality levels for Asian Americans indicated by the unadjusted vital statistics data may be somewhat lower than the actual levels because of data comparability problems. These may be greater for some groups than for others; for example, Filipinos and Japanese have tended to marry out more than have Chinese, so their potential for mixed-race children and eventual adults is greater and therefore so is the potential for death rates that may be too low.

A second reason for some skepticism is the fact that Filipinos are shown to have the lowest mortality among all the groups studied by Yu and her colleagues (1984). If we look at the various factors presumed to affect mortality, there does not seem to be a strong reason to expect such low mortality levels for Filipinos. We might expect a ranking for Filipinos similar to that found in Hawaii in 1980 (Table 3.2), but adjusted death rates less than half those of whites seem a bit low. Perhaps there is a greater tendency toward mismatch problems within the Filipino American population.

However, there is no reason to suppose that Asian American mortality levels, especially those of Chinese and Japanese, are *higher* than those of whites. There is too much evidence in the opposite direction. Rather, I would caution against placing too much reliance on the *size* of the Asian-white differentials reported above. Furthermore, as Lin-Fu (1988) has noted, "The general assumption about the good health status of Asian Pacific Americans as a group tends to mask the serious health problems and needs of some subgroups, such as the Southeast Asian refugees and other recent immigrants" (p. 21).

Summary and Conclusions

At the start of this chapter I posed three questions: What are the levels and patterns of mortality for Asian Americans? How do they compare with those of whites? What are the factors lying behind the observed levels and patterns? I have presented a great deal of information regarding these questions in the preceding pages; is it now possible to answer them?

The path led first through the thicket of data problems. We found that lack of agreement between ethnic classification procedures and definitions of the numerator (deaths) and denominator (individuals at risk) makes it impossible to say that mortality data accurately reflect the actual situation. Studies that "match" numerator and denominator are few, especially for adult mortality, where the research by Kitagawa and Hauser (1973) remains the single national study. Numerous articles and book chapters have presented data on Asian American mortality that cannot be trusted completely because of the matching problem. I must come to conclusions based on these somewhat imperfect data.

My conclusion about adult mortality is that Asian American mortality levels—for the group as a whole and for the three principal subgroups, Chinese, Japanese, and Filipinos—are almost certainly lower than white levels. Data for the separate sexes, for various age groups, and for different causes of death indicate that, although there is much variability across these dimensions, Asian American mortality levels are still relatively low.

As far as infant mortality is concerned, recent computer tapes made available by the National Center for Health Statistics have made it possible for the first time for researchers to calculate infant mortality rates from matched data at the national level. The first results from research using the new tapes show that Asian American infant mortality levels, although not as incredibly low as earlier unmatched data had indicated, are still somewhat lower than white levels, at least for the groups (Chinese, Japanese, and Filipinos) for which data are available and the numbers large enough to trust.

When we seek to discover the factors that lie behind the observed patterns and levels of Asian American mortality, we enter an extremely complicated world. Investigations have proceeded along many dimensions: native-born versus foreign-born and, among the latter, recent arrivals versus long-term residents; sociodemoeconomic characteristics versus cultural behaviors versus genetics versus selection; and cancer versus heart disease versus other causes of death, to name a few.

It seems to be generally conceded that, although genetic predispositions toward certain diseases and conditions may exist among different groups of immigrants from Asia and their descendants, these diseases are relatively unimportant in terms of their contribution to total mortality levels. This does not mean, of course, that individuals afflicted with these diseases are any less anguished or, eventually, any less dead, nor does it detract from the light that studies of these diseases and their changes from area of origin to area of destination can throw upon the disease causation process.

There seems to be no such easy conclusion about the effects of selection on the mortality of immigrants and their descendants. Many researchers make a bow toward selection as a factor that may be operating, but I have found no studies that unequivocally point to effects of selection on mortality. Of course, insofar as selection is on the basis of characteristics, such as income and education, that are known to affect mortality, knowledge of the background of immigrants gives us some clues about selection for health and eventual mortality. More speculative are the arguments about migrants being the healthier members of their particular sociodemoeconomic groups in their areas of origin; it would be practically impossible to carry out a study that examined future mortality levels (or even current health levels) of emigrants and of matched individuals who were not emigrating. The effects of selection on health and mortality of migrants remain so far unquantified, and the effects of selection on the descendants of migrants are even less easy to contemplate.

With regard to the relative importance of sociodemoeconomic characteristics and cultural behavior, one might expect to find clear-cut answers, but such is not the case. Numerous authors state that there are important effects of behavior, whether through diet, support networks, smoking and drinking, or whatever. Researchers studying immigrants find, in general and with exceptions, a pattern in which Asian American disease and mortality levels (of cancers and heart disease in particular) change from the levels of the home country to those found in the United States; these changes are explained, both theoretically and with actual data, in terms of changes in diet and other behavior toward a Westernized model.

The literature does not contain, however, many examples of "controlling for" income, education, and other such factors among Asian Americans and then looking for patterns of disease and death that must be attributable to something beyond these factors. For example, do rich college-educated Chinese Americans have mortality levels different from those of rich college-educated whites? Do middle-class high school-graduate Filipino Americans have mortality levels different from those of middle-class high school-graduate whites?

One of the reasons for the dearth of tests of these questions, of course, is the lack of appropriate data. There are simply no direct data on mortality levels by economic status or most other characteristics (see Yu et al., 1984). If it is hard to get simple matched ethnic-specific numerators and denominators, imagine how much harder it is to get numerators and denominators matched not only for ethnicity but also for income, education, and other factors. Beyond this, of course, there would have to be data on behavior patterns: diet, smoking, exercise, and so forth.[13]

Of course, even if the desire for more information about the relative effects of sociodemoeconomic factors and cultural behavior is not satisfied, that is no reason to back away from naming obvious factors that plainly affect Asian American (and others') mortality levels, regardless of income, education, and so on. If Asian immigrants and their descendants adopt more and more of the majority culture's patterns, in diet, exercise, smoking, and the like, then it is certainly reasonable to expect (and it has already been shown) that Asian American mortality levels and patterns will gravitate toward those of whites, whether the white levels are initially higher (e.g., coronary heart disease) or lower (stomach cancer, compared with Japanese in Japan). Numerous studies show that Asian American behaviors *have* changed and that they *have* come to resemble those of whites more and more. From this evidence, one could predict that Asian American mortality levels *and their differences from those of whites* in the future would come to be dominated by sociodemoeconomic factors and differences.

If immigration from Asia were no longer occurring, this might be the end of the story. However, levels of immigration from Asia continue to be high and are even increasing; it is not likely that the immigration legislation passed in late 1990 will change this. A continuing influx of immigrants will mean a continuing infusion of individuals whose "culture" is not as close to that of the white population as is that of second- and third-generation residents of the same ethnicity. This in turn means health-related behaviors that are different from those of whites and those of earlier immigrants and their descendants, and hence a continuation of differentials between (immigrant) Asian American and white mortality patterns and levels. A modifying factor in this whole equation, however, is that immigrant behaviors may become more and more like those of American whites immediately upon arrival, both because of selection for these behaviors at the origin and because, as some claim, the Asian origin populations themselves are adopting more and more Western habits and tastes.

Notes

1. The 1980 U.S. Census published total population figures for the following groups: Chinese, Filipino, Japanese, Asian Indian, Korean, Vietnamese, Laotian, Thai, Cambodian, Pakistani, Indonesian, and Hmong. Other groups reported were "Bangladeshi, Burmese, Malayan, Okinawan, Pakistani, Sri Lankan, Bhutanese, Borneo, Celebesian, Cernan, Indochinese, Iwo-Jiman, Javanese, Maldivian, Nepali, Sikkim, and Singaporean" (U.S. Bureau of the Census, 1983, Table F). In 1990 there were 6,908,638 Asians counted in the census, including 1,645,472 Chinese, 1,406,770 Filipinos, 847,562 Japanese, 815,447 Asian Indians, 798,849 Koreans, and 614,547 Vietnamese. No other group had as many as 150,000 (U.S. Department of Commerce, 1991).

2. In 1980, the race of the person's mother was used; if this was unavailable, then the first race reported by the individual was used, in this case Chinese.

3. The census also has a question on ancestry that allows multiple responses. However, the Census Bureau does not tabulate ancestry responses by other variables, as it does for race, so the only way to look at characteristics by ancestry is to use the computer tapes (Public Use Micro Sample, or PUMS). Doing this, however, would not avoid the fact about ancestry data that is both its advantage and its disadvantage: One person can belong to more than one ancestry group, so double and triple counting can occur.

4. Helman (1990) presents an excellent discussion of the concept of culture in its relation to health and illness (and hence to mortality).

5. The fact that both numerator and denominator data come from vital statistics does not mean that there are no problems of matching. "Birth attendants (or hospital personnel) complete the birth certificate, and funeral directors generally complete the death certificate. . . . The birth certificate has entries for both the maternal and paternal races; thus, the NCHS criteria for race of the child at birth can be adhered to explicitly. On the other hand, the infant's race at death is assigned according to a single entry on the death certificate, and the races of the parents are not entered onto the death certificate" (Frost & Shy, 1980, p. 974).

6. Asian infant mortality was also lower than for other groups when subdivided into neonatal (first month) and postneonatal (balance of the first year) periods. A further refinement of the research was to look at postneonatal mortality from all causes *except congenital anomalies among normal birth weight infants*. This can be interpreted to be "preventable" mortality and, once again, Asians had the lowest rate (1.8 deaths per 1,000 live births) of any group studied. Whites were next (2.0), followed by blacks (3.9) and American Indians (5.6).

7. These data were based on deaths classified by ethnicity of mother. That is, regardless of the race of the child, the infant mortality rates were calculated by, for example, looking at all births to Chinese women and all infant deaths to those births. This procedure avoids problems of mismatch.

8. That is, for birth weights less than 1,501 grams, the black infant mortality rate was lower than that for Samoans and Koreans; for birth weights of 1,501 to 2,500 grams, the black infant mortality rate was lower than all but that for Hispanics and Chinese; for birth weights of 2,500 to 3,000 grams, black rates were below those for all other groups. Thus the poor position of blacks relative to other groups for total infant mortality rate was in some measure the result of the fact that blacks had relatively low birth weights. "The observed ethnic differential . . . appears to reflect in large measure the effect of birth weight associated with ethnicity" (Park & Horiuchi, 1991, p. 20).

9. That is, if all ethnic groups had equal distribution of births in the various birth weight categories, this would be the ranking.

10. The factors were maternal age, education, marital status, employment, religion, parity, gravidity, history of miscarriage or stillbirth, gestation, sex of baby, occurrence of a major malformation in the child, cigarette and alcohol usage during pregnancy, maternal prepregnant weight and height, length of prenatal care, history of anemia or hypertension, and the occurrence of pregnancy complications.

11. Another effect of support is cited by Weeks and Rumbaut (1988) in their study of infant mortality. They suggest that certain types of family structures and community supports may shape "positive *adaptation* outcomes," which in turn are reflected by surprisingly low (in the light of socioeconomic situations) infant mortality rates (p. 28).

12. Reed et al. (1982) note that, using prevalence data only, "we would have added our support" to the conclusions of Marmot and Syme. However, in "multivariate analyses, there was no association of any measure of acculturation with the incidence of any single clinical group of coronary heart disease" (p. 903). The authors go on to discuss why studies of incidence and prevalence might yield different results; neither, of course, is the same as a study of *mortality*.

13. The situation with regard to determinants of mortality is thus different from the situation with regard to determinants of fertility. Fertility is an individual characteristic that is measured by the census (or a survey) with a question on past fertility. This can be used as a dependent variable in a multivariate equation with selected independent variables chosen from the same data set. Such an approach cannot be used with mortality, because dead people are not included in censuses and surveys. Theoretically, a retrospective question could be asked about the characteristics of individuals who had died in the past year, but such retrospective questions have proven notoriously unreliable even for simple ascertainment of the fact of death, let alone the characteristics of the decedent. Matching of data from death records and population (census) records seems to be the safest approach, but it is extremely difficult. Infant mortality studies, which use the same data source (vital statistics) for both numerator and denominator, are much easier.

References

Adelstein, A. M., & Marmot, M. G. (1989). The health of migrants in England and Wales: Causes of death. In J. K. Cruickshank & D. G. Beevers (Eds.), *Ethnic factors in health and disease* (pp. 35-47). Boston: Wright.

Baker, S. P., O'Neill, B., & Karpf, R. S. (1984). *The injury fact book.* New York: Heath.

Berkman, L. F., & Syme, S. L. (1979). Social networks, host resistance, and mortality: A nine-year follow-up study of Alameda County residents. *American Journal of Epidemiology, 109,* 186-204.

Berry, J. W., Kim, U., Minde, T., & Mok, D. (1987). Comparative studies of acculturative stress. *International Migration Review, 21,* 491-511.

Breslow, L., & Klein, B. (1971). Health and race in California. *American Journal of Public Health, 61,* 763-775.

Buell, P., & Dunn, J. E., Jr. (1965). Cancer mortality among Japanese Issei and Nisei of California. *Cancer, 18,* 656-664.

California Center for Health Statistics. (1983). *California life expectancy: Abridged life tables for California and Los Angeles County, 1979-81* (Data Matters Topical Report No. 83-01031). Sacramento: Author.

Choi, E. S., McGandy, R. B., Dallal, G. E., Russell, R. M., Jacob, R. A., Schaefer, E. J., & Sadowski, J. A. (1990). The prevalence of cardiovascular risk factors among elderly Chinese Americans. *Archives of Internal Medicine, 150,* 413-418.

Dickson, R. I. (1981, March). Nasopharyngeal carcinoma: An evaluation of 209 patients. *Laryngoscope, 91,* 333-354.

Duke University Demographic Studies Center. (1984). *Life tables for 1979-81 by ethnicity.* Unpublished report submitted to the U.S. Department of Health and Human Services Task Force on Minority Health.

Evans, J. (1987). Introduction. In [Special issue on migration and health]. *International Migration Review, 21,* v-xiv.

Frerichs, R. R., Chapman, J. M., & Maes, E. F. (1984). Mortality due to all causes and to cardiovascular diseases among seven race-ethnic populations in Los Angeles County, 1980. *International Journal of Epidemiology, 13*(3), 291-298.

Frost, F., & Shy, K. K. (1980). Racial differences between linked birth and infant death records in Washington State. *American Journal of Public Health, 70,* 974-976.

Fung, K. P., Wong, T. W., & Lau, S. P. (1989). Ethnic determinants of perinatal statistics of Chinese: Demography of China, Hong Kong and Singapore. *International Journal of Epidemiology, 18,* 127-131.

Gardner, R. W. (1984). Life tables by ethnic group for Hawaii, 1980. *Research and Statistics Reports* (Hawaii State Department of Health), *43.*

Gerber, L. M. (1980). The influence of environmental factors on mortality from coronary heart disease among Filipinos in Hawaii. *Human Biology, 52,* 269-278.

Goodman, M. T. (1989). Cancer incidence among Asian Americans. In L. A. Jones (Ed.), *Minorities and cancer* (pp. 35-44). New York: Springer-Verlag.

Gordon, T. (1957). Mortality experience among the Japanese in the United States, Hawaii, and Japan. *Public Health Reports, 72,* 543-553.

Gordon, T. (1967). Further mortality experience among Japanese Americans. *Public Health Reports, 82,* 973-983.

Hackenberg, R. A., Gerber, L., & Hackenberg, B. (n.d.). *Cardiovascular disease mortality among Filipinos in Hawaii: Rates, trends, and associated factors.* Unpublished manuscript.

Haenszel, W., & Kurihara, M. (1968). Studies of Japanese Migrants: I. Mortality from cancer and other diseases among Japanese in the United States. *Journal of the National Cancer Institute, 40,* 43-68.

Hankin, J. H., Kolonel, L. N., Yano, K., Heilbrun, L., & Nomura, A. M. Y. (1983). Epidemiology of diet-related diseases in the Japanese migrant population in Hawaii. *Proceedings of the Nutrition Society of Australia, 8,* 22-40.

Hechter, H. H., & Borhani, N. O. (1965). Longevity in racial groups differs. *California's Health, 22*(15), 121-122.

Helman, C. (1990). Cultural factors in health and illness. In B. R. McAvoy & L. J. Donaldson (Eds.), *Health care for Asians* (pp. 17-27). New York: Oxford University Press.

Hu, J. H., & White, J. E. (1979). Cancer incidence in the western United States: Ethnic differences. *Journal of the National Medical Association, 71,* 345-348.

Kagan, A., Harris, B. R., Winkelstein, W., Jr., Johnson, K. G., Kato, H., Syme, S. L., Rhoads, G. G., Gay, M. L., Nichaman, M. Z., Hamilton, H. B., & Tillotson, J. (1974). Epidemiologic studies of coronary heart disease and stroke in Japanese men living in Japan, Hawaii, and California: Demographic, physical, dietary, and biochemical characteristics. *Journal of Chronic Diseases, 27,* 345-364.

Kasl, S. V., & Berkman, L. (1983). Health consequences of the experience of migration. In L. Breslow et al. (Eds.), *Annual review of public health* (Vol. 4, pp. 69-90). Palo Alto, CA: Annual Reviews.

King, H., & Haenszel, W. (1973). Cancer mortality among foreign-born and native-born Chinese in the United States. *Journal of Chronic Diseases, 26,* 623-646.

King, H., & Locke, F. B. (1980). Cancer mortality risk among Chinese in the United States. *Journal of the National Cancer Institute, 65,* 1141-1148.

King, H., & Locke, F. B. (1987). Health effects of migration: U.S. Chinese in and outside the Chinatown. *International Migration Review, 21,* 555-575.

King, H., Locke, F. B., Li, J.-Y., Pollack, E. S., & Tu, J. T. (1985). Patterns of site-specific displacement in cancer mortality among migrants: The Chinese in the United States. *American Journal of Public Health, 75,* 237-242.

Kitagawa, E. M., & Hauser, P. M. (1973). *Differential mortality in the United States: A study in socioeconomic epidemiology.* Cambridge, MA: Harvard University Press.

Kleinman, J. C. (1990). Infant mortality among minority groups. *Morbidity and Mortality Weekly Reports, 39*(SS-3), 31-40.

Kolonel, L. N. (1980). Cancer patterns of four ethnic groups in Hawaii. *Journal of the National Cancer Institute, 65,* 1127-1139.

Kolonel, L. N. (1988). Variability in diet and its relation to risk in ethnic and migrant groups. In A. D. Woodhead, M. A. Bender, & R. C. Leonard (Eds.), *Phenotypic variations in populations: Relevance to risk assessment* (pp. 129-135). New York: Plenum.

Kolonel, L. N., Hankin, J. H., & Nomura, A. M. Y. (1986). Multiethnic studies of diet, nutrition, and cancer in Hawaii. In Y. Hayashi et al. (Eds.), *Diet, nutrition and cancer* (pp. 29-40). Tokyo/Utrecht: Japan Science Society Press/VNU Science Press.

Kolonel, L. N., Hankin, J. H., Nomura, A. M., & Chu, S. Y. (1981). Dietary fat intake and cancer incidence among five ethnic groups in Hawaii. *Cancer Research, 41,* 3727-3728.

Kolonel, L. N., Hinds, M. W., & Hankin, J. H. (1980). Cancer patterns among migrant and native-born Japanese in Hawaii in relation to smoking, drinking, and dietary habits. In H. V. Gelboin, B. MacMahon, T. Matsushima, T. Sugimura, C. Takayama, & H. Takebe (Eds.), *Genetic and environmental factors in experimental and human cancer* (pp. 327-340). Tokyo: Japan Science Society Press.

Kolonel, L. N., Nomura, A. M. Y., Hinds, M. W., Hirohata, T., Hankin, J. H., & Lee, J. (1983). Role of diet in cancer incidence in Hawaii. *Cancer Research, 43*(Suppl.), 2397s-2402s.

Kolonel, L. N., Nomura, A. M. Y., Hirohata, T., Hankin, J. H., & Hinds, M. W. (1981). Association of diet and place of birth with stomach cancer incidence in Hawaii Japanese and Caucasians. *American Journal of Clinical Nutrition, 34,* 2478-2485.

Kuo, W. H., & Tsai, Y.-M. (1986). Social networking, hardiness and immigrant's mental health. *Journal of Health and Social Behavior, 27,* 133-149.

Li, D. K., Ni, H., Schwartz, S. M., & Daling, J. R. (1990). Secular change in birthweight among Southeast Asian immigrants to the United States. *American Journal of Public Health, 80,* 685-688.

Lin-Fu, J. S. (1988, January-February). Population characteristics and health care needs of Asian Pacific Americans. *Public Health Reports,* 18-27.

Liu, W. (1986). Health services for the Asian elderly. *Research on Aging, 8,* 156-175.

Locke, F. B., & King, H. (1980). Cancer mortality risk among Japanese in the United States. *Journal of the National Cancer Institute, 65,* 1149-1156.

Lung cancer without smoke. (1989, December 22). *Asiaweek,* p. 29.

Marmot, M. G., & Syme, S. L. (1976). Acculturation and coronary heart disease in Japanese Americans. *American Journal of Epidemiology, 104,* 225-247.

Marmot, M. G., Syme, S. L., Kagan, A., Kato, H., Cohen, J. B., & Belsky, J. (1975). Epidemiologic studies of coronary heart disease and stroke in Japanese men living in Japan, Hawaii, and California: Prevalence of coronary and hypertensive heart disease and associated risk factors. *American Journal of Epidemiology, 102,* 514-525.

Mi, M. P. (1971). Optimum birth weight in man. *Excerpta Medica International Congress Series, 223,* 121-122.

Muto, S. (1991, June 28). Lin: Asian Pacific men smoke more than any. *Asiaweek,* pp. 1, 25.

National Cancer Institute. (1986). *Cancer among blacks and other minorities: Statistical profiles* (NIC Publication No. 491-313/44712). Washington, DC: Government Printing Office.

National Center for Health Statistics. (1963). *Vital statistics of the United States, 1960: Vol.2, Part A, mortality.* Hyattsville, MD: Author.

National Center for Health Statistics. (1969). Comparability of marital status, race, nativity, and country of origin on the death certificate and matching census record, United States, May-August 1965. *Vital and Health Statistics,* 2(34).

National Center for Health Statistics. (1985). *United States decennial life tables for 1979-81: Vol. 1, No. 1* (DHHS Publication No. PHS 85-1150-1). Hyattsville, MD: Author.

National Center for Health Statistics. (1991). *Health, United States, 1990* (DHHS Publication No. PHS 91-1232). Hyattsville, MD: Author.

Norris, F. D., & Shipley, P. W. (1971). A closer look at race differentials in California's infant mortality, 1965-67. *HSMHA Health Reports, 86,* 810-814.

Park, C. B. (1991, April 24). *Logit systems in infant mortality and their application.* Paper presented at a seminar presentation at the East-West Population Institute, Honolulu, HI.

Park, C. B., & Horiuchi, B. Y. (1991, March 21-23). *Infant mortality in Hawaii: Birthweight and ethnicity.* Paper presented at the annual meetings of the Population Association of America, Washington, DC.

Polednak, A. P. (1989). *Racial and ethnic differences in disease.* New York: Oxford University Press.

Reed, D., McGee, D., Cohen, J., Yano, K., Syme, S. L., & Feinleib, M. (1982). Acculturation and coronary heart disease among Japanese men in Hawaii. *American Journal of Epidemiology, 115,* 894-905.

Rumbaut, R. G., & Weeks, J. R. (1989). Infant health among Indochinese refugees: Patterns of infant mortality, birthweight and prenatal care in comparative perspective. *Research in the Sociology of Health Care, 8,* 137-196.

Shiono, P. H., Klebanoff, M. A., Graubard, B. I., Berendes, H. W., & Rhoads, G. G. (1986). Birth weight among women of different ethnic groups. *Journal of the American Medical Association, 255,* 48-52.

Stemmermann, G. N., Nomura, A. M. Y., & Kolonel, L. (1987). Cancer among Japanese-Americans in Hawaii. *Gann Monograph on Cancer Research, 33,* 99-108.

Story, M., & Harris, L. J. (1989). Food habits and dietary change of Southeast Asian refugee families living in the United States. *Journal of the American Dietetic Association, 89,* 800-803.

Taffel, S. (1984). Characteristics of Asian Births: United States, 1980. *Monthly Vital Statistics Report, 32*(Suppl. 10).

Trovato, F. (1990). Immigrant mortality trends and differentials. In S. S. Halli, F. Trovato, & L. Driedger (Eds.), *Ethnic demography: Canadian immigrant, racial and cultural variations* (pp. 91-110). Ottawa: Carleton University Press.

Tuberculosis among Asians/Pacific Islanders: United States, 1985. (1987). *Morbidity and Mortality Weekly Report, 36,* 331-334.

U.S. Bureau of the Census. (1983, December). *Asian and Pacific Islander population by State: 1980* (Supplementary Report No. PS80-S1-12). Washington, DC: Government Printing Office.

U.S. Department of Commerce, Economics and Statistics Administration, Bureau of the Census. (1991, June 12). *Census Bureau releases 1990 census counts on specific racial groups* [News release]. Washington, DC: Government Printing Office.

U.S. Department of Health and Human Services. (1985). *Report of the Secretary's Task Force on Black and Minority Health: Vol. 1. Executive summary* (Publication No. 491-313/44706). Washington, DC: Government Printing Office.

U.S. Office of Disease Prevention and Health Promotion. (1987). *ODPHP's prevention fact book: Life expectancy in the United States.* Washington, DC: Government Printing Office.

Weeks, J. R., & Rumbaut, R. G. (1988). *Infant mortality among Indochinese refugees in San Diego County.* Paper presented at the annual meetings of the Population Association of America, San Diego, CA.

Whittemore, A. S. (1989, September). Colorectal cancer incidence among Chinese in North America and the People's Republic of China: Variation with sex, age, and anatomical site. *International Journal of Epidemiology, 18,* 563-568.

Whittemore, A. S., Wu-Williams, A. H., Lee, M., Zheng, S., Gallagher, R. P., Jiao, D., Zhou, L., Wang, X., Chen, K., Jung, D., Teh, C.-Z., Ling, C., Xu, J. Y., Paffenberger, R. S., Jr., & Henderson, B. E. (1990). Diet, physical activity, and colorectal cancer among Chinese in North America and China. *Journal of the National Cancer Institute, 82,* 915-926.

Yano, K., Reed, D. M., & Kagan, A. (1985). Coronary heart disease, hypertension and stroke among Japanese-American men in Hawaii: The Honolulu Heart Program. *Hawaii Medical Journal, 44,* 297-300.

Young, I. (1990). Hereditary disorders. In B. R. McAvoy & L. J. Donaldson (Eds.), *Health care for Asians* (pp. 193-209). New York: Oxford University Press.

Yu, E. (1982). The low mortality rates of Chinese infants: Some plausible explanatory facts. *Social Science and Medicine, 16,* 253-265.

Yu, E. S. H., Chang, C.-F., Liu, W. T., & Kan, S. H. (1984). *Asian-White mortality differentials: Is there excess deaths?* (Special report submitted to the NIH Task Force on Black and Minority Health, Bethesda, Maryland). Chicago: University of Illinois, Pacific/Asian American Mental Health Research Center.

Yu, M. C., Ho, J. H. C., Lang, S. H., & Henderson, B. E. (1986). Cantonese-style salted fish as a cause of nasopharyngeal cancer in Hong Kong. *Cancer Research, 46,* 956-961.

4

Cancer

CHRISTOPHER N. H. JENKINS

MARJORIE KAGAWA-SINGER

Cancer is the second leading cause of death, after cardiovascular diseases, in the United States today. One in four Americans will develop some form of cancer. Compared with other ethnic groups in the United States, however, there are few data available about the epidemiology and control of cancer among Asian Pacific American populations. Major cancer control efforts in public education and the treatment and rehabilitation of cancer patients are being made to reduce the emotional, social, and economic burdens of this disease for individuals and their families. However, specific efforts toward these ends for Asian Pacific American populations have been few (Kagawa-Singer, 1988, 1993).

The objectives of this chapter are to present what is known about cancer in Asian Pacific Americans and to offer suggestions for effective cancer control among these populations. We will first define and describe the disease of cancer and then present what is known about cancer morbidity and mortality in Asian Pacific American populations. We will highlight the significant differences among Asian Pacific American ethnic groups and the differences between these groups and the white population. Following this discussion, we will identify some of the unique cultural factors among Asian Pacific Americans that may facilitate or pose barriers to the prevention, early detection, and treatment of cancer. Finally, we will indicate potential targets and avenues for culturally congruent intervention programs to reduce the burden of the disease in these populations.

Since passage of the Cancer Act of 1971 in the United States, enormous advances have been made in understanding the etiology and course of cancer. Treatments have become more effective and survival of certain cancers has been remarkable. Twenty years ago long-term survival of childhood leukemias was extremely low, as was survival from Hodgkin's disease. Death from cervical cancer was high. Survival rates associated with these three diseases have risen from 5% to 10% to around 90%. Treatments for many other cancers are also increasingly effective. With growing numbers of people surviving cancer and enjoying a satisfactory quality of life, cancer is now listed as one of the *chronic* diseases of U.S. society rather than as an acute, terminal disease. For some of the most common cancers, such as lung, breast, and colon, however, little progress has been made in the overall morbidity and mortality associated with the disease.

In 1984, the National Cancer Institute established the goal of reducing the mortality rate from cancer by half by the year 2000 (Greenwald & Sondik, 1986). This objective is theoretically possible for two reasons. First, from 85% to 90% of cancers are believed to be caused, in part, by behavioral, cultural, and dietary factors. Thus certain cancers can be prevented through the modification of these factors. Second, using existing medical technology, lives can be saved through early detection of cancer, while it is still localized and treatment has the greatest chance for success. Thus cancer control efforts are currently focused on developing, evaluating, and disseminating effective strategies for prevention and early detection.

Cancer, however, has the onerous distinction of symbolically embodying the worst fears of our age: pain, suffering, and death (Sontag, 1977). Prevention and early detection are key elements in control, but, unlike other chronic diseases such as heart disease and diabetes, the emotional aura of fear that surrounds this disease creates unique barriers to the utilization of health care services. Experience with community programs has clearly shown that successful cancer control efforts must be tailored to address the distinct health beliefs and behaviors of different cultural groups.

Cancer: The Disease

Cancer is a collective term for an aberrant process of cell division. Any cell type in the body can become cancerous. The common defect in this process is that the normal mechanisms in the cell that regulate cell proliferation become nonfunctional, and the cell begins to divide and reproduce unchecked. Without treatment to stop the growth of these abnormal cells—surgery, radiation therapy, chemotherapy, and/or biologic modifiers—they will eventually physically press upon surrounding tissues and organs and will usually produce satellite areas of growth called metastases. These metastatic lesions are spread by the bloodstream or by lymphatic circulation to distant parts of the body, where they colonize and continue to grow. Each type of cancer has common sites of metastases. Death results from invasion of cancerous cells into surrounding vital organs and depression of the immune system to a point where the individual is no longer able to resist systemic infections (DeVita, Hellman, & Rosenberg, 1989).

Cancer is ubiquitous worldwide (Muir, Waterhouse, Mack, Shanmugaratnam, & Powell, 1987). The overall incidence of the disease in a population appears fairly consistent when controlled for age (because it occurs more frequently with increasing age) and economic level of development of the country. However, the major anatomic sites of cancer vary significantly by geographic and cultural groups (Schottenfeld & Fraumeni, 1982). Comparative epidemiological studies among countries, studies of migrants, and studies of ethnic groups within particular geographic areas have provided data to support the contention that most cancer can be explained by variations in environment, including diet, smoking, and other lifestyle factors (Bonacini & Valenzuela, 1991; Goodman, Gilbert, & Low, 1984; Haenzel, 1982). Socioeconomic status is a strong risk factor as well. Recent data indicate that poverty is a major risk factor for cancer morbidity and mortality regardless of ethnicity (Freeman, 1989; Rimpela & Pukkala, 1987).

Most significant for policy considerations in the United States, cancer rates among racial or ethnic groups often change when members of a group migrate from their native country to another country. Identifying the reasons for such changes, including those factors that predispose an individual to get cancer as well as those that protect an individual from getting cancer, has clear implications for policy and program planning for cancer prevention and control (Fraumeni, Hoover, Devesa, & Kinlen, 1989; Modan, 1974).

Although the specific causes of most cancers are not well understood, cancer is thought to be caused by three factors: environmental exposure, viral agents, and genetic predisposition. Environmental factors that play a major role in the development of cancer include workplace carcinogens such as asbestos, which has been linked epidemiologically to the development of mesothelioma; ionizing radiation, which has been linked to leukemia, breast cancer, thyroid cancer, and lung cancer; and solar radiation, which has been linked to basal cell skin cancers and melanoma. Other environmental factors include lifestyle behaviors such as cigarette smoking and improper diet. Smoking has been linked to cancer of the lung, mouth, bladder, and other organs. Diets high in fat and low in fiber have been linked to cancer of the colon. Pickled foods have been associated with stomach cancer, and excess alcohol intake has been associated with cancers of the esophagus, tongue, and pharynx (Mettlin, 1992).

Viral infections have been implicated in a growing number of cancers. The human papilloma virus is felt to play a causal role in the development of cancer of the cervix. Those who carry the hepatitis B virus have a greatly increased risk of liver cancer. Helicobacter pylori has been shown to be related to stomach cancer and the Epstein-Barr virus to cancer of the nasopharynx (Nomura et al., 1991). The HTLV-1 and HTLV-2 viruses, endemic in Japan, have been linked to T-cell leukemia (Thomas, 1979).

The third cause, genetic predisposition, appears to account for only 2% of cancer incidence (Desmond, 1987). An individual's risk of contracting some cancers increases if there is a history of that cancer in another blood relative. A woman's breast cancer risk, for example, increases by a factor of two if her mother or sister has had the disease and by a factor of six if both have had it (Page & Asire, 1985). A woman's risk increases by a factor of nine if her mother or sister has had cancer in both breasts before menopause (Anderson, 1972). Children with leukemic siblings have a risk of leukemia four times greater than the risk in the general population (Draper, Heaf, & Kennier-Wilson, 1977).

Although the various factors listed above are strongly implicated in the etiology of the various cancers, the specific triggering mechanism that results in cancer is as yet unknown. The process is dependent upon multiple factors, for not everyone exposed to environmental toxins, viruses, or familial predispositions will actually manifest the disease. Nonetheless, cancer initiation, or carcinogenesis, appears to follow a two-step sequence (DeVita et al., 1989). The *initiation* step probably begins through an environmental assault (e.g., exposure to ionizing radiation or a viral infection) that rearranges the DNA sequencing within a cell. This rearrangement results in deregulation of oncogenes (regulators of cell division) that were perhaps operative in embryonic life. The normal negative feedback signal that controls cell growth is lost, and the cell begins to divide uncontrollably and to invade surrounding tissues. If cells that have undergone this initiation (for example, liver cells that are infected with the hepatitis B virus) are then exposed to a *promoting* factor (such as aflatoxins from food), cancer (in this case, liver cancer) may then develop. The process seems logical, but not everyone in a family with one member who has, say, hepatitis B will be infected, and not all of those infected will develop liver cancer. It is apparent that multiple risk factors are operating, yet because further research is needed, only trends can now be reported.

In order to reduce the morbidity and mortality of cancer, a comprehensive cancer control program contains three strategies that are directed to the two-step process of carcinogenesis. Primary prevention efforts are directed toward preventing the development of the disease. Productive efforts should be directed toward the elimination of cigarette smoking, modification of diet and alcohol intake, and avoidance of exposure to other environmental or occupational carcinogens. For many Asian Pacific American populations, it is especially important to prevent exposure to the hepatitis B virus, a risk factor for liver cancer. Secondary prevention consists of early detection and treatment of the disease at a localized stage in order to maximize positive treatment outcomes. If detected early enough, many cancers can be cured. Tertiary prevention efforts provide optimal treatment and rehabilitation to enhance chances of survival, minimize the morbidity that results from treatment, and maximize the quality of life of the cancer survivor.

Treatments for cancer usually involve a combination of two or more of the following interventions: surgery, radiation therapy, chemotherapy, and use of biologic modifiers. Treatments often extend for 6 months to a year. Public attitudes and beliefs about these treatments, which are often toxic and perceived as mutilating, greatly influence the individual's and family's decisions about accepting the treatments or about completing the full course of treatments once they have begun. These issues are affected by cultural beliefs and will be discussed below, in the section on cultural considerations.

Epidemiology of Cancer in
Asian Pacific Americans

In this section we present what is known about cancer incidence, mortality, stage at diagnosis, and survival among individual Asian Pacific American groups in the United States. At the outset, it is important to acknowledge that cancer data for individual Asian and Pacific Islander groups in the United States are limited; in some cases, they are nonexistent.

In 1985, the U.S. Department of Health and Human Services published a landmark study on the status of minority health in the United States (Heckler, 1985). One index used in this report to measure the burden of disease in an ethnic group was excess mortality, that is, "the difference between the number of deaths actually observed in a minority group and the number of deaths that would have occurred in that group if it experienced the same death rates for each age and sex as the White population" (p. 63). In this section, we will identify cancer sites where Asian Pacific Americans experience excess mortality in relation to the white population and extend the concept to identify sites of excess cancer incidence and lower cancer survival, as well.

In addition, we will report what is known about the prevalence of behavioral risk factors for cancer and utilization of cancer screening procedures among the different Asian Pacific American populations. As national estimates are generally not available, here we will rely on community surveys. Information about risk factor prevalence and cancer screening utilization is important at the national and community levels for planning effective cancer control programs. Finally, we will examine the effect of immigration to the United States on the epidemiology of cancer among Asian Pacific Americans.

Data Sources

To measure the burden of cancer in a population, it is conventional to examine site- and sex-specific rates of incidence, mortality, stage at diagnosis, and five-year relative survival. These data are collected in the United States for different ethnicities by the Surveillance, Epidemiology and End Results (SEER) program of the National Cancer Institute. However, until 1988, the only Asian Pacific American ethnicities for which SEER data are available are Chinese, Japanese, Filipino, and Native Hawaiian. The data are collected from 11 regions around the country that represent about 10% of the U.S. population. SEER data for Chinese, Japanese, and Filipinos are taken from the San Francisco/Oakland registry; data for Native Hawaiians are taken from the Hawaii registry.

Starting in 1988, the SEER program began collecting data for the following additional Asian Pacific American ethnicities: Vietnamese, Laotian, Kampuchean, Hmong, Korean, and Asian Indian/Pakistani. The absence of accurate sex-, age- and county-specific counts for each group, however, precludes calculating cancer incidence and mortality rates for these ethnicities. When these data become available from the 1990 census, rates may be calculated.

In addition, since July 1988 the California Tumor Registry in the California Department of Health Services has gathered cancer data for the entire state of California using the same Asian Pacific ethnicity identifiers as the federal SEER program (Seiffert, Price, & Gordon, 1990). According to the 1990 census, nearly 40% of all Asian Pacific Americans in the United States live in California, more than in any other state (U.S. Bureau of the Census, 1991). California data, therefore, provide a useful surrogate for national Asian Pacific American data. Counts of incident site-specific cancer cases by ethnicity are currently available for years 1988 and 1989 from regional registries of the California Tumor Registry. In this chapter we present SEER data and supplement it, when possible, with data from other sources, including the California data, which may be less reliable but provide preliminary insights into the cancer problem among Asian Pacific Americans.

Incidence

Incidence is the number of new cases of a disease diagnosed during a given time period (usually one year) divided by the total number in a population at risk for that disease. Incidence, therefore, is an estimate of the risk in the population of developing the disease during that time period. For each ethnic group, incidence data can be reported for all anatomic sites combined or for separate anatomic sites, such as lung or liver.

For *all anatomic sites combined*, Chinese, Japanese, and Filipinos of both sexes experience lower cancer incidence rates than whites (Horm, Devesa, & Burhansstipanov, in press). However, certain ethnicities experience excess incidence at certain anatomic sites. Incidence rates for these sites are indicated in bold type in Table 4.1.

Chinese males experience an excess incidence of cancers of the oral cavity and pharynx, other oral cavity, nasopharynx, esophagus, stomach, liver, and gallbladder; Chinese females, of cancers of the oral cavity and pharynx, other oral cavity, nasopharynx, stomach, liver, and cervix uteri. Japanese males experience an excess incidence of cancers of the esophagus, stomach, colon and rectum, liver, and gallbladder. Japanese females experience higher incidence rates of cancers of the oral cavity and pharynx, and, like their male counterparts, of the stomach and liver. Filipino men experience excess incidence of cancers of the oral cavity and pharynx and liver. Filipino females have a higher incidence of cancer of the cervix uteri.

Chinese, Japanese, and Filipinos experience cancer incidence at rates lower than whites at a number of sites. Most notable are lower incidence rates of cancers of the lung, skin, breast, corpus uteri, prostate, urinary bladder, and kidney. Although these rates are lower in comparison to rates in the white population, the suffering caused by these cancers should not be overlooked and the potential to prevent these cancers should be emphasized. In addition, given that many of these cancers are related to lifestyle factors or increasing age, the rates of these cancers may increase dramatically as immigrant Asian Pacific American populations grow older or acculturate to a U.S. lifestyle. For example, the breast cancer rates of Chinese and Japanese women in the United States are significantly higher than those in their native countries. As these populations acculturate, the rates of breast cancer in these groups may approach that of their white American counterparts.

Native Hawaiians, unlike the other Asian Pacific American groups for which we have data, have *higher* cancer incidence rates than whites for *all anatomic sites combined* (Heckler, 1985). Most notably, Native Hawaiians experience excess incidence of cancers of the female breast, cervix uteri, corpus uteri, esophagus, larynx, lung, pancreas, stomach, and multiple myeloma.

Because incidence rates from SEER are available only for Chinese, Japanese, Filipino, and Native Hawaiian ethnic groups, it is

Table 4.1 Average Annual Age-Adjusted[a] Cancer Incidence Rates per
100,000 Population, Malignant Cases Only, for Chinese,
Japanese, and Filipinos Compared With Whites, San Francisco
and Hawaii SEER Areas, 1977 to 1983

	Both Sexes	Male	Female
All sites			
Chinese	247.6	274.0	225.9
Japanese	242.5	289.2	207.4
Filipino	212.4	221.1	178.7
white	349.6	393.5	329.0
Lung and bronchus			
Chinese	40.6	57.4	24.8
Japanese	27.1	45.0	12.6
Filipino	27.3	35.5	16.1
white	53.6	77.5	36.2
Breast			
Chinese	29.8	0.5	59.8
Japanese	30.0	0.4	55.0
Filipino	19.8	0.4	41.3
white	52.6	0.8	46.8
Colon and rectum			
Chinese	40.4	48.8	33.0
Japanese	48.8	62.3	37.5
Filipino	30.3	36.7	18.3
white	49.1	59.6	41.9
Stomach			
Chinese	10.5	13.0	8.4
Japanese	26.6	38.9	17.2
Filipino	7.8	9.3	5.0
white	8.7	13.0	5.5
Prostate			
Chinese	NA	29.6	NA
Japanese	NA	43.8	NA
Filipino	NA	44.0	NA
white	NA	70.7	NA
Liver			
Chinese	9.6	17.0	2.8
Japanese	3.6	6.2	1.4
Filipino	5.4	8.0	2.1
white	2.2	3.5	1.1
Oral cavity and pharynx			
Chinese	15.4	22.8	8.6
Japanese	4.8	7.7	2.5
Filipino	8.9	10.4	7.1
white	13.3	18.7	9.0

(continued)

Table 4.1 Continued

	Both Sexes	Male	Female
Other oral cavity[b]			
Chinese	14.8	22.1	8.0
Japanese	4.3	6.8	2.2
Filipino	7.9	9.2	6.2
white	10.8	14.5	8.0
Nasopharynx			
Chinese	11.1	15.4	7.1
Japanese	0.6	1.2	0.2
Filipino	2.1	2.9	1.1
white	0.5	0.8	0.3
Esophagus			
Chinese	3.3	5.9	0.9
Japanese	2.8	5.6	0.6
Filipino	3.4	4.5	1.6
white	2.9	4.3	2.0
Gallbladder			
Chinese	1.0	1.3	0.8
Japanese	1.5	1.5	1.5
Filipino	1.4	1.4	1.2
white	1.2	0.7	1.6
Cervix uteri			
Chinese	NA	NA	10.3
Japanese	NA	NA	5.9
Filipino	NA	NA	8.6
white	NA	NA	8.3
Pancreas			
Chinese	6.3	6.6	6.1
Japanese	7.1	9.0	5.5
Filipino	4.9	6.1	3.6
white	8.0	9.7	6.8
Melanoma of skin			
Chinese	0.7	0.6	0.9
Japanese	1.2	1.6	1.0
Filipino	1.0	1.1	0.5
white	11.7	13.2	10.6
Corpus uteri			
Chinese	NA	NA	18.0
Japanese	NA	NA	17.7
Filipino	NA	NA	11.3
white	NA	NA	30.6
Ovary			
Chinese	NA	NA	9.2
Japanese	NA	NA	8.8
Filipino	NA	NA	9.7
white	NA	NA	13.5

(continued)

Table 4.1 Continued

	Both Sexes	Male	Female
Urinary bladder			
Chinese	9.0	14.7	3.7
Japanese	8.0	12.0	4.6
Filipino	4.4	5.4	2.9
white	17.2	29.7	8.2
Kidney and renal pelvis			
Chinese	3.5	4.6	2.6
Japanese	3.6	5.7	2.0
Filipino	3.1	4.2	1.8
white	6.0	9.0	3.6
Brain and nervous system			
Chinese	2.4	2.9	2.0
Japanese	2.4	2.8	2.1
Filipino	1.9	2.9	0.5
white	5.4	6.6	4.3
Hodgkin's disease			
Chinese	0.6	0.6	0.7
Japanese	0.5	0.8	0.3
Filipino	1.2	1.4	1.2
white	2.9	3.5	2.4
Non-Hodgkin's lymphoma			
Chinese	8.5	10.3	6.8
Japanese	7.2	8.5	6.2
Filipino	8.3	9.3	7.0
white	11.1	13.0	9.5
Multiple myeloma			
Chinese	1.9	2.4	1.4
Japanese	1.3	1.3	1.4
Filipino	3.2	3.8	2.0
white	3.4	4.2	2.9
Leukemias			
Chinese	4.8	6.3	3.4
Japanese	5.7	7.1	4.5
Filipino	7.1	8.0	5.8
white	9.5	12.6	7.3

NOTES: Excess incidence for Asians/Pacific Islanders in relation to whites is indicated in bold type. NA = not applicable.
a. 1970 U.S. standard.
b. Total oral cavity and pharynx, excluding lip and salivary glands.

useful to examine the California data to gain insights into the cancer burden borne by other Asian and Pacific Islander ethnicities. Although *rates* are not yet available from the California data, it is possible to calculate proportional incidence ratios (PIRs), that is, ratios of the proportion of all cancers accounted for by a particular anatomic site in a population to the same proportion in the white population during a given period of time. For example, if 40% of all cancers among females in a particular ethnic group during a given time period are cancers of the cervix uteri but only 10% of all cancers among white females during the same time period are cancers of the cervix uteri, then the cervical cancer PIR for that ethnic group would be 4.

PIRs at selected sites for Vietnamese, Koreans, Asian Indians, Laotians, Kampucheans, and other Asians are presented in Table 4.2. The data show higher PIRs for some groups at some sites when compared with whites. Although a high PIR may indicate sites that should be targeted for interventions, higher PIRs do not necessarily indicate higher incidence rates.

Several additional cautions should be noted in interpreting these data: The number of site-, sex-, and ethnicity-specific cases recorded for Asian Pacific Americans since 1988 is still relatively small and, therefore, the PIRs calculated here are potentially subject to variability. Furthermore, it can be expected that misclassification errors have resulted in some cancer cases being assigned to incorrect ethnicities, especially because coding of some Asian Pacific American ethnicities began only relatively recently. For example, an individual with the common Korean surname Park, on the basis of the surname only, may be understandably but incorrectly classified as Caucasian. Furthermore, groups such as the Chinese-Vietnamese, that is, individuals of Chinese ancestry born in Vietnam, may be legitimately classified as either Vietnamese or Chinese. In addition, Amerasians or persons of "mixed" ethnicity may present other difficult classification dilemmas.

The proportion of all cancers accounted for by lung cancer is higher among some Asian and Pacific Islander ethnicities than among whites (see Table 4.2). These differences may be explained by the high cigarette smoking prevalence rates, especially among males, of some Asian Pacific immigrant groups, as discussed below.

The proportion of liver cancer among Asian Pacific American males, with the exception of Asian Indians, is dramatically higher for all groups than among whites. This difference is most likely explained by the high prevalence of hepatitis B carrier status, liver fluke infesta-

Table 4.2 Proportional Cancer Incidence Ratios, Asian Pacific Americans in California for Selected Sites

Site	Vietnamese	Korean	Asian Indian	Laotian	Kampuchean	Hmong	Other Asian
Lung	1.0 (42)	1.1 (47)	0.2 (6)	2.3 (6)	1.1 (5)	— (0)	0.7 (60)
Liver (males)	14.5 (17)	12.4 (14)	— (0)	9.6 (1)	25.0 (4)	— (0)	10.1 (22)
Breast (females)	0.4 (22)	0.7 (35)	1.06 (33)	0.6 (1)	0.2 (1)	— (0)	1.4 (115)
Cervix (females)	2.2 (44)	2.6 (45)	1.4 (17)	1.5 (1)	3.7 (6)	— (0)	2.3 (67)
Nasopharynx	24.0 (8)	— (0)	— (0)	100.0 (2)	28.0 (1)	— (0)	14.0 (9)
Colon and rectum	0.7 (33)	0.6 (26)	0.9 (24)	1.1 (3)	0.4 (2)	2.4 (1)	0.6 (51)
Stomach	3.5 (23)	7.6 (50)	1.9 (7)	— (0)	2.5 (1)	— (0)	2.2 (28)
Esophagus	1.9 (5)	2.3 (6)	0.6 (1)	— (0)	— (0)	— (0)	0.8 (4)

SOURCE: California Tumor Registry Regions 1 and 8, 1988-1989; Regions 9 and 10, 1988. Region 10 cancer incidence data have been collected under Subcontract 050F-8710 with the California Public Health Foundation. The contract is supported by the California Department of Health Services as part of its statewide cancer reporting program, mandated by Health and Safety Code Sections 210 and 211.3. The ideas and opinions expressed herein are those of the author, and no endorsement of the State of California, Department of Health Services, or the California Public Health Foundation is intended or should be inferred.
NOTE: Numbers of cases appear in parentheses.

tions, and aflatoxin exposure among Asian immigrants and their high correlation with subsequent development of hepatoma (Centers for Disease Control, 1991; Lam, 1986; Nomura et al., 1991).

The proportion of female breast cancer among Asian Indians parallels the proportion among whites, but for the other Asian and Pacific Islander ethnicities the proportion of breast cancer is dramatically lower. These lower proportions are consistent with lower breast cancer incidence rates for Chinese, Japanese, and Filipinos, as reported above.

Cervical cancer proportions are higher than those for whites for every Asian Pacific American group. Higher cervical cancer proportions may be explained by the relative lack of Pap smear screening among Asian and Pacific Islander immigrants in their countries of origin as well as in the United States, as discussed below. In addition, some have speculated that poor sexual hygiene among Asian Pacific American immigrants in their countries of origin may result in a higher prevalence of the human papilloma virus, which has been linked to the development of cervical cancer (Weisburger & Horn, 1991).

Colorectal cancer proportions are lower than for whites except for Laotians, but stomach cancer proportions are higher. Vietnamese and Korean esophageal cancer proportions are higher than for whites, whereas Asian Indian, Laotian, Kampuchean, and other Asian proportions are lower. The "other Asian" category includes Thais, Malaysians, Indonesians, and Burmese.

Stage at Diagnosis

Although the terminology for the stage of the disease at the time of diagnosis varies by the site of cancer, its cell type, and current practice, cancer can be classified into four stages at diagnosis: *in situ*, confined to an area less than or equal to 1 to 3 cm and a thickness of one cell layer; *localized*, restricted to a single anatomical area with no gross lymph node involvement; *regional*, contained within an anatomical region with lymph node involvement; and *distant*, which includes metastatic sites distant from the primary or original site. With this information, we can calculate the proportion of cancer at a particular site that is diagnosed at in situ, localized, regional, and distant stages. It is important to have data regarding the stage of the disease at the time of diagnosis, because the stage indicates the degree of spread of the disease. As mentioned above, the more localized the disease, the better the chance for cure. Some groups of Asian Pacific Americans with potentially curable cancers are diagnosed with late-stage disease.

When compared with whites, for example, on the average, Japanese, Chinese, Vietnamese, Filipino, and Korean women are diagnosed with cervical cancer at later stages (Figure 4.1). The comparisons for breast cancer (Figure 4.2), however, show less dramatic differences between whites and Asian Pacific Americans. Vietnamese, Chinese, and Japanese women, on the average, present with earlier-stage breast cancer than do whites, whereas Filipino and Korean women present at a later stage. Detection at a later stage may mean higher mortality and lower survival rates. Culturally appropriate cancer screening programs may result in the detection of cancer among Asian Pacific Americans at an earlier, more treatable stage.

Mortality

The mortality rate is calculated by dividing the number of persons who have died of a disease during a given time period (usually

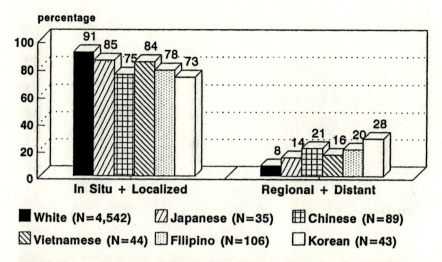

Figure 4.1. Cervical Cancer Stage at Diagnosis, Asian Pacific American Ethnicities and Whites, California

SOURCE: Data from the California Tumor Registry, Regions 1 and 8, 1988-1989; Regions 9 and 10, 1988 only.
NOTE: Total percentage may be less than 100 because unstaged cases are omitted.

a year) by the total number in the population during that period. As with incidence rates, mortality rates can also be reported for all anatomic sites combined or for separate sites.

National SEER data show that mortality rates from cancer at *all anatomic sites combined* are lower among Chinese, Japanese, and Filipinos than among whites (Horm et al., in press). However, when the data are disaggregated by anatomic site, rates exceed the comparable white rates for certain sites and for certain groups. Mortality rates are shown in Table 4.3.

Chinese males experience excess mortality of cancers of the oral cavity and pharynx, other oral cavity, nasopharynx, esophagus, stomach, and liver; Chinese females experience excess cancer mortality at the same sites, with the exception of esophagus and the addition of cervix uteri. Japanese males experience excess deaths from cancers of the nasopharynx, stomach, liver, and gallbladder; Japanese females, from cancers of the stomach and liver. Filipino males experience excess mortality from cancers of the nasopharynx and liver; Filipino females, from cancer of the nasopharynx only.

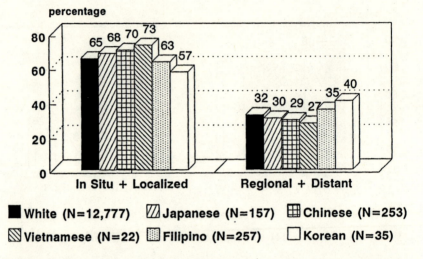

Figure 4.2. Breast Cancer Stage at Diagnosis, Asian Pacific American Ethnicities and Whites, California Females

SOURCE: Data from the California Tumor Registry, Regions 1 and 8, 1988-1989; Regions 9 and 10, 1988 only.
NOTE: Total percentage may be less than 100 because unstaged cases are omitted.

Native Hawaiians, however, have, as with incidence rates, higher cancer mortality rates than whites for all sites combined (Heckler, 1985). Specifically, Native Hawaiians experience excess mortality from cancers of the female breast, cervix uteri, rectum, esophagus, larynx, lung, pancreas, stomach, and multiple myeloma.

Chinese, Japanese, and Filipinos experience lower cancer mortality rates than whites at a number of sites (Table 4.3). Most notable are lower incidence rates of cancers of the colon and rectum, lung, skin, breast, corpus uteri, prostate, urinary bladder, and kidney.

Five-Year Relative Survival Rates

Five-year relative survival rates represent the percentage of persons with cancer who remain alive 5 years after diagnosis, after adjusting for age, race, and other causes of mortality. As shown in Table 4.4, for *all sites combined,* Chinese and Filipinos of both sexes and Japanese males have lower 5-year relative survival rates than

Table 4.3 Average Annual Age-Adjusted[a] Cancer Mortality Rates per 100,000 Population for Chinese, Japanese, and Filipinos Compared With Whites, San Francisco and Hawaii SEER Areas, 1977 to 1983

	Both Sexes	Male	Female
All sites			
Chinese	125.0	158.0	93.5
Japanese	108.0	138.6	84.8
Filipino	72.0	84.0	48.2
white	164.2	209.8	133.5
Lung and bronchus			
Chinese	31.7	45.2	18.6
Japanese	19.8	34.0	8.7
Filipino	14.5	20.0	6.9
white	41.6	69.6	21.0
Breast			
Chinese	6.1	0.2	12.0
Japanese	5.8	—	10.2
Filipino	3.9	0.2	7.8
white	15.0	0.2	26.8
Colon and rectum			
Chinese	17.9	23.8	12.4
Japanese	16.8	21.8	13.0
Filipino	7.9	9.8	4.2
white	21.4	25.7	18.4
Stomach			
Chinese	7.6	10.1	5.3
Japanese	17.9	24.3	13.2
Filipino	3.5	4.0	2.6
white	5.2	7.6	3.6
Prostate			
Chinese	NA	7.4	NA
Japanese	NA	8.4	NA
Filipino	NA	8.7	NA
white	NA	21.1	NA
Liver			
Chinese	10.1	16.4	3.8
Japanese	3.4	4.9	2.1
Filipino	3.5	5.3	1.3
white	1.9	2.7	1.3
Oral cavity and pharynx			
Chinese	5.4	8.0	2.7
Japanese	1.7	2.8	0.8
Filipino	2.4	3.0	1.2
white	3.3	5.2	1.8

(continued)

Table 4.3 Continued

	Both Sexes	Male	Female
Other oral cavity[b]			
Chinese	5.3	7.8	2.6
Japanese	1.6	2.6	0.7
Filipino	2.2	2.8	1.0
white	3.0	4.7	1.6
Nasopharynx			
Chinese	4.1	6.3	1.9
Japanese	0.4	0.5	0.2
Filipino	0.8	1.0	0.4
white	0.2	0.4	0.2
Esophagus			
Chinese	2.8	4.7	0.9
Japanese	2.1	3.8	0.8
Filipino	1.8	2.6	0.3
white	2.6	4.5	1.2
Cervix uteri			
Chinese	NA	NA	3.3
Japanese	NA	NA	2.2
Filipino	NA	NA	1.9
white	NA	NA	3.2
Gallbladder			
Chinese	0.7	0.5	0.9
Japanese	1.1	0.9	1.2
Filipino	0.6	0.6	0.6
white	0.9	0.6	1.2
Pancreas			
Chinese	6.4	7.6	5.3
Japanese	7.0	8.3	6.0
Filipino	3.5	4.5	2.1
white	8.4	10.4	6.8
Melanoma of skin			
Chinese	0.2	0.4	0.2
Japanese	0.2	0.3	0.1
Filipino	0.3	0.3	0.3
white	2.2	2.8	1.6
Corpus uteri			
Chinese	NA	NA	2.7
Japanese	NA	NA	2.4
Filipino	NA	NA	1.7
white	NA	NA	3.9
Ovary			
Chinese	NA	NA	3.8
Japanese	NA	NA	4.4
Filipino	NA	NA	2.6
white	NA	NA	8.1

(continued)

Table 4.3 Continued

	Both Sexes	Male	Female
Urinary bladder			
Chinese	1.7	2.6	0.9
Japanese	1.8	2.3	1.5
Filipino	1.4	1.6	0.7
white	3.8	6.8	1.9
Kidney and renal pelvis			
Chinese	1.7	2.4	1.1
Japanese	1.6	2.5	1.0
Filipino	0.8	1.1	0.5
white	3.2	4.6	2.1
Brain and nervous system			
Chinese	1.3	1.5	1.1
Japanese	1.3	1.4	1.1
Filipino	1.1	1.3	0.7
white	4.2	5.0	3.4
Hodgkin's disease			
Chinese	0.3	0.5	0.1
Japanese	0.1	0.1	0.0
Filipino	0.3	0.3	0.2
white	0.9	1.1	0.7
Non-Hodgkin's lymphoma			
Chinese	2.8	3.1	2.5
Japanese	3.5	4.2	3.0
Filipino	3.4	3.8	2.6
white	5.2	6.3	4.4
Multiple myeloma			
Chinese	1.4	1.8	1.1
Japanese	1.3	1.7	1.0
Filipino	1.5	1.9	0.6
white	2.4	3.0	2.0
Leukemias			
Chinese	4.1	5.2	3.1
Japanese	3.5	4.9	2.4
Filipino	4.1	5.0	2.3
white	6.7	8.9	5.2

NOTES: Excess mortality for Asians/Pacific Islanders in relation to whites is indicated in bold type. NA = not applicable; Dash indicates that there were no cases.
a. 1970 U.S. standard.
b. Total oral cavity and pharynx, excluding lip and salivary glands.

whites (Horm et al., in press). Japanese women, however, have higher 5-year relative survival rates than white women.

The data for individual anatomic sites show that Chinese males have lower survival rates for cancers of the colon and rectum, liver, pancreas, and prostate, and the leukemias; Chinese females, for cancers of the liver, pancreas, lung and bronchus, corpus uteri, and urinary bladder, and non-Hodgkin's lymphoma and the leukemias. Japanese males have lower survival rates for cancers of the oral cavity and pharynx, esophagus, liver, pancreas, and lung and bronchus, and non-Hodgkin's lymphoma and the leukemias; Japanese females, for cancers of the liver, lung and bronchus, corpus uteri, and urinary bladder, and non-Hodgkin's lymphoma and the leukemias. Filipino males have lower survival rates for cancers of the oral cavity and pharynx, other oral cavity, colon and rectum, prostate, urinary bladder, kidney, and renal pelvis, and non-Hodgkin's lymphoma and the leukemias; Filipino females, for cancers of the colon and rectum, pancreas, lung and bronchus, breast, and corpus uteri, and non-Hodgkin's lymphoma and the leukemias.

Native Hawaiians have poorer survival rates for all sites combined than whites (Heckler, 1985). Specifically, Native Hawaiians have lower survival rates from cancers of the urinary bladder, female breast, cervix uteri, colon, larynx, lung and bronchus, and prostate and from multiple myeloma.

Chinese, Japanese, and Filipinos experience higher 5-year relative survival rates than whites at a number of sites. Most notable are higher survival rates for cancers of the nasopharynx, stomach, breast, colon and rectum, cervix, and ovary.

Although, as an aggregate group, Chinese, Japanese, and Filipinos have lower cancer incidence and mortality rates than whites for all anatomic sites combined, their survival experience is generally poorer than that of whites. In other words, overall, Asian Pacific Americans may be less likely to develop cancer and, overall, Asian Pacific Americans may be less likely to die from cancer. But those Asian Pacific Americans who do develop cancer are less likely to survive. Especially noteworthy is that 5-year relative survival rates among some Asian Pacific American groups for cancers of the colon and rectum and breast, for example, are poorer even though mortality rates at these sites are lower when compared with those of whites.

Prevalence of Cancer Risk Factors

Published national data show that the prevalence of cigarette smoking, a risk factor for cancer of the lung and other organs, is lower among the *aggregate* Asian Pacific population than among

Table 4.4 Five-Year Relative Survival Rates for Cancer Cases Diagnosed From San Francisco/Oakland and Hawaii SEER Registries, 1975 to 1984, for Chinese, Japanese, and Filipinos Compared With Whites at the Same Sites (in percentages)

	Both Sexes	Male	Female
All sites			
Chinese	47.5	38.9	56.2
Japanese	53.1	44.4	61.6
Filipino	46.1	38.9	56.7
white	52.9	46.1	58.7
Lung and bronchus			
Chinese	15.1	15.0	15.4
Japanese	14.3	13.4	16.8
Filipino	13.2	14.3	10.1
white	15.7	13.8	18.9
Breast			
Chinese	80.9	—	80.8
Japanese	85.4	—	85.4
Filipino	73.6	—	73.7
white	78.3	90.2	78.3
Colon and rectum			
Chinese	53.1	48.7	58.8
Japanese	61.7	60.8	62.8
Filipino	44.8	42.5	51.4
white	54.4	54.2	54.6
Stomach			
Chinese	21.6	17.8	26.6
Japanese	29.8	28.1	32.5
Filipino	18.8	21.2	0.0
white	16.3	14.3	18.8
Prostate			
Chinese	NA	72.5	NA
Japanese	NA	80.5	NA
Filipino	NA	71.7	NA
white	NA	73.0	NA
Liver			
Chinese	2.0	1.4	4.1
Japanese	1.5	1.5	0.0
Filipino	6.7	5.0	—
white	4.2	3.2	6.1
Oral cavity and pharynx			
Chinese	55.7	54.3	58.5
Japanese	44.4	41.7	51.6
Filipino	46.6	40.6	58.4
white	50.2	49.6	51.1

(continued)

Table 4.4 Continued

	Both Sexes	Male	Female
Other oral cavity[a]			
Chinese	54.6	53.8	56.2
Japanese	45.1	42.9	50.5
Filipino	45.0	39.1	56.8
white	42.6	39.3	47.6
Nasopharynx			
Chinese	56.6	55.9	57.7
Japanese	45.1	—	—
Filipino	47.5	46.3	—
white	41.1	43.1	35.5
Esophagus			
Chinese	11.5	7.0	—
Japanese	5.8	4.8	—
Filipino	3.4	6.5	—
white	5.8	6.3	4.8
Gallbladder			
Chinese	—	—	—
Japanese	16.2	—	14.9
Filipino	—	—	—
white	8.8	3.0	10.8
Pancreas			
Chinese	0.0	0.0	0.0
Japanese	2.6	0.9	4.8
Filipino	5.2	3.8	0.0
white	2.1	2.2	2.1
Corpus uteri			
Chinese	NA	NA	86.1
Japanese	NA	NA	84.1
Filipino	NA	NA	79.9
white	NA	NA	86.9
Melanoma of skin			
Chinese	—	—	—
Japanese	81.0	—	—
Filipino	—	—	—
white	83.2	78.5	88.3
Cervix uteri			
Chinese	NA	NA	74.6
Japanese	NA	NA	70.2
Filipino	NA	NA	73.0
white	NA	NA	69.0
Ovary			
Chinese	NA	NA	43.3
Japanese	NA	NA	43.5
Filipino	NA	NA	44.7
white	NA	NA	37.4

(continued)

Table 4.4 Continued

	Both Sexes	Male	Female
Urinary bladder			
Chinese	78.5	83.9	**56.8**
Japanese	80.8	85.6	**70.1**
Filipino	**58.4**	**64.9**	—
white	77.5	79.0	73.5
Kidney and renal pelvis			
Chinese	60.7	58.9	—
Japanese	63.1	61.4	66.7
Filipino	**47.0**	**44.3**	—
white	53.1	54.6	50.0
Brain and nervous system			
Chinese	35.9	25.5	—
Japanese	40.6	26.5	57.4
Filipino	29.6	28.4	—
white	25.1	22.8	28.3
Hodgkin's disease			
Chinese	—	—	—
Japanese	—	—	—
Filipino	**43.5**	—	—
white	73.5	69.7	78.7
Non-Hodgkin's lymphoma			
Chinese	50.3	51.4	**48.7**
Japanese	**41.1**	**38.5**	**43.9**
Filipino	**33.8**	**32.9**	**35.1**
white	49.9	47.9	52.1
Multiple myeloma			
Chinese	**20.5**	—	—
Japanese	37.6	—	—
Filipino	**17.1**	**7.8**	—
white	25.4	26.1	24.6
Leukemias			
Chinese	**19.8**	**22.1**	**16.4**
Japanese	**26.0**	**22.0**	31.4
Filipino	**22.3**	**21.9**	**22.5**
white	32.8	33.7	31.6

NOTES: Lower survival for Asians/Pacific Islanders in relation to whites is indicated in bold type. NA = not applicable. Dashes indicate instances in which there were too few cases for a reliable estimate of the five-year relative survival rate.
a. Total oral cavity and pharynx, excluding lip and salivary glands.

whites. Table 4.5 shows comparative cigarette smoking prevalence data for Asian Pacific Americans compared with whites from the National Health Interview Survey (NHIS; National Center for

Table 4.5 Prevalence of Cigarette Smoking Among U.S. Whites and
Asian Pacific Americans

	Year	Male	Female
Whites (NHIS)	1991	30.9	28.6
Whites (CPS)	1991	27.0	23.3
Aggregated Asian Pacific American data			
Asians (NHIS)	1991	24.9	11.9
Asian Pacific Islanders (CPS)	1991	22.1	10.5
Disaggregated Asian Pacific American data			
Vietnamese	1991	35.0	0.4
Filipinos	1991	20.0	6.3
Chinese	1989	28	1
Koreans	1989	33	2
Laotians	1985	72	—[a]
Kampucheans	1982	70.7	12.9
Hmong	1982	26.0	1.7
Sino-Vietnamese	1982	54.5	1.7

SOURCES: For whites (NHIS) and Asians (NHIS), National Center for Health Statistics (1991); for whites and Asians/Pacific Islanders (CPS), National Heart, Lung and Blood Institute (1991); for Vietnamese and Chinese, Centers for Disease Control (1992c); for Filipinos, Jang (1991); for Koreans, Han et al. (1989); for Lao, Levin (1985); for Kampucheans, Hmong, and Sino-Vietnamese, Rumbaut (1989).
NOTE: a. Women were not surveyed

Health Statistics, 1991) and the Current Population Survey (CPS) conducted by the U.S. Bureau of the Census (National Heart, Lung and Blood Institute, 1991). These data show that smoking rates among Asian Pacific Americans are lower than rates among whites. Cigarette smoking rates among Asian Pacific American females, especially, are considerably lower than among their white counterparts.

Disaggregated Asian Pacific American data from community surveys, however, show considerable variation in smoking rates by ethnicity. Some groups, especially recently immigrated Vietnamese, Chinese, Korean, Laotian, Kampuchean, and Sino-Vietnamese males, have smoking rates that are considerably higher than white rates. The community smoking survey data again illustrate how important health status differences can be discerned if each Asian and Pacific Islander ethnicity is examined separately rather than as an aggregate Asian Pacific group.

Carriers of the hepatitis B virus have a risk of liver cancer that is more than 200 times that in the noninfected population (Beasley & Hwang, 1984). Although the prevalence of hepatitis B carrier status is less than .05% in the general U.S. population, the rates among immigrants to the United States from Asia, where the disease is endemic, range from 10% to 14% (Jenkins, McPhee, Bird, & Bonilla, 1990; Mettlin & Dodd, 1991; National Cancer Institute, 1987). Hepatitis B is 100 times more contagious than the human immunodeficiency virus (HIV).

An important liver cancer prevention strategy is the screening of pregnant women for hepatitis B carrier status and the provision of immunoprophylaxis to infants born to women who are found to be carriers of the virus. A number of screening programs are in place, but compliance with immunoprophylaxis protocols is sometimes poor. For example, in 1984 to 1985, at one San Francisco Bay Area county hospital, 89% of pregnant immigrant Asian and Pacific Islander women were screened for hepatitis B. However, only 37% of the infants born to hepatitis B carrier mothers in this hospital completed the recommended three-dose immunoprophylaxis protocol (Klontz, 1986).

More recently, the Centers for Disease Control (1991) has published guidelines that call for the universal immunization of all infants against hepatitis B. However, the cost of the three-dose immunizations (approximately $120) is likely to remain a barrier to successful implementation of the universal immunization guidelines among Asian Pacific Americans. In addition, the supplies of vaccine and the staff available in clinics that administer the vaccines are limited (Hammer, 1992).

Screening

Screening guidelines for the early detection of cancer in asymptomatic individuals have been established by the National Cancer Institute (1987) and the American Cancer Society (Mettlin & Dodd, 1991). Early cancer detection and treatment have been associated with lower mortality and higher survival rates. Although the two sets of guidelines differ somewhat in the recommended frequencies and ages at which screening is advised, they both recommend regular Papanicolaou tests, pelvic examinations, clinical breast examinations and mammography for women, and digital rectal examinations, stool occult blood tests, and sigmoidoscopy for both sexes.

Table 4.6 Compliance With Cancer Screening Recommendations Among
Asian Pacific Americans and U.S. Whites (in percentages)

Population, Year	Pap Smear Never	Pap Smear Over-due	Breast Exam Never	Breast Exam Over-due	Mammo-graphy Never	Mammo-graphy Over-due	Rectal Exam Never	Rectal Exam Over-due	Stool Blood Test Never	Stool Blood Test Over-due
					Procedure					
Chinese, 1989	45	—	—	—	68	—	—	—	—	—
Koreans, 1989	—	65[a]	—	71[b]	—	—	—	—	—	—
Vietnamese, 1991	51	62	47	57	48	55	70	—	62	—
Hawaiian, 1987	—	—	—	—	55[c]	78[c], 73[d]	—	—	—	—
Asian Pacific Islander, 1990	—	—	—	—	71	—	—	—	—	—
Whites, California, 1990, and United States, 1987	5[e]	34[e]	12[e]	31[e]	30[e]	38[e]	42[f], 43[g]	81[f], 77[g]	63[f], 63[g]	83[f], 80[g]

SOURCES: For Chinese, Centers for Disease Control (1992a); for Koreans, Han et al. (1989); for Vietnamese, Centers for Disease Control (1992b); for Hawaiians, Tash et al. (1988); for Asian Pacific Americans, Jones (1990); for whites, California, California Department of Health Services (1990); for whites, United States, Brown, Potosky, Thompson, and Kessler (1990).
NOTES: Dashes indicate no data available.
a. Women age ≥18 who did not have a Pap smear in the last year.
b. Women age ≥18 who did not have a breast exam in the last year.
c. Hawaiian women of any ethnicity, age ≥50.
d. Hawaiian women of any ethnicity, ages 40-49.
e. California women.
f. U.S. men, age ≥40.
g. U.S. women, age ≥40.

Table 4.6 presents a summary of results available from community surveys among Asian Pacific American groups regarding compliance with cancer screening guidelines. When compared with whites, all Asian Pacific American populations have lower compliance for all procedures. As can be seen from the table, there are many Asian and Pacific Islander ethnicities for which there are no data on compliance with certain cancer screening recommendations.

Using a modified Behavioral Risk Factor Survey instrument, investigators at Asian Health Services, a community clinic in Oakland, California, conducted Chinese-language face-to-face surveys of 296 Chinese households in 1989 (Centers for Disease Control,

1992a). They found that Chinese women were less likely to have ever had mammograms or Pap smears than were women in the general California population. Chinese women with less than eighth-grade education or who did not speak English fluently were less likely to have ever had mammograms than their Chinese counterparts who were more highly educated or spoke English more fluently.

Han et al. (1989) conducted a Korean- and English-language bilingual mail survey of 345 Korean households in Los Angeles County in 1989. They found that the frequency of having had a Pap smear in the past year was highest among the reproductive age group, ages 30 to 44, but declined thereafter. Frequency of having had a breast examination within the last year was highest among the 45 to 64 age group but lower among both younger and older women.

Using a modified Behavioral Risk Factor Survey instrument, investigators at the University of California, San Francisco, surveyed 1,011 Vietnamese in California in the Vietnamese language using a computer-assisted telephone interview method in 1991 (Centers for Disease Control, 1992b). They found that women were significantly less likely to have had a Pap smear if they had less than a college education, were unemployed, were unmarried, had lower household incomes, or were more recent immigrants. Furthermore, women who were unmarried, had lower household incomes, or were more recent immigrants were significantly less likely to have had clinical breast examinations. Lower income and more recent immigration were also significantly associated with never having had a mammogram.

In an earlier study, the same authors conducted Vietnamese-language face-to-face interviews with 215 Vietnamese individuals in the San Francisco area in 1987 (Jenkins et al., 1990). They observed that respondents who reported that their regular physicians were Vietnamese were less likely to have had rectal examinations or stool occult blood tests than were respondents with non-Vietnamese physicians. The authors speculated that reluctance to disrobe, especially among Vietnamese women, and physician deference to a patient's modesty may act as barriers to some cancer screening procedures.

In Hawaii, investigators using the Behavioral Risk Factor Survey instrument surveyed 1,862 adults of all ethnicities using random-digit dialing techniques in 1987 (Tash, Chung, & Yasunobu, 1988). Among the 181 women surveyed who were of Hawaiian or part-

Hawaiian ethnicity, 73% had heard of mammograms, compared
with 92% of their Caucasian counterparts in Hawaii. Among women
of any ethnicity age 50 or more, 55% had never had mammograms,
compared with national data for white women of 18% (Wirthlin
Group, 1992).

It should be noted that there are no effective screening procedures
available for some cancers that commonly strike Asian Pacific Americans (e.g., cancers of the liver, pancreas, stomach, esophagus, and
corpus uteri). Moreover, because symptoms of these cancers may
appear only after the disease has advanced to a relatively late stage,
these cancers may have very poor prognosis. Thus health care practitioners should be alert to a possible cancer diagnosis when a patient
presents with vague complaints of discomfort that could be early signs
of cancer at these common sites. These complaints may be mistaken
for part of the Asian and Pacific Islander cultural tendency to somatize
emotional complaints and may be treated symptomatically, without
diagnostic workup.

Implications of Migration Studies for Cancer Control

Migration studies compare cancer rates between members of a
group in a country of origin and members of that same group in a host
country to which they have immigrated. Investigators also compare
successive generations of immigrants in the host country and ob-
serve the successive changes in cancer rates and the concomitant
acculturation changes that occur in the group. These studies are
important in clarifying the role of nongenetic determinants in the
etiology of cancer. Identification of the changes in environmental
exposures and lifestyle habits that are correlated with changes in
cancer incidence among immigrants has significant implications
for the prevention of cancers for Asian Pacific American groups
specifically, but the findings may also be applicable for cancer
prevention in general.

Migration studies among Asian Pacific immigrant groups to the
United States that document the effect of immigration on cancer
epidemiology are limited to studies of Chinese and Japanese. The
incidence rates of the following cancers have been shown to rise
among Chinese and Japanese when they emigrate from their respective countries of origin to the United States: prostate, corpus
uteri, breast, colon, rectum, and pancreas (Thomas, 1979). For ex-

ample, migration studies show that when Chinese move to the United States, their prostate cancer incidence rates increase more than 11-fold, although the rates remain less than half those found among males in the general U.S. population (Yu, Randall, Gao, Gao, & Wynder, 1991). Colon cancer incidence rates among Chinese Americans are three times higher than rates among Shanghai Chinese (Yu et al., 1991).

In addition, female breast cancer incidence rates have risen more than threefold among Chinese immigrants while still remaining below white rates (Yu et al., 1991). A similar increase in breast cancer incidence has been noted among Japanese immigrants to the United States; during the period from 1968 to 1971 the breast cancer incidence ratio among Japanese women in Miyagi, Japan, was 0.18 (using the rate among whites in San Francisco for the same period as the reference, 1.00), whereas during the same period the ratio was 0.59 among their Japanese counterparts in San Francisco (Thomas, 1979). Further evidence of this increase in successive generations of migrants are the higher breast cancer death rates for Nisei (second-generation Japanese Americans) than among Issei (first-generation Japanese Americans). More recently, it has been shown that Japanese women who immigrate to the United States at younger ages have a higher breast cancer incidence rate than those who immigrate at an older age (Shimizu et al., 1991).

Colorectal and breast cancer have been related to diets rich in animal fat (Armstrong & Doll, 1975; Goodwin & Boyd, 1987). Traditional diets in China and Japan are lower in fat than is the typical U.S. diet. In Japan, for example, fat accounts for only 10% to 15% of calories in the traditional diet (mostly unsaturated fat derived from fish oils) compared with the Western diet, in which fat makes up 40% of calories (Weisburger, 1991). The total dietary fat intake of Americans is 2.7 times that consumed by Chinese (Yu et al., 1991). The evidence is growing that the increased incidence of colorectal and breast cancers among Chinese and Japanese immigrants to the United States may be the result of immigrants' adoption of American dietary practices as they acculturate.

Diet may also affect breast cancer rates through hormonal influences. The high-fat diet of girls in the United States may cause them to reach the critical fat-to-lean body mass ratio necessary for the onset of menarche earlier than girls in China. Earlier onset of menarche and later menopause is related to higher incidence of breast cancer. Some have speculated that with early onset of menarche the breast tissue of women is exposed to the stimulation of estrogen for a longer period of time, thus increasing the likelihood of mutations or translocations of genetic material. In China, the average age of puberty is 17, whereas in the United States the average age of puberty has steadily been decreasing to its present level of 12.8 years of age (Harris, Lippman, Veronesi, & Willett, 1992).

The incidence rates for the following cancers decline for Chinese and Japanese when they immigrate to the United States: liver, cervix uteri, stomach, and esophagus (Thomas, 1979). Declines in liver cancer may be caused by two factors: better control and lower prevalence of the hepatitis B virus, and improved food handling and storage, resulting in less exposure to aflatoxins. Declines in cancer of the cervix may be the result of increased rates of Pap smear screening and the detection of precancerous lesions that may then be excised. Cervical cancer rates may also decline as immigrants adopt better sexual hygiene practices or barrier contraception methods, thereby reducing the transmission of the human papilloma virus, which has been associated with cervical cancer.

Diets low in fresh fruits and vegetables and high in dried, salted fish, pickled vegetables, and smoked fish (common in many Asian diets but rare in the United States) have been shown to raise the risk of stomach cancer (Howson, Hiyama, & Wynder, 1986). Declines in stomach cancer may therefore be the result of favorable dietary changes among Chinese and Japanese immigrants to the United States as they acculturate to the American diet. Esophageal cancer also has a dietary etiology and has been linked to consumption of food and alcoholic beverages contaminated with carcinogenic nitros-compound-forming yeasts and molds ("Leads in Oesophageal Cancer," 1974). Declines in esophageal cancer may be the result of better food preservation methods in the United States.

Clearly, the field of migration studies offers fertile ground for insights into the causes of cancer. Future research should focus on such large immigrant populations as Filipinos, Koreans, Vietnamese, Laotians, and Kampucheans, which have not yet been studied. In order to perform such studies, however, it will be necessary to develop rigorous cancer incidence, mortality, and behavioral risk factor data in the countries of origin so that comparisons can be made among foreign-born, migrant, and U.S.-born groups. For such data to be collected, it will be necessary to conduct behavioral risk factor surveillance and to establish national tumor registries in the countries of origin.

Cultural Considerations in
the Treatment and Rehabilitation of
Asian Pacific American Cancer Patients

We have focused thus far on the epidemiological data to describe the burden of cancer on Asian Pacific Americans. We turn now to a consideration of the emotional and social impact of the cancer experience. We will show how the individual's cultural background fundamentally influences how that person will interpret and utilize cancer control efforts.

Enormous emotional, existential, and practical problems arise for individuals and their families when they are confronted with a diagnosis of cancer. Negotiating the health care system to obtain treatment, for example, requires sophistication, perseverance, and understanding of the implicit culturally framed structure in which health care is provided. Many individuals, regardless of ethnicity, do not have the skills to enter the health care system. Even those who are able to enter are often overwhelmed by the demands and restrictions made upon them for decisions and choices. The perseverance and assertiveness required to obtain good care are characteristics not usually found in Asian Pacific American families when dealing with people in authority or institutions. Instead, they put their trust in their family physician and expect him or her to do whatever is in their best interest; their responsibility is to follow the doctor's recommendations as closely as possible. Asserting their desires to expedite treatment or to change doctors with whom they are dissatisfied would most often not even be considered as options. Thus Asian Pacific American patients are often viewed as "compliant" by Western providers.

An unchallenging and accepting demeanor may not always be in the patient's best interest. For example, such a patient may be less likely to complain of symptoms, and treatment, therefore, may be delayed. On the other hand, being compliant may also be a factor in the better survival rates found among Asian Pacific Americans than for whites for some cancers (Young, Ries, & Pollack, 1984). These patients may endure the negative side effects of treatments and receive higher overall doses of treatment over longer periods of time and thereby may obtain more complete eradication of microdisease sites.

Although the epidemiological findings presented above clearly indicate that ethnicity affects cancer incidence, mortality, and survival, a

Western ethnocentric bias is implicit in the majority of psychosocial studies conducted by Western and Western-trained researchers. This research overlooks the variations in cultural beliefs and behaviors that define ethnicity. This bias assumes that the desired outcomes and means for adaptation to cancer and its treatment are similar for all populations.

Although a patient's cultural background influences the entire cancer experience for the patient and the family, very little effort has been made to study the specific effects of cultural beliefs and behaviors on the emotional and physical response to cancer of differing ethnic groups. This is especially true for Asian Pacific Americans. The general health beliefs and behaviors of many traditional Asian and Pacific Islander cultures are based upon a paradigm that is very different from the Western biomedical paradigm (Kitano, 1990; Marr, 1987). Both paradigms are equally rational and "scientific" within the context of the belief system, but areas of inconsistency can create miscommunication and misunderstanding (Kleinman, 1980; Muecke, 1983).

Culture influences beliefs about the meaning of cancer; emotional and physical responses to the treatments; side effects of the treatments; perception of pain and attitudes toward suffering, death, and dying; patterns of decision making; and patterns of family communication used to cope with the entire experience (Gordon, 1990; Long & Long, 1982). Only one study has been conducted to explore the impact of cancer on an Asian Pacific American cancer patient population (Kagawa-Singer, 1988). This study supports the premise that culture frames the entire cancer experience, from the threat posed by the cancer to the problems created by the disease for the patient and family, and finally to the means used by the patients and their social networks to cope with the disease and its treatments. More research attention must be aimed toward exploration of the ramifications of cultural indicators in order to develop intervention programs that will effectively enhance the outcomes for prevention, early detection, and treatment of cancer.

Classification of Cultural Factors Affecting Cancer Control

Cultural factors affecting cancer control can be classified into two categories: structural and conceptual. Each of these two categories can be further classified into those that inhibit and those that facilitate cancer control.

Structural factors, such as accessibility of care, affordability of care, and whether or not the signs and symptoms of cancer and the treatments prescribed by a physician are understandable to the individual and family, affect all individuals faced with cancer. Specific examples of structural factors affecting Asian Pacific American individuals of limited acculturation are whether or not health care providers of the same ethnic group are available, whether or not patients understand spoken and written English, whether or not health education materials are available in the appropriate language or at the appropriate literacy level, whether or not respectful communication and behavior are displayed by providers, and whether or not providers have sufficient knowledge of the culture to provide appropriate care. The last two factors overlap with the second category: conceptual issues.

Conceptual issues include the specific knowledge, attitudes, beliefs, and values of a particular ethnic group toward cancer in general and, specifically, toward preventive health care practices, early cancer detection procedures, and the various cancer treatment options. We cannot describe these factors here for each of the 60 Asian Pacific American groups (partly because they are not known). However, these factors are important determinants of whether or not cancer control efforts will be considered appropriate, desirable, or relevant by a particular population. Understanding the conceptual issues for each ethnic group is essential for planning effective cancer control programs.

However, we cannot wait until studies are conducted to describe the specific beliefs and behaviors about cancer for the major Asian Pacific American groups before we provide care. It is possible to deliver health care now using current knowledge about these groups. Many ethnic community clinics, for example, have developed successful methods for addressing many of the structural barriers listed above. To provide easier access, clinics are physically located within the communities they serve. Care is made more affordable through income-dependent, sliding fee scales for those patients without health insurance. Finally, these clinics utilize health care staff who speak the language and understand the culture of the patient. When bilingual providers are unavailable, highly trained translators are utilized. Greater ethnic specificity in the planning and delivery of health care services will be possible as information becomes available from evaluations of intervention and treatment programs tailored to particular ethnic groups.

In the meantime, it is known that cancer has a very negative connotation in Asian Pacific American communities, as it does in every other culture. Although it is commonly believed that Asian families are a strong source of support in a positive sense, these same cultural norms can also function to isolate the patient and family from support available from outside the family. Whether this is adaptive or maladaptive, however, depends upon whether or not the patient and family can meet their desired needs optimally through the traditional norms of beliefs and behaviors. We will discuss the ramifications of this possible behavior below.

To design effective interventions, we must know the beliefs about the causes of cancer for the major Asian Pacific American groups. Beliefs about etiology determine beliefs about appropriate interventions for the disease. For example, cancer is felt by some to be caused by hereditary defects. In more traditional families, such a belief can cause the offspring in families with a cancer history to be viewed as less marriageable. Others believe that cancer is a punishment for transgressions in this life or in past lives. This belief can result in shunning of the cancer patient by the community. Both beliefs may result in reluctance to make a cancer diagnosis in a family member known to the community.

Most Japanese and Chinese American patients interviewed by Kagawa-Singer (1988) felt that their cancer was a result of *karma*, caused by lifestyle choices made in the past, such as imprudent diets or smoking. Their response to these self-inflicted cancers was one of acceptance, and their efforts were directed toward doing all they could to rid themselves of the disease so they would not be a burden on their families. Among study subjects, compliance with the prescribed treatment regimen was extremely high (greater than 95%).

Social support is another important area of study in cancer care. American patients appear to utilize support from a wide network of friends and professional services. Asian Pacific American patients seem to use much smaller networks of support, mainly immediate family and possibly one or two very close friends (Kagawa-Singer, 1988, 1993). Community members who are not part of the significant social network of the patient and family can be reticent to offer assistance because, for instance, as noted above, the patient and family may be felt to have brought on their own suffering. Asian

Pacific Americans are also reluctant to enter where they are not invited. Individuals and families are socialized to take care of such private matters by themselves and to bear the consequences alone. Thus community members may be reluctant to offer help when it is not asked for. Community members may fear insulting the patient and family by intimating that the family is not capable of enduring this hardship on its own. This practice may be functional in the native country or in traditional enclaves where family networks are relatively cohesive, but it may become dysfunctional in American society, where the extended family is not always in geographic proximity and economic and social norms encourage women to work outside the home. Traditionally, women are the caretakers of the sick. If a woman is working, she is torn between a career (or possible loss of her job and health insurance coverage) and familial obligations. She may also become a target for community derision because she does not fulfill her culturally expected roles of caretaker and nurturer.

Much of Western cancer psychosocial support efforts aim to encourage the individual to be self-sufficient and autonomous in his or her decision making, even when in the sick role. However, such efforts may create distress in Asian Pacific Americans, rather than reduce it as intended. Self-sufficiency and autonomy are values that are diametrically opposed to the Asian Pacific cultural ethos of group identity, dependency, and consensus modes of decision making (Kagawa-Singer, 1988). Efforts to promote more individualistic values can create discomfort in Asian Pacific Americans and raise barriers to health education and treatment. The Western duality of mind and body is also an unfamiliar concept to most Asian Pacific Americans, whose concept of the individual is more integrated and interdependent. Cancer control efforts are often implicitly designed to address one or the other of the duality, and the resultant message is either incomprehensible or irrelevant to Asian Pacific Americans.

We will now examine whether certain Asian Pacific structural or conceptual factors may help to explain the poorer 5-year relative survival rates discussed above. Access to health care is a structural issue. Many Asian Pacific American groups have less access to health care services in general and cancer screening services in particular, and thus may be diagnosed at later stages, when the possibility of survival and cure is lower. Beliefs about cancer etiology may cause those Asian Pacific Americans who discover cancer themselves to delay seeking diagnosis and treatment from a physician or, once diagnosed, to be less likely to adhere to treatment protocols. Beliefs that cancer is a form of retribution (Ito, 1982) or other punishment for past transgressions can make them reluctant to seek treatment publicly. This reluctance may account for the late stage at diagnosis for cervical cancer among Japanese, Chinese, Vietnamese, Filipino, and Korean women in California, as shown in Figure 4.1.

Asian Pacific American patients may also first seek alternative, indigenous healers as the first line of treatment or as parallel services. For example, investigators have reported the case of a Cambodian family whose adolescent son developed brain cancer (Eisenbruch & Handelman, 1990). Believing that the tumor was caused by bad karma, the parents requested that two Buddhist monks conduct a ceremony in their home to increase their son's merit and thereby improve his karma and prognosis. At the same time, however, the boy was taken to a nearby hospital for surgery and radiation therapy. Some of the techniques used by alternative practitioners may be helpful; some may not. Little research has been done in the area of alternative medications and treatments (U.S. Congress, 1990).

There may also be a higher prevalence of cell types with poorer prognosis for some tumors among some Asian Pacific ethnicities, and responses to treatment regimens may differ because of basic biological differences in pharmacokinetics and pharmacodynamics. No research has yet been conducted to test differential response to cancer chemotherapeutic agents, yet there is a growing awareness of clinical reports of greater sensitivity to medications by Asian and Pacific Islanders (Kalow, 1989; Lin & Findler, 1983; Singer, 1992; Zhou, Koshakji, Silberstein, Wilkinson, & Wood, 1989). It is apparent that further research is needed to explore these differences.

Summary and Implications

Asian Pacific American populations now constitute a significant segment of the U.S. population. Heretofore, little attention has been given to the study of the burden of cancer on these populations. The numbers of Asian Pacific American individuals in most studies have been too small to be statistically significant as a separate group. Thus they have often been aggregated within a category labeled "other," and their visibility lost. When cancer data have been obtained for Asian Pacific Americans as an aggregate group, cancer incidence and mortality rates have been found to be lower when compared with white rates. When the data are separated by ethnic group and anatomic site, however, the cancer incidence and mortality rates at many sites are higher than rates among the white population. Although Asian Pacific Americans suffer from the enormity of the cancer experience—as do all other groups in the United States—they have fewer support services.

Asian Pacific Americans have not been targeted as an underserved group for two reasons: the illusion created by the aggregate data that these groups are not at risk, and the erroneous belief that they are capable of taking care of their own and therefore do not need social service assistance. To understand adequately the problem of cancer among Asian Pacific Americans and to plan effective intervention programs, it is first essential to have accurate disaggregated data on each ethnic group. Aggregated data are inadequate, because they mask important variations in rates and risk factors within and between particular Asian Pacific subgroups. Next, data are needed for each group on the cultural values, knowledge, attitudes, beliefs, and behaviors that may facilitate or pose special barriers to access to high-quality cancer care.

Specific cancer control efforts can be instituted immediately. For primary prevention, certain groups within the Asian Pacific American population are at high risk and should be targeted for screening and early detection programs. These groups offer enormous opportunities for cancer control. For example, within a generation, effective hepatitis B immunoprophylaxis programs directed at Asian Pacific American groups could reduce liver cancer from its position as one of the most common cancer killers of Asian Pacific Americans to the relatively rare form of cancer it is among whites. The current levels of cigarette smoking, especially among some male Asian Pacific American groups, portend an epidemic of lung cancer and other tobacco-related cancers in the future. It is essential, therefore, to direct culturally appropriate smoking prevention and cessation programs toward these communities. In addition, it would be wise to encourage immigrant Asian Pacific American communities to maintain their traditional low-fat dietary practices and to refrain from adopting American high-fat dietary habits.

Research shows that the etiology of cancer is multifactorial; the environment, viruses, genetic makeup, and diet and other lifestyle habits are all involved. As Asian Pacific Americans acculturate and adopt the diet and behaviors of mainstream Americans with successive generations, their epidemiological profile grows more similar to that of whites and less similar to that of their counterparts living in their native countries.

Migration studies that focus on those Asian Pacific American groups whose cancer rates are lower than those among whites could yield useful information about the etiology and control of cancer. The information obtained from these studies would benefit the American population as a whole and move us toward achieving the objective of halving the mortality rate associated with this disease by the year 2000.

Secondary prevention strategies should target Asian Pacific American communities to improve access to and utilization of cancer screening services. The public health impact of cervical cancer, which appears to be proportionally higher among some Asian Pacific American groups than among whites, could be greatly reduced through regular Papanicolaou testing. Mortality rates for breast and colon cancers, which are rising rapidly among some Asian Pacific American groups, could be reduced through early detection and screening. Practitioners also need to be alert to the signs and symptoms of cancers of the nasopharynx, esophagus, pancreas, liver, and stomach, which, although relatively rare in the white population, are more common among the various Asian Pacific American ethnic groups.

In designing primary and secondary cancer prevention programs for Asian Pacific American communities, it is important to bear in mind that each community is culturally and linguistically different from the others. To plan an effective program, therefore, it is important that we gather information from each targeted group about the cultural values, knowledge, and attitudes that may enable or pose special barriers to behavioral change and utilization of health care services.

For communities with recent immigrants, programs must be carried out in their language. Education and screening programs should be conducted in each ethnic community with bilingual, bicultural staff. Educational materials should be produced in the patients' language and at an appropriate level of literacy (Jones & Kay, 1992; Michielutte, Bahnson, & Beal, 1990). Health education materials that have been directly translated from English into an Asian language are usually ineffective. Instead, materials must be developed that contain the necessary information but that are framed and presented in a manner that is culturally sensitive to the target population.

Cultural beliefs and behaviors significantly affect how individuals meet adversity. Practitioners and researchers interested in understanding the burden of cancer on Asian Pacific American populations must know the nature of the threat posed by cancer, the cultural modes of communication for the patient and family with health care practitioners, the significant roles the patient holds in his or her life, and how the cancer interferes with fulfillment of these roles.

Finally, those who develop interventions must understand health beliefs and practices within the cultural contexts in which they have meaning. The fabric woven of these beliefs and behaviors provides strength and security to its members. Single beliefs and practices lose their meaning when taken out of context, and programmatic efforts to reduce the negative impact of cancer will not have their intended effect unless program designers understand and work within the cultural context as an equally valid interpretation of experience.

Administrators, educators, and practitioners now have the infrastructure available to support research and the delivery of cancer control programs of high quality for Asian Pacific Americans. Since 1980 the U.S. Bureau of the Census has used multiple identifiers for the Asian Pacific American population, enabling us to find the target populations. The U.S. government has funded two national agencies to study mental and physical health and treatment outcomes in the Asian Pacific American population. A national organization, the Asian and Pacific Islander American Health Forum, collects the available information and disseminates it to researchers and legislators. And several consortia of community clinics have developed models of culturally appropriate health care services for Asian Pacific American populations. Efforts must now be made to use the integrated view of culturally congruent care to implement effective programs and research to reduce cancer morbidity and mortality for Asian Pacific American cancer patients. The alternative is unacceptable.

References

Anderson, D. E. (1972). A genetic study of human breast cancer. *Journal of the National Cancer Institute, 48,* 1029.

Armstrong, B., & Doll, R. (1975). Environmental factors and cancer incidence and mortality in different countries with special reference to dietary practices. *International Journal of Cancer, 15*, 617-631.

Beasley, R. P., & Hwang, L. Y. (1984). Hepatocellular carcinoma and hepatitis B virus. *Seminars in Liver Diseases, 4*, 13-121.

Bonacini, M., & Valenzuela, J. E. (1991). Changes in the relative frequency of gastric adenocarcinoma in Southern California. *Western Journal of Medicine, 154*, 172-174.

Brown, M. L., Potosky, A. L., Thompson, G. B., & Kessler, L. G. (1990). The knowledge and use of screening tests for colorectal and prostate cancer: Data from the 1987 National Health Interview Survey. *Preventive Medicine, 19*, 562-574.

California Department of Health Services. (1990). [Unpublished data from the California Behavioral Risk Factor Survey].

Centers for Disease Control. (1991). Hepatitis B virus: A comprehensive strategy for eliminating transmission in the United States through universal childhood vaccination. *Morbidity and Mortality Weekly Report, 40*, 1-25.

Centers for Disease Control. (1992a). Behavioral risk factor survey of Chinese: California, 1989. *Morbidity and Mortality Weekly Report, 41*, 266-270.

Centers for Disease Control. (1992b). Behavioral risk factor survey of Vietnamese: California, 1992. *Morbidity and Mortality Weekly Report, 41*, 69-72.

Centers for Disease Control. (1992c). Cigarette smoking among Chinese, Vietnamese, and Hispanics: California 1989-1991. *Morbidity and Mortality Weekly Report, 41*, 362-387.

Desmond, S. (1987). Diet and cancer: Should we change what we eat? Medical Staff Conference, University of California, San Francisco. *Western Journal of Medicine, 146*, 73-78.

DeVita, V. T., Jr., Hellman, S., & Rosenberg, S. A. (Eds.). (1989). *Cancer: Principles and practice of oncology* (3rd ed.). Philadelphia: J. B. Lippincott.

Draper, G. J., Heaf, M. M., & Kennier-Wilson, L. M. (1977). Occurrence of childhood cancers among sibs and estimation of familial risks. *Journal of Medical Genetics, 14*, 81-90.

Eisenbruch, M., & Handelman, L. (1990). Cultural consultation for cancer: Astrocytoma in a Cambodian adolescent. *Social Science and Medicine, 31*, 1295-1299.

Fraumeni, J. F., Jr., Hoover, R. N., Devesa, S. S., & Kinlen, L. J. (1989). Epidemiology of cancer. In T. DeVita, Jr., S. Hellman, & S. A. Rosenberg (Eds.), *Cancer: Principles and practice of oncology* (3rd ed., pp. 196-235). Philadelphia: J. B. Lippincott.

Freeman, H. P. (1989). Cancer in the economically disadvantaged. *Cancer, 64*(Suppl.), 324-334.

Goodman, M. J., Gilbert, F. I., Jr., & Low, G. (1984). Screening for breast cancer in Hawaii: Further implications. *Hawaii Medical Journal, 43*, 356-360.

Goodwin, P. J., & Boyd, N. F. (1987). Critical appraisal of the evidence that dietary fat intake is related to breast cancer risk in humans. *Journal of the National Cancer Institute, 79*, 473.

Gordon, D. R. (1990). Embodying illness, embodying cancer. *Culture, Medicine and Psychiatry, 14*, 275-297.

Greenwald, P., & Sondik, E. J. (1986). *Cancer control objectives for the nation: 1986-2000* (NIH Publication No. 86-2880). Washington, DC: Government Printing Office.

Haenzel, W. (1982). Migrant studies. In D. Schottenfeld & J. F. Fraumeni, Jr. (Eds.), *Cancer epidemiology and prevention* (pp. 194-207). Philadelphia: W. B. Saunders.

Hammer, M. (1992, October 5). Hepatitis B vaccination off to a slow start. *Nurseweek*, 5(24), 1, 8.

Han, E. E. S., Kim, S. H., Lee, M. S., Miller, J. S. K., Rhee, S., Song, H., & Yu, E. Y. (1989). *Korean Health Survey: A preliminary report*. Los Angeles: Korean Health Education, Information and Referral Center.

Harris, J. R., Lippman, M. E., Veronesi, U., & Willett, W. (1992). Breast cancer. *New England Journal of Medicine*, 327, 219-328.

Heckler, M. M. (1985). *Report of the Secretary's Task Force on Black and Minority Health: Vol. 1. Executive summary*. Washington, DC: U.S. Department of Health and Human Services.

Horm, J. W., Devesa, S. S., & Burhansstipanov, L. (in press). Cancer incidence, survival and mortality among racial and ethnic minority groups in the United States. In D. Schottenfeld & J. F. Fraumeni, Jr. (Eds.), *Cancer epidemiology and prevention*. New York: Oxford University Press.

Howson, C. P., Hiyama, T., & Wynder, E. L. (1986). Decline of gastric cancer: Epidemiology of an unplanned triumph. *Epidemiology Review, 8*, 1-27.

Ito, K. (1982). Illness as retribution. *Culture, Medicine and Psychiatry, 6*, 385-403.

Jang, M., (1991). [Preliminary data]. San Francisco: Asian and Pacific Islander American Health Forum.

Jenkins, C. N. H., McPhee, S. J., Bird, J. A., & Bonilla, N.-T. (1990). Cancer risks and prevention behaviors among Vietnamese refugees. *Western Journal of Medicine, 153*, 34-39.

Jones, E. G., & Kay, M. (1992). Instrumentation in cross cultural research. *Nursing Research, 41*(3), 186-188.

Jones, L. (1990, August 24). Breast cancer test surveyor encouraged. *Los Angeles Times*, p. B4.

Kagawa-Singer, M. (1988). *Bamboo and oak: Differences in adaptation to cancer by Japanese-American and Anglo-American cancer patients*. Unpublished doctoral dissertation, University of California, Los Angeles.

Kagawa-Singer, M. (1993). *A review of the cross-cultural literature on psychosocial cancer care*. Unpublished manuscript.

Kalow, W. (1989). Race and therapeutic drug response [Editorial]. *New England Journal of Medicine, 320*, 588-590.

Kitano, H. H. L. (1990). Values, beliefs, and practices of the Asian-American elderly: Implications for geriatric education. In M. S. Harper (Ed.), *Minority aging: Essential curricula content for selected health and allied health professions* (DHHS Publication No. HRS P-DV-90-4) (pp. 341-348). Washington, DC: Government Printing Office.

Kleinman, A. (1980). *Patients and healers in the context of culture*. Berkeley: University of California Press.

Klontz, K. C. (1986, May 23). Analysis of a program for the prevention of perinatal hepatitis B. *California Morbidity*, p. 20.

Lam, N. S. (1986). Geographical patterns of cancer mortality in China. *Social Science and Medicine, 23*, 241-247.

Leads in oesophageal cancer [Editorial]. (1974). *Lancet, 2*, 504.

Levin, B. L. (1985). *Cigarette smoking habits and characteristics in the Laotian refugee: a Perspective pre- and post-resettlement*. Paper presented at the Refugee Health Conference, San Diego, CA.

Lin, K. M., & Finder, E. (1983). Neuroleptic dosage for Asians. *American Journal of Psychiatry, 140*, 490-491.

Long, S., & Long, B. D. (1982). Curable cancer and fatal ulcers: Attitudes toward cancer in Japan. *Social Science and Medicine, 16,* 2101-2108.

Marr, D. G. (1987). Vietnamese attitudes regarding illness and healing. In N. G. Owen (Ed.), *Death and disease in Southeast Asia: Explorations in social, medical and demographic history* (pp. 162-186). Singapore: Oxford University Press.

Mettlin, C. (1992). Research in cancer prevention and detection. *Current Issues in Cancer Nursing Practice Updates, 1*(4), 1-10.

Mettlin, C., & Dodd, G. D. (1991). The American Cancer Society guidelines for the cancer-related checkup: An update. *Cancer, 41,* 279-282.

Michielutte, R., Bahnson, B. S., & Beal, P. (1990). Readability of the public education literature on cancer prevention and detection. *Journal of Cancer Education, 5,* 55-61.

Modan, B. (1974). Role of ethnic background in cancer development. *Israeli Journal of Medical Science, 74,* 1112-1116.

Muecke, M. A. (1983). Caring for Southeast Asian refugee patients in the USA. *American Journal of Public Health, 73,* 431-438.

Muir, C., Waterhouse, J., Mack, T., Shanmugaratnam, K., & Powell, J. (1987). *Cancer incidence in five continents* (Vol. 5). Lyon: International Agency for Research on Cancer.

National Cancer Institute. (1987). *Working guidelines for early cancer detection: Rationale and supporting evidence to decrease mortality* (Monograph, Division of Cancer Prevention and Control, Early Detection Branch). Washington, DC: Author.

National Center for Health Statistics. (1991). *Health, United States, 1990* (DHHS Publication No. PHS 91-1232). Hyattsville, MD: Author.

National Heart, Lung and Blood Institute. (1991, July). *Infomemo.* Bethesda, MD: Public Health Service.

Nomura, A., Stemmermann, G. N., Chyou, P. H., Kato, I., Perez-Perez, G. I., & Blaser, M. J. (1991). Helicobacter pylori infection and gastric carcinoma among Japanese Americans in Hawaii. *New England Journal of Medicine, 325,* 1132-1136.

Page, H. S., & Asire, A. J. (1985). *Cancer rates and risks* (NIH Publication No. 85-691). Washington, DC: Government Printing Office.

Rimpela, A. H., & Pukkala, E. I. (1987). Cancer of affluence: Positive social class gradient and rising incidence trend in some cancer forms. *Social Science and Medicine, 24,* 601-606.

Rumbaut, R. G. (1989). Portraits, patterns, and predictors of the refugee adaptation process: Results and reflections from the IHARP panel study. In D. W. Haines (Ed.), *Refugees as immigrants: Cambodians, Laotians, and Vietnamese in America.* Totowa, NJ: Rowman & Littlefield.

Schottenfeld, D., & Fraumeni, J. F., Jr. (Eds.). (1991). *Cancer epidemiology and prevention.* Philadelphia: W. B. Saunders.

Seiffert, J. E., Price, W. T., & Gordon, B. (1990). The California tumor registry: A state-of-the-art model for a regionalized, automated, population-based registry. *Topics in Health Record Management, 11,* 59-73.

Shimizu, H., Ross, R. K., Bernstein, L., Yatani, R., Henderson, B. E., & Mack, T. M. (1991). Cancers of the prostate and breast among Japanese and white immigrants in Los Angeles County. *British Journal of Cancer, 63,* 963-966.

Singer, P. A. (1992). Will postpartum recurrence of Grave's hyperthyroidism become a thing of the past? [Editorial]. *Journal of Clinical Endocrinology and Metabolism, 75*(1), 5A-5B.

Sontag, S. (1977). *Illness as metaphor.* New York: Random House.

Tash, E., Chung, C. S., & Yasunobu, C. (1988). *Hawaii's health risk behaviors, 1987.* Honolulu: Hawaii State Department of Health, Health Promotion and Education Branch.

Thomas, D. B. (1979). Epidemiologic studies of cancer in minority groups in the western United States. *National Cancer Institute Monographs, 53,* 103-113.

U.S. Bureau of the Census. (1991, June 12). [Press release CB91-215].

U.S. Congress, Office of Technology Assessment. (1990). *Unconventional cancer treatments* (Publication No. OTA-H-405). Washington, DC: Government Printing Office.

Weisburger, J. H. (1991). Causes, relevant mechanisms, and prevention of large bowel cancer. *Seminars in Oncology, 18,* 316-336.

Weisburger, J. H., & Horn, C. L. (1991). The causes of cancer. In A. I. Holleb, D. J. Fink, & G. P. Murphy (Eds.), *Clinical oncology* (pp. 80-98). Atlanta, GA: American Cancer Society.

Wirthlin Group. (1992, January). *Breast cancer survey for the American Cancer Society.* Paper presented at the National Breast Summit.

Young, J. L., Ries, L. G., & Pollack, E. S. (1984). Cancer patient survival among ethnic groups in the United States. *Journal of the National Cancer Institute, 43,* 341-351.

Yu, H. E., Randall, E. H., Gao, Y.-T., Gao, R., & Wynder, E. L. (1991). Comparative epidemiology of cancers of the colon, rectum, prostate and breast in Shanghai, China versus the United States. *International Journal of Epidemiology, 20,* 76-81.

Zhou, H.-H., Koshakji, R. P., Silberstein, D. J., Wilkinson, G. R., & Wood, A. J. J. (1989). Racial differences in drug response: Altered sensitivity to clearance of propranolol in men of Chinese descent as compared with American whites. *New England Journal of Medicine, 320,* 365-370.

5

Hepatitis B

HIE-WON LEE HANN

With the recent identification of the previously elusive non-A, non-B transfusion-associated hepatitis virus, hepatitis C (Choo et al., 1989; Kuo et al., 1989), there are now five classical hepatitis viruses, designated A, B, C, D, and E. Hepatitis B virus (HBV) is perhaps the most thoroughly studied virus with regard to epidemiology, pathogenesis, transmission, and preventive measures. Of the five hepatitis viruses, HBV is the only DNA virus; the rest are RNA viruses. Hepatitis A and E appear in epidemic form and spread mainly through fecal-oral routes (Ramalingaswami & Purcell, 1988). Hepatitis B, C, and D appear sporadic or endemic in form and are transmitted mainly via blood-borne routes. Hepatitis D virus (HDV) is a defective RNA agent, capable of replicating and surviving only in the presence of Hepatitis B surface antigen (Rizzetto et al., 1982). HDV may coinfect with HBV or superinfect a chronic HBV carrier.

HBV has strong implications for Asian Pacific Americans. Indeed, the virus is responsible for a majority of hepatocellular carcinoma (HCC) and for a significant portion of chronic liver disease such as chronic active hepatitis and cirrhosis among Asians (Beasley, 1988; Hann, Kim, London, Whitford, & Blumberg, 1982). HBV is distributed worldwide and perpetuated among humans through a large reservoir of chronic carriers. More than 200 million persons around the world, 5% of the entire population, are chronically infected with HBV (i.e., are HBV carriers) (Zuckerman, 1983). However, the distribution of HBV carriers is skewed; 75% of these 200 million carriers live in Asia.

Since the discovery of HBV surface antigen (HBsAg) in 1965 by Blumberg, Alter, and Visnich (1965), subsequent studies have demonstrated that chronic infection with HBV may lead to the development of chronic hepatitis (chronic persistent and chronic active), postnecrotic cirrhosis, and HCC. There is a striking epidemiological correlation between the incidence of HCC and the prevalence of chronic HBV carrier state. Globally, HBV is probably responsible for 75% to 95% of HCC (Beasley, 1988). HCC is rare in the United States and Western Europe, but it is one of the leading cancers in the world, perhaps the most common cancer (Beasley, 1988). HCC is the most prevalent malignant neoplasm in much of Asia, especially China, and sub-Saharan Africa (Beasley, 1988; Zuckerman, 1983). In Taiwan, HCC is the most common malignant neoplasm, accounting for 20% of all cancers and is the second leading cause of death (Beasley, Lin, Hwang, & Chien, 1981). In China alone, approximately 100,000 people die every year from HCC in a population of 850 million (Li & Shiang, 1980). According to a 1988 report of the Korean Ministry of Health, HCC is the second most common malignancy, next to stomach cancer, in Korea, and liver cirrhosis is the leading cause of death for males over 40 years of age. Similarly high death rates from HCC have been observed among the black population of Africa. Half of the world's population lives in areas of high incidence for HCC. Worldwide, more than 250,000 persons per year succumb to HBsAg(+) HCC (Cook-Mozafferi & Van Rensburg, 1984; Szmuness, 1978; Zuckerman, 1983).

Studies have shown that about 90% of infected individuals develop antibodies against HBsAg (anti-HBs) and become protected from infection by HBV. The other 5% to 10% of infected persons remain chronically infected with the virus. Those who have persistent HBsAg in their blood (for more than six months) are termed *chronic carriers* and become the source of infection of other individuals who do not have immunity against HBV.

However, if HBV transmission occurs during the perinatal period, up to 90% of infected infants will remain chronic carriers of HBV (Rizzetto et al., 1982; Stevens, Beasley, Tsui, & Lee, 1975). Indeed, more than 40% of chronic carriers in Korea are infected at birth through maternal transmission. Also, surveys have shown that 90% of HBV carriers in Taiwan are infected during childhood, approximately half by their mothers at birth (Beasley et al., 1982; Stevens et al., 1975).

Many newborns infected neonatally who become chronic HBV carriers may develop chronic hepatitis B, cirrhosis, and HCC later in life. A prospective study in Taiwan of 18 asymptomatic HBsAg carrier children of 4 to 9 years of age showed evidence that some pathologic changes of the liver following perinatal infection started early (Chang, Hwang, Hsu, Lee, & Beasley, 1988). These changes included either mild nonspecific histologic changes (mild mononuclear cell infiltration in the portal tracts), which were seen in 15 of the children, or chronic persistent hepatitis, which was observed in 3 of the children. Shiraki, Yoshihara, Kawana, Yasui, and Sakurai (1977) reported histologic observations in two young children (ages 15 and 28 months old) born to HBV carrier mothers with abnormal serum biochemical tests. They found mild portal fibrosis with lymphocytic infiltration in one child and mild infiltration with minimal fibrosis in portal tracts in the other child. Furthermore, Maggiore, DeGiacomo, Marzani, Sessa, and Scotta (1983) described 11 infants with abnormal liver biochemical tests owing to HBV infection; although 8 of the 11 were born to asymptomatic HBV carrier mothers, 5 of the 11 had chronic persistent hepatitis, 5 chronic active hepatitis (2 with cirrhosis), and 1 chronic lobular hepatitis. On the other hand, Piccinino, Sagnelli, Manzillo, and Pasquale (1977) report the histologic findings on 20 HBV carrier children: normal liver in 6, nonspecific lesions in 6 and minimal granuloma in 1, minimal hepatitis in 5, and resolving hepatitis in 2. Whether these children were infected perinatally or during childhood was unknown.

In the United States alone, there are more than 200,000 cases of new HBV infection annually; of these, 12,000 to 20,000 become chronic HBV carriers each year (Advisory Committee on Immunization Practices, 1985). Furthermore, with the large wave of immigration from Asia, the newly arriving Asians have brought with them their high HBV carrier rate (5% to 20% compared with 0.2% in the United States) and the increased risk of chronic liver disease and HCC.

Characteristics of Hepatitis B Virus

Hepatitis B virus is a 42 nm (in diameter) double-stranded DNA virus belonging to the hepadna virus (hepatotropic DNA virus) family, which includes similar viruses that infect woodchucks, squirrels, and ducks (Marion, Oshiro, Renergy, Scullard, & Robinson, 1980; Mason, Seal, & Summers, 1980; Summers, Smolec, & Snyder, 1978). The intact

Table 5.1 Antigen and Antibody System of HBV

Antigen	Antibody
Hepatitis B surface antigen (HBsAg)	Antibody to HBsAg (anti-HBs)[a]
Hepatitis B core antigen (HBcAg)	Antibody to HBcAg (anti-HBc)
Hepatitis B e Antigen (HBeAg)	Antibody to HBeAg (anti-HBe)

NOTE: a. Protective antibody.

virus, referred to as the Dane particle, has an outer coat component of hepatitis B surface antigen and an inner core component of hepatitis B core antigen (HBcAg) (Almeida, Rubenstein, & Scott, 1971; Blumberg et al., 1965; Dane, Cameron, & Briggs, 1970). During hepatitis B infection, a breakdown product of core, hepatitis B e antigen (HBeAg) circulates in the blood and signifies viral replication in the liver and a relatively increased state of infectivity (Magnius & Epsmark, 1972; Yoshizawa, Machida, Miyakawa, & Mayumi, 1979).

The hepatitis B viral genome is approximately 3,200 base pairs in length, is partially double-stranded, and uses a retroviral method of replication (Summers & Mason, 1982). The viral genome contains genes that code for HBsAg, HBcAg, and DNA polymerase. In addition, there are pre-S regions that code for proteins thought to be involved in the process of viral attachment to the hepatocytes during infection. An additional X gene codes for a protein whose function has not been fully defined (Tiollais, Charnay, & Vyas 1981; Tiollais, Pourcel, & Dejean, 1985; Tiollais & Wain-Hopson, 1984). The antigen and antibody systems are shown in the Table 5.1.

HBsAg. This antigen is the marker that indicates the presence of the HBV. It is detected in the serum during both acute and chronic infection with the virus. This antigen circulates not only as the surface component of the whole virus but also as isolated particles containing only surface antigen shaped as 20 nm spheres and tubules (20 nm in width, with variable length). HBsAg is made in excess of the whole virus and thus readily detected in the serum of the infected person; it is the most important marker for HBV infection.

HBcAg. This antigen is not found free in the serum. In most cases, it induces antibody response so effectively that the antibody (anti-HBc) is usually detected in the serum.

HBeAg. This is a soluble protein, probably a subcomponent of core antigen (HBcAg) (Yoshizawa et al., 1979) and found only in HBsAg positive serum. HBeAg in the serum generally indicates the presence of high levels of virus, DNA polymerase activity, intact whole virus, Dane particles, and suggests high infectivity.

Anti-HBs. This is the protective antibody. If a person acquires anti-HBs through natural infection, anti-HBc is also present. If a person develops antibodies after hepatitis B vaccine that contain only HBsAg, anti-HBs alone is present in the serum.

Anti-HBc. This antibody indicates past or present infection with HBV. It is not a protective antibody. Anti-HBc is almost always present with HBsAg (especially in chronic carriers) and also appears with anti-HBs in the serum of individuals who have recovered from natural infection.

   Anti-HBc may appear alone without HBsAg or anti-HBs in a few different situations: (a) during the immediate recovery stage from HBV infection, the so-called window period, at which time anti-HBc is in the form of IgM and anti-HBs will soon appear in the serum of the patient, (b) long after HBV infection, (c) in the low carrier state, or (d) after exposure to the virus with incomplete immune response. These individuals produce anti-HBs, although generally of lower titer than those without anti-HBc, after hepatitis B vaccination (Hann, Stahlhut, et al., 1989; Hann, Stahlhut, & Maddrey, in press).

Anti-HBe. This antibody is not protective either. Anti-HBe appears after HBeAg disappears, and this conversion indicates decrease of viral concentration, DNA polymerase, and infectivity. Anti-HBe is present in the serum with either HBsAg or anti-HBs. The conversion from HBeAg to anti-HBe takes place at the height of clinical illness in the case of acute symptomatic forms with biochemical evidence of hepatitis. The conversion is a favorable prognostic sign that may suggest the resolution of clinical illness and viral infection. However, in chronic carriers, the conversion takes place with or without symptoms and/or biochemical change, and the presence of anti-HBe with HBsAg indicates a late stage of HBV carrier status. Table 5.2 shows the serological markers of HBV infection frequently seen in Asian Americans and the interpretations.

Table 5.2 Serological Markers of HBV Infection and the Interpretations

	HBsAg	Anti-HBs	Anti-HBc[a]	HBeAg	Anti-HBe	Interpretation
1	+	−	+	+	−	chronic carrier of relatively shorter duration, frequently seen in relatively younger people
2	+	−	+	−	+	chronic carrier of relatively longer duration, frequently seen in relatively older people
3	+	+	+	−	−	still called a carrier
4	−	+	+	−	+	natural immunity
	−	+	+	−	−	natural immunity
5	−	+	−	−	−	immunity after HBV vaccination
6	−	−	+	−	−	(a) long after HBV infection; (b) immediate recovery from HBV infection, usually this time, IgM-anti-HBc, so-called window period; (c) "low carrier" state; (d) exposure to the virus, but incomplete immune response (can be vaccinated; they produce anti-HBs, but in general lower titer than those negative for anti-HBc)

NOTES: a. IgG-Anti-HBc. b. Hann et al., 1989; Hann, Stablhut, & Maddrey, 1991.

Host Responses to HBV Infection

Adults

When adults are exposed to HBV, they respond in one of three patterns: acute symptomatic hepatitis, self-limited and subclinical hepatitis B infection, or development of the chronic HBsAg carrier state (Hoofnagle, 1981) (see Table 5.3).

Table 5.3 Patterns of Host Responses to HBV Infection

Pattern	Incidence (%)
Acute symptomatic hepatitis	30-40
Self-limited, subclinical infection	50
Chronic carrier state	5-10[a]

NOTE: a. If infected at birth, nearly 90%.

Acute Symptomatic Hepatitis. Some 30% to 40% of people respond this way. Patients have jaundice, malaise, feverishness, nausea, and abdominal pain. Several weeks after exposure, HBsAg appears first in serum, followed by HBeAg, DNA polymerase, and HBV-DNA, indicating active viral replication in the liver. Anti-HBc also appears at this time, in IgM class (IgM anti-HBc). Within several weeks, HBeAg, DNA polymerase, and HBV-DNA will disappear. After clinical recovery, HBsAg disappears within several months, and anti-HBs appears. Anti-HBs is a long-lived antibody and is a useful marker of recovery and immunity. Anti-HBc also persists in serum but gradually changes into IgG class of anti-HBc, which remains indefinitely.

Self-Limited and Subclinical Hepatitis B Infection. This pattern of host response is seen in about 50% of adults exposed to HBV. They do not develop clinically apparent hepatitis but rather experience transient subclinical infections, having a silent seroconversion producing anti-HBs (Hoofnagle, Seeff, Bales, Gerety, & Tabor, 1978). HBsAg appears in low titer and for a brief period, perhaps 2 weeks, of antigenemia, followed by the appearance of anti-HBs. Anti-HBc and anti-HBe also appear and may last for a long time. Symptoms are mild, nonspecific, or absent. This pattern of host response is common and accounts for the presence of anti-HBs in the sera of people who do not recall histories of having clinical hepatitis.

Development of the Chronic HBsAg Carrier State. Some 5% to 10% of adults infected with hepatitis B virus become chronic carriers of HBV (remaining HBsAg[+] for more than 6 months). HBsAg develops during the late incubation period of the disease and persists for months or years, or for life. Anti-HBc appears soon afterward and persists with HBsAg. HBeAg appears with or shortly after the appearance of HBsAg, rises to high titer, and persists (Aikawa et al., 1987; Krugman et al., 1979). HBeAg persists in serum for variable amounts of time, ranging from a year to a decade or longer. HBeAg eventually disappears, followed by the appearance of anti-HBe.

Infants Born to Carrier Mothers

Depending on the mother's infectivity status, the transmission rate of HBV to the newborn varies. For infants born to HBeAg(+) mothers, the perinatal infection rate is 90% to 100%; for infants born to HBeAg(−) and anti-HBe(+) mothers, the infection rate is 10% to 20% (Beasley et al., 1983; Okada et al., 1976; Shiraki, Yoshihara, Sakurai, Eto, & Kawana, 1980; Stevens, Neurath, Beasley, & Szmuness, 1979). The risk for chronic infection is inversely related to age at HBV infection. Perinatal infection of newborns leads to an almost 90% carrier rate. For those who are infected during childhood, the chronic carrier rate ranges from 29% to 40% (Stevens et al., 1975).

The Hepatitis B Carrier State
and Hepatocellular Carcinoma

Chronic infection with HBV may lead to the development of chronic hepatitis (chronic persistent and chronic active), cirrhosis, and HCC. Of chronic HBsAg carriers, 40% of men and 15% to 20% of the women will die of long-term sequelae of HBV infection, such as chronic active hepatitis, cirrhosis, and HCC (Beasley, 1988; Beasley et al., 1981).

The causal association of HBV infection and HCC has been well documented by a large prospective study carried out in Taiwan by Beasley et al. (1983). They recruited 22,707 Taiwanese male government workers, ages 40 to 60 years, during the period 1975 to 1978 (Table 5.4). As of 1986, with an average follow-up of 8.9 years, there were 161 cases of HCC among these people, 152 from the 3,454 HBsAg(+) carriers and 9 from the 19,253 HBsAg(−) persons. Even those 9 patients were all anti-HBc(+); 7 were anti-HBs(+).

From a clinical viewpoint, persons with chronic infection with HBV, so-called chronic HBsAg carriers, can be divided into two groups: those with chronic liver disease, often referred to as having chronic hepatitis B, and those with no obvious liver disease, referred

Table 5.4 Prospective Study of Asymptomatic HBV Carriers and
              Controls: Taiwan

HBV Status at Recruitment	Population at Risk	HCC	HCC/ 100,000/year	Relative Risk
HBsAg(+)	3,454	152	494.5	98.4
HBsAg(−)	19,253	9	5.3	
Total	22,707	161	79.7	

SOURCES: Beasley et al. (1981), Beasley (1988).
NOTE: Entry to study, November 3, 1975 to June 30, 1978. Last follow-up, 1986 (average 8.9 years).

to as being asymptomatic or as in a "healthy" carrier state (Hoofnagle,
Shafritz, & Popper, 1987). However, even patients with chronic hepatitis B often do not have symptoms and are incidentally found to
have abnormal liver function and underlying liver disease during
investigations following the HBV screening that revealed their
HBsAg(+) status.

HCC is sometimes detected in persons who appear clinically
healthy, and the presence of preceding chronic HBV infection is
often not evident. However, more than 80% of HCC patients have
an underlying but silent cirrhosis (Beasley, 1988; Popper, Shafritz,
& Hoofnagle, 1987). It is likely that those with already ongoing
chronic liver disease carry a greater risk of developing HCC than
those who are "healthy" carriers. The pathway from the "healthy"
carrier state to chronic hepatitis, cirrhosis, or HCC is not established (Popper et al., 1987).

Popper et al. (1987) hypothesize that integration of HBV-DNA
into host chromosomes in acute or chronic hepatitis, or during the
"healthy" carrier state, corresponds to an initiation event similar to
that described in chemical carcinogenesis. This initiation itself may
not result in transformation or any significant histological alteration.
However, episodic necroinflammatory reactivation or superinfection may induce regeneration and cirrhosis, and, by stimulating
mitosis, these alterations may render the integrated viral DNA and
its flanking sequences susceptible to a molecular biologically demonstrated disarrangement. This last process can initiate transformation and progression to HCC. Such events are clinically reflected in
exacerbations seen in patients with persistent HBV infection (Popper
et al., 1987).

Table 5.5 Natural History of Chronic HBV Infection Acquired Neonatally

Phase	Clinical and Serological Features
1 (age ≤ 20 years) Replicative stage	mild unrecognized clinical illness minor histologic activity; HBV-DNA level high; HBeAg(+)
2 (age 20-40 years) Low replicative stage	remission and relapse chronic active hepatitis common; HBV-DNA level low; loss of HBeAg, 20-30%/year; anti-HBe(+), 15-20%/year
3 (age 40 years) Nonreplicative stage	clinical remission histologic activity subsides; HBV-DNA undetectable; anti-HBe(+); cirrhosis 2%/year; HCC 1%/year

Natural History of HBV Carriers

Age at HBV infection influences greatly the natural history of infected individuals. Studies have indicated that the majority of chronic HBV carriers among Asian Americans acquired infection at birth or during early childhood (Dienstag, 1982). The natural history of persons who acquired HBV infection neonatally is summarized from the prospective study of Liaw, Lin, Sheen, Chen, and Chu (1988) in Taiwan (see Table 5.5).

HBV Infection in Asian Americans

As of 1990, there were more than 6.5 million Asian Americans; by the year 2,000, they are expected to total 9.9 million, representing 4% of the U.S. population. According to the 1989 U.S. Census, the proportions of foreign-born (immigrant) Asian Americans in the six largest groups were 28% of Japanese, 63% of Chinese, 66% of Filipinos, 70% of Asian Indians, 82% of Koreans, and 91% of Vietnamese. Studies have shown that foreign-born Asian Americans have higher HBsAg carrier rates than those born in the United States (London, 1990). Although Asian Americans represent less than 3% of the total U.S. population at present, they contribute a significant number of carrier pools in the United States. Estimated prevalence rates of hepatitis B chronic carriers in selected populations

Table 5.6 Estimated Prevalence of Hepatitis B Chronic Carriers in
Selected Populations in the United States

Population	Prevalence (%)	Number of Chronic Carriers
Asian Americans	8-15	480,000
Alaskan Eskimos	14	6,720
Sub-Saharan Africans	6-14	4,400
Pacific Islanders	5-10	20,800
Haitians	7	6,510
Drug addicts, intravenous	7	52,500
Institutionalized for mental retardation	7	9,800
Medical personnel	1	23,000
CDC's highest-risk group	7	604,000
CDC's recommended screening group	4	755,000
U.S. population	0.2	1,000,000

SOURCE: Arevalo and Washington (1988). Data for Asian Americans, Alaskan Eskimos, sub-Saharan Africans, Pacific Islanders, Haitians, and U.S. population are adapted from 1980 U.S. Census data. Data for drug addicts, institutionalized persons, and medical personnel from Hoofnagle and Alter (1984). Data for CDC (Centers for Disease Control) groups from Advisory Committee on Immunization Practices (1984).

in the United States are shown in Table 5.6 (Arevalo & Washington, 1988).

HBV infection is a common problem in the Asian Pacific American population. Chronic HBV carrier rates from 5% to 15% have been reported in the Chinese, Korean, Filipino, Southeast Asian, and Pacific Islander American populations (Franks et al., 1989; Hann, London, McGlynn, & Blumberg, 1987; London, 1990; McGlynn, London, Hann, & Sharrar, 1986; Stevens et al., 1985; Szmuness et al., 1978). Perinatal transmission is the most common mode of HBV transmission. The remainder of carriers are infected during earlier childhood, and a lesser number during the teenage years. HBV test results of Asian Americans at different locations are summarized in Table 5.7.

Stevens et al. (1985) screened a large number of pregnant Asian American women for HBV (results are shown in Table 5.8). Approximately half of these HBsAg(+) mothers were also HBeAg(+). Perinatal transmission of the virus will occur in the majority of infants born to HBeAg(+) mothers. Therefore prevention of perinatal transmission is of utmost importance in the Asian American population.

Table 5.7 Estimates of HBsAg Prevalence in Selected Population of
Asian Americans

Population	HBsAg (%)	Source
Chinese men in New York City	9	Szmuness et al. (1978)
Asian women in California	9	Stevens et al. (1985)
Southeast Asians in Georgia	11	Franks et al. (1989)
Asians in Philadelphia area		London (1990)
Ethnic Chinese (Vietnamese, Laotian,		
Cambodian)	15	
Vietnamese	13	
Laotians	11	
Hmong	11	
Chinese	10	
Khmer	10	
Other Southeast Asians	9	
Koreans	6	

Recently, Franks et al. (1989) studied 257 Southeast Asian children who were born in the United States. Of 31 children born to
HBsAg(+) mothers, 17 (55%) had been infected with HBV. However,
of 226 children born to uninfected HBsAg(−) mothers, 15 (6.6%)
were infected—more than 10 times the 0.5% prevalence of HBV
infection among white children in the same age range in the general
population (McQuillan et al., 1989). The risk of infection was greatest (26%) among children living in households with other HBV
carrier children but not so much with their fathers or other adult

Table 5.8 Prevalence of HBsAg and HBeAg in Pregnant Asian American
Women, by Country of Birth

Country of Birth	Number Tested	HBsAg(+) (%)	HBeAg(+) (%)
China, Taiwan, Hong Kong	7,162	11.4	3.7
Cambodia, Laos, Vietnam	3,688	11.5	5.3
Korea	1,623	5.5	2.9
Philippines	1,478	5.1	0.8
Japan	612	1.8	0.0
United States	637	2.0	0.7
Other, unknown	3,642	5.7	1.3
Total	18,842	8.7	3.0

SOURCE: Stevens et al. (1985).

Table 5.9 Prevalence of HBsAg in Korean Americans in Philadelphia,
New Jersey, New York, Baltimore, and Washington, DC

Age	Number	HBsAg(+) (%) Males	Females
≤20	1,280	5.1	4.6
21-40	2,385	9.9	5.8
≥41	3,197	7.4	5.2
Total	6,862	7.5	5.2

carriers. A total of 3.9% of children with no infected household members were HBsAg(+). Thus Franks et al. conclude that child-to-child transmission within and between households may also play an important role in transmission of virus during early childhood.

During the past few years, the Liver Disease Prevention Center at Thomas Jefferson University Hospital has screened close to 7,000 Korean Americans residing in the vicinities of Philadelphia, New Jersey, New York, Baltimore, and Washington, D.C. The HBV test results are shown in Table 5.9. The identified HBsAg carriers were further evaluated for the presence of liver diseases. Most of the newly identified carriers were unaware of their HBV infection and had not had symptoms of liver disease except fatigue in some cases, which they attributed to long work hours. They also denied having had clinical hepatitis. The first 139 people were investigated for the presence of liver disease by abdominal ultrasound or magnetic resonance imaging, physical examination, liver biochemical tests, and liver biopsy if indicated. The results are shown in Table 5.10. These findings surprised both patients and physicians. However, such findings are not uncommon among Asian immigrants, especially males over 30 years of age with family histories of chronic liver disease or HCC.

A 34-year-old Korean man who had been working hard in his business since immigration 5 years before noticed one day that his abdomen appeared somewhat swollen, but he ignored it. One week later his legs became swollen and he felt fullness in his stomach. On his first visit to Jefferson, his abdominal ultrasound, physical examination, and liver function evaluation revealed that he had already advanced liver cirrhosis with ascites. Also, he and two younger brothers were found to be chronic HBV carriers. One brother was

Table 5.10 Identified Asymptomatic HBV Carriers and Their Liver
Disease Status

Diagnosis	Number	Percentage
Chronic hepatitis	57	42
Liver cirrhosis	17	11
Healthy carriers (normal liver function, normal physical exam, normal abdominal ultrasound or MRI)	65	47
Total	139	100

noted to have chronic hepatitis and the other early cirrhosis of the liver. Neither had had any symptoms except for occasional fatigue.

A 56-year-old Korean man was found to have chronic active hepatitis B 5 years before, when he developed increasing fatigue. After a few months' rest he returned to work, knowing that his liver enzymes had not returned to normal. He lived well for the next 4 years, until 2 months prior to his hospital visit, when he felt increasing fatigue. Three weeks later he developed severe indigestion, epigastric pain, ascites, and fever. CT scan showed multiple masses and a markedly nodular liver. Laparoscopic liver biopsy confirmed HCC. His alpha-fetoprotein (AFP) at that time was 152,730 ng/ml. He died within 2 months.

A 41-year-old Korean man, a known chronic HBV carrier, had been followed by his physician regularly in California. His 47-year-old brother died of HCC the year before. In March his abdominal ultrasound showed a 3 cm mass. Biopsy of this mass indicated a regenerating nodule. In July the man did not feel well. Abdominal CT scan at this time showed a 10 cm mass and additional small masses in the liver. The man died within 2 months.

It is important for physicians to recognize these points when they see Asian American patients who have immigrated to the United States. Whether the patient has chronic hepatitis B and/or cirrhosis or is a "healthy" carrier, the individual needs to be followed at regular intervals for the appearance of HCC.

On the other hand, it is important to understand that not all HBV carriers are at equal risk of developing serious liver disease and liver cancer. Among chronic HBV carriers, 40% to 50% of the men and 15% of the women will eventually develop and die of cirrhosis or HCC (Beasley, 1988; Beasley et al., 1981); the rest will remain free

162   HEALTH STATUS

Table 5.11   Risk Factors for HCC Among HBsAg(+) Carriers

Cirrhosis
Male sex
Age 40 years
Asian background
Serum ferritin 300 ng/ml (sustained)
Chronic hepatitis
IgM anti-HBc
Alcoholism

---

of serious liver disease. It would be useful for both doctor and patient to identify, while the patient is relatively young, the risk group to which the individual carrier belongs.

With a need for early detection of HCC in these HBsAg(+) carriers, it is particularly important to identify persons at highest risk for development of HCC. Table 5.11 shows the suggested risk factors. Obviously, patients with cirrhosis are at high risk. Also, patients of Asian background are most likely to have been infected early in life.

Males have a higher incidence rate for HCC (male:female ratio is 4:1) (Beasley, 1988). The biological basis for the sex difference in the risk for HCC is not well understood. Male hormones (Beasley, 1988), differences in body iron storage (Hann, Kim, London, & Blumberg, 1989; Israel, McGlynn, Hann, & Blumberg, 1989), and differences in behavior (drinking, smoking) (Ohnishi, Terabayashi, Unuma, Takahashi, & Okuda, 1987) might be contributory factors.

HCC occurs most commonly later in life, after the age of 40. Among male HBV carriers over 40 years of age, 40% to 50% will eventually develop and die of cirrhosis or HCC (Beasley, 1988).

Sustained serum ferritin levels of greater than 300 ng/ml, suggesting relatively higher iron storage, have been noted to be a risk factor. In a longitudinal follow-up study of 249 patients with chronic hepatitis B and cirrhosis in Korea, Hann, Kim, et al. (1989) observed that chronic HBsAg carrier males with sustained serum ferritin greater than 300 ng/ml had a 50% chance of developing HCC, compared with a 20% risk of HCC for carrier males with lower serum ferritin levels. Increased level of IgM anti-HBc was associated with the development of HCC (Sjogren, Lemon, Chung, Sun, & Hoofnagle, 1984).

HBV and HCC in Asian Americans

Given that the HBV infection rate is high in Asian Americans, it is to be expected that there is also higher incidence of HCC in this population. Only a few studies have been undertaken concerning HCC cases in Asian Americans. Two U.S. studies from the 1970s indicated that the death rate among Chinese American males was at least 10 times higher than that of whites (Fraumeni & Mason, 1974; Szmuness et al., 1978). A follow-up study of more than 7,000 men of Japanese ancestry in Hawaii revealed that 18 had died of HCC and 63% of the HCC patients had been HBsAg(+) (Nomura, Stemmermann, & Wasnich, 1982). Family clustering of HBV infection in the family members of Asian patients with HCC has been reported (Tong, Weiner, Ashcavai, & Vyas, 1979). Recently, Tong, Schwindt, Lo, and Co (1991), in a prospective study of 207 HBsAg(+) Asian American patients for an average follow-up period of 3.3 years, observed 8 cases of HCC. The 207 patients studied had chronic liver diseases; asymptomatic HBsAg(+) people with normal liver tests and normal physical examinations were not included in the study. The estimated death rate from HCC in Tong et al.'s (1991) series with chronic hepatitis B patients was 33,865/100,000. This is much higher than those reported in Taiwan by Beasley (1988) (495/100,000) and by Liaw et al. (1986) (826/100,000 for all ages and 2,768/100,000 for patients over age 35 years). Beasley's study included asymptomatic carriers and Liaw's group studied patients with chronic hepatitis B.

Treatment

The time interval between HBV infection and the development of serious liver disease and HCC is usually more than 40 years. During the interim, HBV carriers may remain "healthy," asymptomatic, with or without underlying progressive chronic liver disease, or may develop symptomatic liver disease such as chronic active hepatitis and/or cirrhosis.

There is no effective treatment for healthy carriers at the present time, except regular follow-up for the early detection of HCC in adult carriers.

For those with chronic active hepatitis who have elevated ALT, HBeAg, and HBV-DNA in their sera, alpha-interferon is the most widely used drug at present. Recently a multicenter trial of 169 patients with chronic hepatitis B using recombinant alpha-interferon has been completed in the United States (Perrillo et al., 1990). Nearly 40% of patients cleared HBeAg, and 50% showed sustained loss of HBV-DNA in response to a 16-week treatment of alpha-interferon, 5 million units daily. Moreover, in about 10% of patients, HBsAg disappeared from the serum.

However, the results of this study may have little relevance for most Asian HBsAg carriers, because the patients were mostly Caucasians (only four were Asians) who were likely to have been infected in adulthood, suggesting their shorter duration of chronic HBV infection. For Asian patients, most of whom are infected perinatally or in early childhood, interferon therapy has not been as encouraging. Studies in Hong Kong have demonstrated low rates of HBeAg seroconversion (10% to 15%) in both pediatric and adult Chinese HBsAg carriers in controlled trials of alpha-interferon (Lai et al., 1987; Lok, Lai, Wu, & Leung, 1988). Once the drug was discontinued, no increase in the spontaneous conversion rate of HBeAg to anti-HBe or HBsAg to anti-HBs was observed when compared with the controls.

Nevertheless, there is encouraging news from recent Asian studies of HBV patients. In a preliminary study in Hong Kong by Lok et al. (1989) Chinese patients with increased serum aminotransferase levels (twofold or greater) showed a 56% response rate with interferon therapy, which is comparable to rates observed in the United States and Western Europe. Similar high response rates have been reported in Japan, Taiwan, and Malaysia (Kim, 1989; Liaw et al., 1988). It is important to point out that patients in these studies had substantially increased enzyme levels. Therefore Asian adults with similar laboratory indicators of disease to those observed in Caucasian patients may have comparable response rates to interferon.

The most serious consequence of chronic HBV infection is the development of HCC. Several centers in various parts of the world are attempting to detect HCC at early stages, when surgical resection of small asymptomatic tumors may result in long-term survival. Reports from China, Taiwan, and Alaska show that 50% to 75% of patients who had small tumors, less than 4 cm, resected have survived 5 years, in contrast to 5% survival among those who did not benefit from surgery (Heyward et al., 1985; Tang, 1985). Elsewhere, particularly in Japan (Okuda et al., 1985), early surgical intervention has not been as successful. The reasons for the differences in outcomes are not known.

In order to detect small tumors at the earliest possible stage of the disease, it is important for physicians to monitor HBV carriers, especially those with the risk factors (see Table 5.11) for developing HCC, at regular intervals using imaging studies such as abdominal ultrasound and/or magnetic resonance imaging, liver chemistry, liver tumor markers (serum alpha-fetoprotein and ferritin), and careful physical examination.

AFP is a fetal serum protein; its reappearance in mice with hepatoma has been documented by Abelev, Perova, Khramkova, Posttnikova, and Irlin (1963) and in patients with liver cancer by Tatarinov (1963, 1964). Since then the useful role of AFP in diagnosing advanced HCC has become well recognized (Alpert, Uriel, & de Nechaud, 1968; Chen & Sung, 1977; Kew, 1974; O'Connor, Tatarinov, Abelev, & Uriel, 1970; Tatarinov, 1964). Its use as a tool for early detection of HCC has been tested by several investigators (Chen et al., 1982; Kubo, Okuda, Musha, & Nakashima, 1978; Obata et al., 1980; Okuda et al., 1975; Tang, Ying, & Gu, 1982). However, AFP is not often elevated in early HCC and also is slightly but significantly elevated in patients with chronic hepatitis and cirrhosis. Taketa (1990) recently reviewed the controversy as to the specificity of AFP in HCC. Currently, serum levels of AFP at the time of HCC diagnosis are taking on less importance as a result of the advanced imaging and biopsy techniques available for the diagnosis of HCC.

Ferritin has been evaluated as a diagnostic tumor marker with certain malignancies in the past. These include HCC (Chapman et al., 1982; Hann, Kim, et al., 1982; Kew et al., 1978; Niitsu et al., 1975; Taketa, 1990), neuroblastoma (Hann, Levy, & Evans, 1982; Hann, Stahlhut, & Millman, 1984), breast cancer (Marcus & Zinberg, 1975), lung cancer (Gropp, Havemann, & Lehmann, 1978), and Hodgkin's disease (Jones, Miller, Worwood, & Jacobs, 1973). HCC cells synthesize ferritin, as demonstrated by a culture of HCC cells and release of ferritin into the medium (Hann, Stahlhut, & Hann, 1990). Also, nude mice bearing human HCC showed the presence of human ferritin circulating in the murine serum, indicating that the circulating ferritin was derived from the HCC (Hann et al., 1984).

Ferritin is elevated in serum (300 ng/ml) in about 68% of patients with HCC (Chapman et al., 1982; Hann, London, Blumberg, Stahlhut, & Kim, 1982; Kew et al., 1978; Niitsu et al., 1975). However, increased serum ferritin is also seen in chronic hepatitis and cirrhosis, although not as high as in HCC (Chapman et al., 1982; Hann, London, et al., 1982). Therefore, neither AFP nor ferritin is a completely satisfactory tumor marker for HCC. However, when both markers are used in a longitudinal follow-up, they are helpful measurements. Tatsuta, Yamamura, Iishi, Kasugai, and Okuda (1986) have observed that the combination of AFP and ferritin measurements in serum is useful for the early detection of HCC. Nakano, Kumada, Sugiyama, Watahiki, and Takeda (1984) report that sensitivity for diagnosis of HCC increased by serial and simultaneous determination of ferritin and AFP because high ferritin levels were observed more often on low AFP-producing HCC.

In a study of Chinese HCC patients, Zhou, Stahlhut, Hann, and London (1988) report that a correct diagnosis of HCC was made in 38% of patients (54/142) by measuring ferritin (300 ng/ml) alone and in 83.8% (119/142) by measuring AFP (500 ng/ml) alone, but in 92.3% (131/142) by the measurement of a combination of these two markers.

Imaging studies are needed if AFP level is $\geq$ 25 ng/ml and sustained above this level for 1 month while liver enzyme (ALT) remains normal. This is similar to the criterion used by the Alaskan Native Hepatitis B Control Programme (Heyward et al., 1982; McMahon et al., 1987). For ferritin, based on the report by Hann, Kim, et al. (1989), an imaging study is needed if serum ferritin levels are $\geq$ 300 ng/ml for more than 6 months to 1 year while ALT remains normal.

Prevention

The medical consequences of chronic HBV infection and the pathogenesis of HCC are shown in Figure 5.1. There are two ways to approach HBV: (a) through primary prevention, that is, through immunization, whether of all uninfected individuals or of all infants born to HBV carrier mothers; and (b) secondary prevention, through follow-up every 6 months with HBV carriers for early detection of HCC.

The ultimate goal is to eliminate HBV infection by immunization of all susceptible individuals. Two HBV vaccines are currently available in the United States: Recombivax-B, produced by Merck, Sharp and Dohme; and Engerix B, by Smithkline French. Both are effective vaccines.

Summary

Since the recent identification of the long sought non-A, non-B transfusion-associated hepatitis virus and designation of the virus

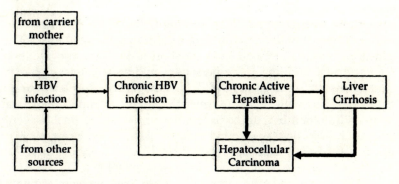

Figure 5.1. Pathogenesis of HCC

as hepatitis C virus (HCV), there are at present five human hepatitis viruses, A, B, C, D, and E. Of these, HAV and HEV are transmitted via fecal-oral routes and are highly infectious but do not cause chronic liver diseases or carrier status. On the other hand, HBV, HCV, and HDV are transmitted mostly via blood and blood-borne products and are less infectious, but they cause chronic liver diseases and carrier status. Furthermore, HBV and HCV are associated with hepatocellular carcinoma. HDV is a defective virus, able to survive only in the presence of HBsAg.

The most significant of all hepatitis viruses for humans is HBV. HBV is responsible for 80% of HCC in the world. Annually 250,000 people die of HCC (100,000 in China alone). Chronic persistent infection with HBV is causally associated with development of HCC. There are 300 million HBV-infected people (HBV carriers) in the world, and 75% of these carriers live in Asia. HCC is one of the leading cancers in Asia.

Prospective studies show that HBV carriers (HBsAg[+]) have 100 times greater risk of developing HCC than do noncarriers. Reasons for the high HBV carrier rate for Asians are thought to include perinatal infection of newborns by healthy carrier mothers and horizontal transmission of the virus in overcrowded living conditions. It appears that children infected early in life continue to have persistent infection with HBV, and some of them develop chronic active (or persistent) hepatitis, cirrhosis, and eventually HCC during adulthood.

Because this process takes approximately 40 years and those at high risk for HCC can first be identified by HBV testing, it is extremely important that all Asian Pacific Americans be tested for HBV. For those (especially adults) found to be carriers (HBsAg[+]), full evaluation of liver status should be performed, including abdominal ultrasound, physical examination, and liver function tests. If these evaluations show normal findings, these persons would be called asymptomatic carriers. For those noted to have chronic hepatitis, especially chronic active hepatitis with HBeAg(+) (meaning high viral replication), treatment with alpha-interferon can be employed, depending on the severity of liver disease. For those found to have cirrhosis, symptomatic management can be offered. Most important, patients in the above categories would be known to be at increased risk of developing HCC. Therefore, it would be extremely important to follow these patients at regular intervals (twice annually or more often) by repeating liver function tests, liver tumor markers (alpha-fetoprotein and ferritin), and abdominal ultrasound (at least once a year). If detected early, HCC can be treated by surgical resection with great success. If HCC is detected late and is inoperable, the survival rate is extremely low. In the future, liver transplantation may become an important modality for advanced liver cirrhosis and HCC. However, at present rates of survival after transplant remain relatively poor because of reinfection of HBV in the newly grafted liver. Risk factors for HCC among HBsAg(+) carriers are summarized in Table 5.11. Finally, those who are uninfected (HBsAg[−], anti-HBs[−]) should be immunized with a hepatitis B vaccine.

It is my hope that the above strategies will be applied nationwide and worldwide to eliminate new cases of HBV infection and to save the lives of patients at risk of HCC.

References

Abelev, G. I., Perova, S. D., Khramkova, N. I., Posttnikova, Z. A., & Irlin, I. S. (1963). Production of embryonal alpha-globulin by transplantable mouse hepatomas. *Transplant Bulletin, 1,* 174-180.

Advisory Committee on Immunization Practices. (1984). Postexposure prophylaxis of hepatitis B. *Morbidity and Mortality Weekly Report, 33,* 285-290.

Advisory Committee on Immunization Practices. (1985). Recommendations for protection against viral hepatitis. *Morbidity and Mortality Weekly Report, 34,* 313-315.

Aikawa, T., Sairenji, H., Furuta, S., Kiyosawa, K., Shikata, T., Imai, M., Miyakawa, Y., Yanase, Y., & Mayumi, M. (1987). Seroconversion from HBeAg to anti-HBe in acute hepatitis B virus infection. *New England Journal of Medicine, 298,* 439-442.

Almeida, J. D., Rubenstein, D., & Scott, E. J. (1971). New antigen-antibody system in Australia: Antigen positive hepatitis. *Lancet, 2,* 1225-1227.

Alpert, M. E., Uriel, J., & de Nechaud, B. (1968). Alpha-1-fetoprotein in the diagnosis of human hepatoma. *New England Journal of Medicine, 278,* 984-986.

Arevalo, J. A., & Washington, E. (1988). Cost-effectiveness of prenatal screening and immunization for hepatitis B virus. *Journal of the American Medical Association, 259,* 365-369.

Beasley, R. P. (1988). Hepatitis B virus: The major etiology of hepatocellular carcinoma. *Cancer, 61,* 1942-1956.

Beasley, R. P., Hwang, L. Y., Lin, C. C., Leu, M. L., Stevens, C. E., Szmuness, E., & Chen, K. P. (1982). Incidence of hepatitis B virus infections in preschool children in Taiwan. *Journal of Infant Development, 146,* 198-204.

Beasley, R. P., Hwang, L. Y., Stevens, C. E., Lin, C.-C., Hsieh, F.-J., Wang, K.-Y., Sun, T.-S., & Szmuness, W. (1983). Efficacy of hepatitis B immune globulin for prevention of perinatal transmission of the hepatitis B virus carrier state: Final report of a randomized double-blind, placebo-controlled trial. *Hepatology, 3,* 135-141.

Beasley, R. P., Lin, C.-C., Hwang, L. Y., & Chien, C.-S. (1981). Hepatocellular carcinoma and hepatitis B virus: A prospective study of 22,707 men in Taiwan. *Lancet, 2,* 1129-1132.

Blumberg, B. S., Alter, J. H., & Visnich, S. (1965). A "new" antigen in leukemia sera. *Journal of the American Medical Association, 191,* 541-545.

Chang, M. H., Hwang, L. Y., Hsu, H. C., Lee, C. Y., & Beasley, R. P. (1988). Prospective study of asymptomatic HBsAg carrier children infected in the perinatal period: Clinical and liver histologic studies. *Hepatology, 8,* 374-377.

Chapman, R. W., Bassendine, M. F., Laulight, M., Gorman, A., Thomas, H. C., Sherlock, S., & Hoffbrand, A. V. (1982). Serum ferritin and binding of serum ferritin to concanavalin A as a tumor marker in patients with primary liver cell cancer and chronic liver disease. *Digestive Diseases and Sciences, 27,* 111-116.

Chen, D. S., & Sung, J. L. (1977). Serum alpha-fetoprotein in hepatocellular carcinoma. *Cancer, 40,* 779-783.

Chen, D. S., Sung, J. L., Sheu, J. C., Lai, M. Y., Lee, C. S., Su, C. T., Tsang, Y. M., How, S. W., Wang, T. H., Yu, J. Y., Yang, T. H., Wang, C. Y., & Hsu, C. Y. (1982). Small hepatocellular carcinoma: A clinicopathological study in thirteen patients. *Gastroenterology, 83,* 1109-1119.

Choo, Q.-L., Kuo, G., Weiner, A. J., Overby, L. R., Bradley, D. W., & Houghton, M. (1989). Isolation of a cDNA clone derived from a blood-borne non-A, non-B viral hepatitis genome. *Science, 244,* 359-361.

Cook-Mozafferi, P., & Van Rensburg, S. (1984). Cancer of the liver. *British Medical Bulletin, 40,* 342-345.

Dane, D. S., Cameron, C. H., & Briggs, M. (1970). Virus-like particles in serum of patients with Australia antigen associated hepatitis. *Lancet, 2,* 695-698.

Dienstag, J. L. (1982). The epidemiology of hepatitis B. In I. Millman, T. Eisentein, & B. S. Blumberg (Eds.), *Hepatitis B: The virus, the disease and the vaccine* (pp. 55-65). New York: Plenum.

Franks, A. L., Berg, C. J., Kane, M. A., Browne, B. B., Sikes, R. K., Elsea, W. R., & Burton, A. (1989). Hepatitis B virus infection among children born in the United States to Southeast Asian refugees. *New England Journal of Medicine, 321,* 1301-1305.

Fraumeni, J. F., & Mason, T. J. (1974). Cancer mortality among Chinese Americans, 1950-69. *Journal of the National Cancer Institute, 52,* 659-665.

Gropp, C., Havemann, K., & Lehmann, F. (1978). Carcinoembryonic antigen and ferritin in patients with lung cancer before and during therapy. *Cancer, 42,* 2802-2808.

Hann, H. L., Kim, C. Y., London, W. T., & Blumberg, B. S. (1989). Increased serum ferritin in chronic liver disease: A risk factor for primary hepatocellular carcinoma. *International Journal of Cancer, 43,* 376-379.

Hann, H. L., Kim, C. Y., London, W. T., Whitford, P., & Blumberg, B. S. (1982). Hepatitis B virus and primary hepatocellular carcinoma: Family studies in Korea. *International Journal of Cancer, 30,* 47-51.

Hann, H. L., Levy, H. M., & Evans, A. E. (1982). Serum ferritin as a guide to therapy in neuroblastoma. *Cancer Research, 40,* 1411-1413.

Hann, H. L., London, W. T., Blumberg, B. S., Stahlhut, M. W., & Kim, C. Y. (1982). Isoferritins in the sera of patients with primary hepatocellular carcinoma (PHC). *Proceedings of the American Society of Clinical Oncologists, 1, 8.*

Hann, H. L., London, W. T., McGlynn, K., & Blumberg, B. S. (1987). Prevention of hepatitis B and primary liver cancer in Asian populations in the United States. In T. Phan & M. Katcher (Eds.), *Proceedings of The Next Decade, the 1986 Conference on Refugee Health Care Issues and Management* (pp. 95-109). Madison: Wisconsin Division of Health, Refugee Health Program.

Hann, H. L., Stahlhut, M. W., & Hann, C. L. (1990). Effect of iron and deferoxamine on cell growth and in vitro ferritin synthesis in human hepatoma cell lines. *Hepatology, 11,* 566-569.

Hann, H. L., Stahlhut, M. W., London, W. T., Menduke, H., Chon, C. Y., Millman, I., & Blumberg, B. S. (1989). Serum ferritin and antibody (Ab) response to hepatitis B vaccine. *Gastroenterology, 96,* A605.

Hann, H. L., Stahlhut, M. W., & Maddrey, W. C. (1991). Host factors influencing antibody response to hepatitis vaccine. *Gastroenterology, 100,* A751.

Hann, H. L., Stahlhut, M. W., & Millman, I. (1984). Human ferritins present in the sera of nude mice transplanted with human neuroblastoma or hepatocellular carcinoma. *Cancer Research, 44,* 3898-3901.

Heyward, W. L., Bender, T. R., Lanier, A. P., Francis, D. P., McMahon, B. J., & Maynard, J. E. (1982). Serologic markers of hepatitis B virus and alpha-fetoprotein levels preceding primary hepatocellular carcinoma in Alaskan Eskimos. *Lancet, 2,* 889-891.

Heyward, W. L., Lanier, A. P., McMahon, B. J., Fitzgerald, M. A., Kilkenny, S., & Paprocki, T. R. (1985). Early detection of primary hepatocellular carcinoma among persons infected with hepatitis B virus. *Journal of the American Medical Association, 254,* 3052-3054.

Hoofnagle, J. H. (1981). Serologic markers of hepatitis B virus infection. *Annual Review of Medicine, 32,* 1-11.

Hoofnagle, J. H., & Alter, H. (1984). Chronic viral hepatitis. In G. N. Vyas, J. L. Dienstag, & J. H. Hoofnagle (Eds.), *Viral hepatitis and liver diseases* (pp. 97-113). New York: Grune & Stratton.

Hoofnagle, J. H., Seeff, L. B., Bales, Z. B., Gerety, R. J., & Tabor, E. (1978). Serologic responses in hepatitis B. In G. N. Vyas, S. N. Cohen, & R. Schmid (Eds.), *Viral hepatitis* (pp. 219-242). Philadelphia: Franklin Institute.

Hoofnagle, J. H., Shafritz, D. A., & Popper, H. (1987). Chronic type B hepatitis and the "healthy" HBsAg carrier state. *He, UKpatology, 7,* 758-763.

Israel, J., McGlynn, K., Hann, H. L., & Blumberg, B. S. (1989). Iron related markers in liver cancer. In M. de Souza & J. Brock (Eds.), *Iron in immunity, cancer and inflammation* (pp. 301-316). Chichester, UK: John Wiley.

Jones, P. A. E., Miller, F., Worwood, M., & Jacobs, A. (1973). Ferritin in leukemia and Hodgkin's disease. *British Journal of Cancer, 27,* 212-217.

Kew, M. C. (1974). Alpha-fetoprotein in primary liver cancer and other diseases. *Gut, 15,* 814-821.

Kew, M. C., Torrance, J. D., Derman, D., Simon, M., MacNab, G. M., Charlton, R. W., & Bothwell, T. H. (1978). Serum and tumor ferritin in primary liver cancer. *Gut, 19,* 294-299.

Kim, B. S. (1989). Intron A in the treatment of chronic hepatitis B in Asian adults. In *Alpha-2b interferon in the treatment of viral hepatitis: Proceedings of a symposium held at the 8th Asian-Pacific Congress of Gastroenterology, Seoul, S. Korea* (pp. 20-25). Princeton, NJ: Excerpta Medica.

Krugman, S., Overby, L. R., Mushahwar, I. K., Ling, C. M., Froesner, G. G., & Deinhardt, F. (1979). Viral hepatitis, type B: Studies on natural history and prevention re-examined. *New England Journal of Medicine, 300,* 101-107.

Kubo, Y., Okuda, K., Musha, H., & Nakashima, T. (1978). Detection of hepatocellular carcinoma during a clinical follow-up of chronic liver disease: Observation in 31 patients. *Gastroenterology, 74*, 578-582.

Kuo, G., Choo, Q.-L., Alter, H. J., Gitnick, G. L., Redeker, A. G., Purcell, R. H., Miyamura, T., Dienstag, J. L., Alter, M. J., Stevens, C. E., Tegtmeier, G. E., Bonino, F., Colombo, M., Lee, W.-S., Kuo, C., Berger, K., Shuster, J. R., Overby, L. R., Bradley, D. W., & Houghton, M. (1989). An assay for circulating antibodies to a major etiologic virus of human non-A, non-B hepatitis. *Science, 244*, 362-364.

Lai, C. L., Lok, A. S. F., Lin, H. J., Wu, P. C., Yeoh, E. K., & Yeung, C. Y. (1987). Placebo-controlled trial of recombinant alpha-interferon in Chinese HBsAg carrier children. *Lancet, 2*, 877-880.

Li, F. P., & Shiang, E. L. (1980). Cancer mortality in China. *Journal of National Cancer Institute, 65*, 217-221.

Liaw, Y. F., Lin, S.-M., Sheen, I. S., Chen, T.-J., & Chu, C.-M. (1988). Treatment of chronic type B hepatitis in Southeast Asia. *American Journal of Medicine, 85*, 147-154.

Liaw, Y. F., Tai, D. I., Chu, C. M., Lin, D. Y., Sheen, I. S., Chen, T. J., & Pao, C. C. (1986). Early detection of hepatocellular carcinoma in patients with chronic type B hepatitis. *Gastroenterology, 90*, 263-267.

Lok, A. S. F., Lai, C. L., Wu, P. C., Lau, J. Y. N., Leung, E. K. Y., & Wong, L. S. K. (1989). Treatment of chronic hepatitis B with interferon: Experience in Asian patients. *Seminars in Liver Diseases, 9*, 249-253.

Lok, A. S. F., Lai, C. L., Wu, P. C., & Leung, E. K. Y. (1988). Long-term follow-up in a randomized controlled trial of recombinant alpha-interferon in Chinese patients with chronic hepatitis B virus infection. *Lancet, 2*, 298-302.

London, W. T. (1990). Prevention of hepatitis B and hepatocellular carcinoma in Asian residents in the United States. *Asian Journal of Clinical Science Monograms: Hepatitis B Virus Infections, 11*, 49-57.

Maggiore, G., DeGiacomo, C., Marzani, D., Sessa, F., & Scotta, M. S. (1983). Chronic viral hepatitis B in infancy. *Journal of Pediatrics, 103*, 749-752.

Magnius, L. O., & Epsmark, J. A. (1972). New specificities in Australia antigen positive sera distinct from the le Bouvire determinants. *Journal of Immunology, 109*, 1117-1121.

Marcus, D. M., & Zinberg, N. (1975). Measurement of serum ferritin by radioimmunoassay: Results in normal individuals and patients with breast cancer. *International Cancer Institute, 55*, 791-795.

Marion, P. L., Oshiro, L. S., Renergy, D. C., Scullard, G. H., & Robinson, W. S. (1980). A virus of beechy ground squirrels which is related to hepatitis B virus of man. *Proceedings of the National Academy of Sciences, 77*, 2941-2945.

Mason, W. S., Seal, G., & Summers, J. (1980). A virus of Peking ducks with structural and biological relatedness to human hepatitis B virus. *Journal of Virology, 35*, 829-836.

McGlynn, K., London, W. T., Hann, H.-W., & Sharrar, R. G. (1986). Prevention of primary hepatocellular carcinoma in Asian populations in the Delaware Valley. *Advances in Cancer Control: Health Care Financing and Research* (pp. 237-246). New York: Alan R. Liss.

McMahon, B. J., Rhoades, E., Heyward, W. L., Tower, E., Ritter, D., Lanier, A. P., Wainwright, R. B., & Helminiak, C. (1987). A comprehensive program to reduce the incidence of hepatitis B virus infection and its sequelae in Alaskan natives. *Lancet, 2*, 1134-1136.

McQuillan, G. M., Townsend, T. R., Fields, H. A., Carroll, M., Leahy, M., & Polk, B. F. (1990). Seroepidemiology of hepatitis B virus infection in the United States: 1976 to 1980. *American Journal of Medicine, 87*(Suppl. 3A), 5S-10S.

Nakano, S., Kumada, T., Sugiyama, K., Watahiki, H., & Takeda, I. (1984). Clinical significance of serum determination for hepatocellular carcinoma. *American Journal of Gastroenterology, 79*, 623-627.

Niitsu, Y., Ohtsuka, S., Kohgo, Y., Watanabe, N., Koseki, J., & Urushizaki, I. (1975). Hepatoma ferritin and tumor and serum. *Tumor Research, 10,* 31-41.

Nomura, A., Stemmermann, G. N., & Wasnich, R. D. (1982). Presence of hepatitis B surface antigen before primary hepatocellular carcinoma. *Journal of the American Medical Association, 247,* 2247-2249.

Obata, H., Hayashi, N., Motoike, Y., Hisamitsu, T., Okuda, H., Kobayashi, S., & Nishioka, K. (1980). A prospective study on the development of hepatocellular carcinoma from liver cirrhosis with persistent hepatitis B virus infection. *International Journal of Cancer, 25,* 741-747.

O'Connor, G. T., Tatarinov, Y. S., Abelev, G. I., & Uriel, J. (1970). A collaborative study for the evaluation of a serological test for primary liver cancer. *Cancer, 25,* 1091-1098.

Ohnishi, K., Terabayashi, H., Unuma, T., Takahashi, A., & Okuda, K. (1987). Effects of habitual alcohol intake and cigarette smoking on the development of hepatocellular carcinoma. *Alcoholism: Clinical and Experimental Research, 11,* 45-48.

Okada, K., Kamiyama, I., Inomata, M., Imai, M., Miyakawa, Y., & Mayumi, M. (1976). E antigen and anti-e in the serum of asymptomatic carrier mothers as indicators at positive and negative transmission of hepatitis B virus to their infants. *New England Journal of Medicine, 294,* 746-749.

Okuda, K., Kotoda, K., Obata, H., Hayashi, N., Hisamitsu, T., Tamaya, M., Kubo, Y., Yakushiji, F., Nagata, E., Shigenobu, J., & Shimokawa, Y. (1975). Clinical observations during a relatively early stage of hepatocellular carcinoma, with special reference to serum alpha-fetoprotein levels. *Gastroenterology, 69,* 226-234.

Okuda, K., Phtsuki, T., Obata, H., Tomimatsu, M., Okazaki, N., Hasegawa, H., Nakajima, Y., & Ohnishi, K. (1985). Natural history of hepatocellular carcinoma and prognosis in relation to treatment: Study of 850 patients. *Cancer, 56,* 918-928.

Perrillo, R. P., Schiff, E. R., Davis, G. L., Bodenheimer, H. C., Lindsay, K., Payne, J., Dienstag, J. L., O'Brien, C., Tamburro, C., Jacobson, I. M., Sampliner, R., Feit, D., Lefkowitch, J., Kuhns, M., Meschievitz, C., Sanghri, B., Albrecht, J., Gibas, A., & the Hepatitis Interventional Therapy Group. (1990). A randomized controlled trial of interferon alpha-2b, alone and following prednisone withdrawal, in the treatment of chronic hepatitis B. *New England Journal of Medicine, 323,* 295-301.

Piccinino, F., Sagnelli, E., Manzillo, G., & Pasquale, G. (1977). Liver histology in 34 HBsAg long-term healthy carriers. *Acta Hepato-gastroenterology, 23,* 148-154.

Popper, H., Shafritz, D. A., & Hoofnagle, J. (1987). Relation of the hepatitis B virus carrier state to hepatocellular carcinoma. *Hepatology, 7,* 764-772.

Ramalingaswami, V., & Purcell, R. H. (1988). Waterborne non-A, non-B hepatitis. *Lancet, 2,* 571-573.

Rizzetto, M., Bonino, R., Sakuma, K., Takahara, T., Okuda, L., Tsuda, F., & Mayumi, M. (1982). Prognosis of hepatitis B surface antigen carriers in relation to routine liver function tests: A retrospective study. *Gastroenterology, 83,* 114-117.

Shiraki, K., Yoshihara, N., Kawana, T., Yasui, H., & Sakurai, M. (1977). Hepatitis B surface antigen and chronic hepatitis in infants born to asymptomatic carrier mothers. *American Journal of Diseases of Children, 131,* 644-647.

Shiraki, K., Yoshihara, N., Sakurai, M., Eto, T., & Kawana, T. (1980). Acute hepatitis B in infants born to carrier mothers with the antibody to hepatitis Be antigen. *Journal of Pediatrics, 97,* 768-774.

Sjogren, M. H., Lemon, S. M., Chung, W. K., Sun, H. S., & Hoofnagle, J. H. (1984). IgM antibody to hepatitis B core antigen in Korean patients with hepatocellular carcinoma. *Hepatology, 4,* 615-616.

Stevens, C. E., Beasley, R. P., Tsui, J., & Lee, W.-C. (1975). Vertical transmission of hepatitis B antigen in Taiwan. *New England Journal of Medicine, 292,* 771-774.

Stevens, C. E., Neurath, R. A., Beasley, R. P., & Szmuness, W. (1979). HBeAg and anti-HBe detection by radioimmunoassay: Correlation with vertical transmission of hepatitis B virus in Taiwan. *Journal of Medical Virology, 3*, 237-241.

Stevens, C. E., Toy, P. T., Tony, M. J., Taylor, P. E., Vyas, G. N., Nair, P. V., Guduralli, M., Krugman, S. (1985). Perinatal hepatitis B virus transmission in the United States: Prevention by passive-active immunization. *Journal of the American Medical Association, 253*, 1740-1745.

Summers, J., & Mason, W. S. (1982). Relation of the genome of a hepatitis B-like virus by reverse transcription of an RNA intermediate. *Cell, 29*, 403-415.

Summers, J., Smolec, J. M., & Snyder, R. (1978). A virus similar to human hepatitis B virus associated with hepatitis and hepatoma in woodchucks. *Proceedings of the National Academy of Sciences, 75*, 4533-4537.

Szmuness, W. (1978). Hepatocellular carcinoma and the hepatitis B virus: Evidence for a causal association. *Progress in Medical Virology, 24*, 40-69.

Szmuness, W., Stevens, C. E., Ikram, H., Much, M. I., Harley, E. J., & Hollinger, B. (1978). Prevalence of hepatitis B virus infection and hepatocellular carcinoma in Chinese-Americans. *Journal of Infectious Diseases, 137*, 822-829.

Taketa, K. (1990). Alpha-fetoprotein: Re-evaluation in hepatology. *Hepatology, 12*, 1420-1432.

Tang, Z. Y. (1985). Prognosis of hepatocellular carcinoma and factors influencing it. In Z. Y. Tang (Ed.), *Subclinical hepatocellular carcinoma* (pp. 79-187). New York: Springer-Verlag.

Tang, Z. Y., Ying, Y. Y., & Gu, T. J. (1982). Hepatocellular carcinoma: Changing concepts in recent years. In H. Popper & F. Schaffner (Eds.), *Progress in liver disease* (Vol. 7, pp. 637-647). New York: Grune & Stratton.

Tatarinov, Y. S. (1963). The discovery of fetal globulin in patients with primary cancer of the liver. In *First International Biologochemistry Congress of the USSR*. Moscow: Academy of Sciences USSR.

Tatarinov, Y. S. (1964). Presence of embryospecific alpha-globulin in the serum of patients with primary hepatocellular carcinoma. *Voprosy Meditsinskoi Khimii, 10*, 90-91.

Tatsuta, M., Yamamura, H., Iishi, H., Kasugai, H., & Okuda, S. (1986). Value of serum alpha-fetoprotein and ferritin in the diagnosis of hepatocellular carcinoma. *Oncology, 43*, 306-310.

Tiollais, P., Charnay, P., & Vyas, G. N. (1981). Biology of hepatitis B virus. *Science, 213*, 406-411.

Tiollais, P., Pourcel, C., & Dejean, A. (1985). The hepatitis B virus. *Nature, 317*, 489-495.

Tiollais, P., & Wain-Hopson, S. (1984). Molecular genetics of the hepatitis B virus. In F. V. Chiari (Ed.), *Advances in hepatitis research* (pp. 9-20). New York: Masson.

Tong, M. J., Schwindt, R. R., Lo, G. H., & Co, R. L. (1991). Chronic hepatitis and hepatocellular carcinoma in Asian-Americans. In E. Tabor, A. Bisceglie, & R. Purcell (Eds.), *Advances in applied biotechnology: Series 13. Etiology, pathology and treatment of hepatocellular carcinoma in North America* (pp. 15-23). New York: Academic Press.

Tong, M. J., Weiner, J. M., Ashcavai, M. W., & Vyas, G. N. (1979). Evidence for clustering of hepatitis B virus infection in families of patients with primary hepatocellular carcinoma. *Cancer, 44*, 2338-2342.

Yoshizawa, H., Machida, A., Miyakawa, Y., & Mayumi, M. (1979). Demonstration of hepatitis B e antigen in hepatitis core particles obtained from the nucleus of hepatocytes infected with hepatitis B virus. *Journal of General Virology, 42*, 513-519.

Zhou, X. D., Stahlhut, M. W., Hann, H. L., & London, W. T. (1988). Serum ferritin in hepatocellular carcinoma. *Hepato-gastroenterology, 35*, 1-4.

Zuckerman, A. J. (1983). World Health Organization Report of a W.H.O. scientific group. *Lancet, 1*, 463-465.

6

Obesity and Diabetes

DOUGLAS E. CREWS

Diabetes and obesity have been established as major health problems among Pacific Islander Americans. Whether residing on their home islands or the U.S. mainland, Samoans, Native Hawaiians, and Micronesians are noted for their frequent obesity and non- insulin-dependent diabetes mellitus (NIDDM) (Crews, 1988a; Crews, Bindon, & Ozeran, 1991; Pawson & Janes, 1981; Zimmet, 1979), as are several other Pacific Islander populations such as the Maori and Naruans (see Baker, 1984; King & Zimmet, 1988). Conversely, the extent and prevalence of obesity and diabetes among Asian Americans have not been well documented. Underlying mechanisms that lead to increases in obesity and NIDDM when Asian Pacific Americans adopt lifestyles similar to those of Anglo Americans have yet to be established.

The main purpose of this chapter is to review data documenting prevalence rates of obesity and diabetes in Asian Pacific American populations and to place these rates in context with those from other migrant and nonmigrant groups. Prior to describing the data, I will briefly review aspects of the epidemiology and etiology of obesity and diabetes. In the third section, I examine some correlates and outcomes of obesity and NIDDM among Asian Pacific Americans. I then discuss barriers to care, along with several factors that may lead to late presentation of Asian Pacific Americans for treat-

AUTHOR'S NOTE: I would like to thank Claire K. Hughes, M.S., R.D., and Laura Newell-Morris, Ph.D., for their many insightful and useful comments on an earlier version of this chapter.

ment, and some strategies for health promotion, disease prevention, and medical interventions. Sections that follow examine factors
that may have combined to prevent research on obesity and diabetes from proceeding as rapidly in Asian Pacific American communities as in Anglo, African and Hispanic American communities,
reveal some strategies for health promotion and disease prevention
and give directions for future research; the final section provides a
brief chapter summary.

Unfortunately, as federal health and demographic data on Asian
Pacific Americans are infrequently reported by ethnicity and most
state agencies fail to classify various Asian Pacific Americans by
their individual race/ethnic identities (Asian and Pacific Islander
American Health Forum, 1991), published epidemiological reports
on the prevalence and incidence of obesity and diabetes in Asian
Pacific Americans are relatively rare. Thus accomplishing the stated
tasks of this chapter is not as simple as articulating them. Whatever
data have been reported frequently are specific to geographically
isolated groups of long-term Asian Pacific residents in Honolulu,
California, or Seattle, Washington. Thus the majority of data on
obesity and diabetes in Asian Pacific populations are not from U.S.
residents, but from populations in their homelands and migrants
to destinations such as the United Kingdom, Tanzania, Singapore,
Mauritius, and Fiji. The purpose here is not to provide an exhaustive review of all available literature but to draw attention to the
extent of these related health problems in Asian Pacific Americans
and to emphasize areas where data are lacking.

Obesity and Diabetes

Obesity is often defined as a disease of energy metabolism. The
common belief is that obesity in present-day populations is a by-
product of modern lifestyles and dietary practices that include
psychosocial stress, excess food or energy consumption, and/or
deficient energy expenditure. Although its exact inheritance pattern is not known, obesity also is recognized as having a genetic
basis (Bouchard, 1991; Garn, Bailey, & Block, 1979; Garn, Sullivan,
& Hawthorne, 1989; Newman et al., 1987; Selby et al., 1989). A
central or masculine (e.g., trunk, upper body) pattern of fat distribution may be a more important promoter of conditions such as diabetes
and cardiovascular diseases than is absolute amount of overweight

(Vague, 1956; Vague, Björntrop, Guy-Grand, Rebuffe-Scrive, & Vague, 1985). Visceral fat, in particular, may be an important factor in the development of a diabetogenic lipid and lipoprotein profile. It is metabolically active and is associated with greater insulin resistance compared with subcutaneous fat (Dowse et al., 1991; Kissebah, Peiris, & Evans, 1988; Knowler, Pettit, Savage, & Bennett, 1981; McKeigue, Shah, & Marmot, 1991; Osei, 1990; Selby et al., 1989).

Diabetes mellitus includes a heterogeneous group of related disorders. Currently, two major types of diabetes mellitus, along with several less frequent types—gestational diabetes, metabolic diabetes, malnutrition-related diabetes, maturity onset diabetes of youth, and tropical diabetes—are commonly recognized. The two major types are insulin-dependent diabetes mellitus (IDDM) and noninsulin-dependent diabetes mellitus (NIDDM), following international nomenclature (World Health Organization, 1985). Previously these were described as Type I and Type II, or juvenile- and adult-onset diabetes, respectively. Diabetes mellitus is typified by glucose intolerance, an overabundance of glucose in the blood, and a deficit of insulin activity (insulin facilitates the passage of glucose into muscle and fat cells) in response to a glucose load (Foster, 1989; World Health Organization, 1985). Although the precise etiology of neither IDDM nor NIDDM is established, IDDM is now thought to result at least in part from an autoimmune reaction, likely occurring as the result of a genetic-based variability in immune function, and an environmental trigger, perhaps viral infection (see Lipton & LaPorte, 1989). The etiology of NIDDM remains somewhat more of a mystery. At present it is unclear whether the apparent deficit in insulin that appears to be associated with NIDDM is absolute (not enough insulin) or relative (an inability to use insulin). Furthermore, although recent data suggest that insulin resistance is a manifest characteristic of NIDDM (see Osei, 1990), lack of conversion of proinsulin to insulin may also typify some types of NIDDM (see Temple et al., 1989).

Although both genetic and environmental determinants have been hypothesized to influence the onset of NIDDM, no consistent genetic associations have been established (Cox, Epstein, & Spielman, 1989). For instance, insulin-receptor and apolipoprotein genes have been found to be associated with development of NIDDM in Chinese Americans (Xiang et al., 1989) but not in other populations. Takeda and colleagues (1986) failed to find a significant association between the class 3 restriction fragment length polymorphism (RFLP) of the 5' portion of the human insulin gene (RFLPs are polymorphisms of size detected when certain "restriction enzymes" cut DNA at a particular sequence of bases) and diabetes in a Japanese sample; however, in an unrelated study, this same class 3 allele was observed at an elevated frequency among nonobese Japanese patients with NIDDM and a family history of NIDDM (Nomura et al., 1986). Such results indicate that even within a single ethnic group variable associations of genotypes with the NIDDM phenotype may be observed, results that should not be surprising given the heterogeneous nature of NIDDM.

Epidemiologically, the closest correlates of declining glucose tolerance, the *sine qua non* of NIDDM, are obesity and age. Obesity and NIDDM are closely linked as disorders of energy balance and both show statistically significant associations with insulin levels (Ohno, Ikeda, & Abe, 1990), as does age. The suggestion is that obesity, especially accompanied by a central body distribution of adipose tissue (fat), is a promoting factor for NIDDM in certain individuals. Asian Pacific Americans appear to be at increased risk for both obesity and NIDDM when they migrate to or are born in the United States or adopt "Western" lifestyles *in situ*. This review is designed to describe the current state of knowledge regarding obesity and NIDDM in Asian Pacific Americans throughout the United States and its territories. Aspects of IDDM are not reviewed. The frequency of IDDM has recently been assessed in a series of international surveys, and this condition appears to be rare in Pacific Island and East Asian populations (Rewers, LaPorte, King, & Tuomilehto, 1988). This is not to suggest that IDDM could not also increase in prevalence among Asian Pacific individuals as they adopt lifeways similar to those of their Anglo counterparts, but that these issues need to be examined in a format that emphasizes IDDM in these cases.

Prevalence and Mortality Studies

Obesity: Prevalence

Asian Pacific Americans

Two Pacific Islander populations, Samoans and Native Hawaiians, are among the most obese peoples in the world (see Tables 6.1 and 6.2). In each population, both men and women show average body mass indices (BMI = weight (kg)/height (m)^2) that exceed those currently used to define obesity in the general U.S. popula-

Table 6.1 Average Body Mass Index[a] in Various Adult Populations

Population	Body Mass Index Men	Women	Sample Description (Source)
Western Samoan	26	28	ages 20+ (Pawson, 1986)
Hawaii Samoan	31	33	ages 20+ (Pawson, 1986)
California Samoan	35	34	ages 20+ (Pawson, 1986)
American Samoan	30	33	ages 20+ (Crews, 1988b)
Native Hawaiian	31	30	ages 20-59 (Aluli, 1991)
Japanese American	24	22	adults (Klatsky & Armstrong, 1991)
Filipino American	24	23	adults (Klatsky & Armstrong, 1991)
Chinese American	23	21	adults (Klatsky & Armstrong, 1991)
Other Asian American	24	22	adults (Klatsky & Armstrong, 1991)
U.S. white	27	28	ages 20-74 with diabetes (Harris et al., 1987)
U.S. black	29	30	ages 20-74 with diabetes (Harris et al., 1987)
Klong Toey, Thailand	10	11	adults (Bunnag et al., 1990)
Singapore Chinese	22	22	ages 18-69 (Hughes et al., 1990)
Singapore Malay	23	25	ages 18-69 (Hughes et al., 1990)
Singapore Indian	23	25	ages 18-69 (Hughes et al., 1990)
London European	26	25	ages 40-69 (McKeigue et al., 1991)
London South Asian	26	27	ages 40-69 (McKeigue et al., 1991)
London Afro-Caribbean	26	—	ages 40-69 (McKeigue et al., 1991)

NOTES: Terms used to describe ethnic groups were used in the original publications.
a. BMI = weight (kg)/height (m)^2.

tion (approximately 27-28 kg/m^2; Najjar & Rowland, 1987) (Table 6.1). Data presented in Table 6.2 suggest that Native Hawaiian men are more obese than Samoan men. However, greater than 20% of ideal weight was the threshold used to establish obesity in the Hawaiian sample, whereas a BMI ≥ 30 kg/m^2 was used in the Samoan sample. Application of a BMI of 27 kg/m^2 in the Samoan sample classifies approximately 65% of men and 76% of women as obese, proportions that slightly exceed prevalence rates in Native Hawaiians. In both populations, younger cohorts are more obese than older ones. For example, in Native Hawaiians BMI averages 32 kg/m^2 in men and women aged 40 to 49 years, and 71% of women and 68% of men are classified as obese (Aluli, 1991). In cross-sectional studies among Samoan Americans, height, weight, and BMI generally increase with level of modernization, determined by place of residence in American Samoa, Hawaii, or California (Table 6.1).

Table 6.2 Obese in Various Adult Populations

Population	Percentage Obese Men	Women	Sample Description (Source)
American Samoan	46	66	ages 20+ (Crews, 1988b)
Native Hawaiian	66	63	ages 20-59 (Aluli, 1991)
Japanese American	38	18	adults (Klatsky & Armstrong, 1991)
Filipino American	42	26	adults (Klatsky & Armstrong, 1991)
Chinese American	27	13	adults (Klatsky & Armstrong, 1991)
Other Asian American	27	15	adults (Klatsky & Armstrong, 1991)
U.S. white	24	25	ages 20-74 (Aluli, 1991)
U.S. black	26	45	ages 20-74 (Aluli, 1991)
U.S. white	28	25	ages 35-44 (Pi-Sunyer, 1990)
U.S. white	30	30	ages 45-54 (Pi-Sunyer, 1990)
U.S. black	41	41	ages 35-44 (Pi-Sunyer, 1990)
U.S. black	41	61	ages 44-54 (Pi-Sunyer, 1990)
Klong Toey, Thailand	10	11	adults (Bunnag et al., 1990)
Singapore Chinese	17	21	ages 18-69 (Hughes et al., 1990)
Singapore Malay	22	52	ages 18-69 (Hughes et al., 1990)
Singapore Indian	14	42	ages 18-69 (Hughes et al., 1990)

NOTE: Terms used to describe ethnic groups were used in the original publications.

Among Korean men obesity increases with length of residence in the United States; among Korean women a less marked increase occurs (Han, 1990). Moreover, affluent Korean men tend to be more obese than the less affluent, although affluent Korean women tend to be leaner than their counterparts, findings reminiscent of data from U.S. whites (see Garn, 1993). Obesity is also more frequent among Japanese American men aged 45 to 69 who reside in Hawaii and California than among their counterparts in Japan (Curb & Marcus, 1991a, 1991b). Caloric intakes of Japanese American men are similar to those of their counterparts in Japan; however, the percentage of calories from fat among those in Japan are half those of Hawaiian Japanese men. Among second-generation Japanese American (Nisei) men, body fatness and fat distribution are significantly associated with impaired glucose tolerance (IGT) and NIDDM (Newell-Morris, Treder, Shuman, & Fujimoto, 1989). In a recent study of Chinese, Filipino, Japanese, and other Asian Pacific Americans residing in California, U.S.-born and Hawaiian-born men showed greater levels of adiposity than their homeland counterparts and all samples of Asian Pacific men show a similar trend of greater adiposity in those who are more educated (Klatsky & Armstrong,

Table 6.3 Average Waist/Hip Ratios in Various Adult Populations

Population	Waist/Hip Ratio Men	Women	Sample Description (Source)
London Sikh	0.98	—	ages 40-69, divided by language and religion (McKeigue et al., 1991)
London Punjabi Hindu	0.98	—	ages 40-69, divided by language and religion (McKeigue et al., 1991)
London Gujarati Hindu	0.97	—	ages 40-69, divided by language and religion (McKeigue et al., 1991)
London Muslim	0.98	—	ages 40-69, divided by language and religion (McKeigue et al., 1991)
London British	0.93	—	ages 40-69, divided by language and religion (McKeigue et al., 1991)
London European	0.94	0.76	ages 40-69, divided by ethnicity (McKeigue et al., 1991)
London South Asian	0.98	0.85	ages 40-69, divided by ethnicity (McKeigue et al., 1991)
London Afro-Caribbean	0.94	—	ages 40-69, divided by ethnicity (McKeigue et al., 1991)

NOTE: Terms used to describe ethnic groups were used in the original publication.

1991), the pattern seen in U.S. whites and Korean Americans. These combined data can be interpreted as suggesting that changed lifestyles and environments in the United States combine to promote increased obesity in Asian Pacific Americans and that these changes likely are associated with the higher levels of IGT and NIDDM.

Non-U.S. Asian Populations

Additional data on obesity in migrant Asians is available from several communities outside the United States. In a combined sample of South Asians from London, men differed little in average BMI or waist/hip ratio, a measure of the degree to which adipose tissue shows a masculine (i.e., central, trunk) distribution, from Europeans. A waist/hip ratio of 1.0 in men or 0.8 in women is considered to indicate central or abdominal obesity and to be a risk factor for diabetes and other chronic diseases. The London European men, however, showed the lowest average waist/hip ratio (Table 6.3). South Asian women showed higher average BMI and greater waist/hip ratio than their European counterparts (Tables 6.1 and 6.3). For South Asians residing in London, men approach this level, 0.98, and women exceed it, 0.85 (Table 6.3). In London, even normoglycemic South Asians exhibit a syndrome of hyperinsulinemia, central obesity, high plasma triglycerides, and low HDL-cholesterol that is not observed in comparable samples of either white or black London residents (McKeigue et al., 1991). Not surprisingly, the frequency of NIDDM and IGT combined among London South Asians (19%) was 3.8 times that of their white counterparts (5%).

Among Thais residing in the Klong Toey area of Bangkok, Thailand, a region of slums and government housing at the low end of the affluence spectrum, obesity is much rarer than observed in migrant Asian or in U.S. populations (Table 6.2) (Bunnag, Sitthi-Amorn, & Chandraprasert, 1990). This sample likely represents people with a higher-fiber, lower-fat, and lower-calorie diet, and may therefore be more representative of the baseline level of obesity to be expected in more traditional nonmigrant Asian populations. Among most migrant Asian groups the prevalence of obesity exceeds that of their nonmigrant compatriots. Among Chinese, Malays, and Indians who have migrated to Singapore obesity is common among both men and women, 17% and 21%, 22% and 52%, and 14% and 42%, respectively (Hughes et al., 1990)—prevalence rates that, except for the Chinese, exceed rates observed in the U.S. white female population but are about equal to rates observed among African Americans (Table 6.2). Unfortunately, similar or comparable data are not available for most Asian Pacific ethnic groups. However, based on the available evidence, the hypothesis is strongly supported that obesity is likely increasing as a health problem among both short- and long-term Asian Pacific residents of the United States, as it is among Japanese Americans in California and Hawaii (Curb & Marcus, 1991a) and Seattle, Washington (Newell-Morris et al., 1989); Korean men (Han, 1990); Samoans in American Samoa, Hawaii, and California (Crews, 1988a; Pawson & Janes, 1981); and Native Hawaiians (Aluli, 1991).

Diabetes: Prevalence

Prevalence and mortality rates for NIDDM above those in the Anglo American population have been documented for several Asian Pacific groups (Baker & Crews, 1986; Crews, Bindon, & Ozeran, 1991; Crews & MacKeen, 1982; Davidson, 1986). Unfortunately, such data are limited to but few of the many U.S. Asian Pacific ethnic groups and are available for but few geographic regions of the

United States. Significantly more data on NIDDM are available for overseas Asian Pacific groups in the United Kingdom, Fiji, Mauritius, Singapore, and Tanzania and in their native Asian and island homelands than are available for Asian Pacific people who actually reside in the United States.

Japanese Americans

In 1986, the Office of Minority Health reported that, "of the 12 Asian groups enumerated in the 1980 census, Japanese Americans are the only group in which detailed studies of the impact of diabetes have been undertaken" (p. 271). Among Japanese American men aged 40 and older the prevalence rate of diabetes is 10% to 14%, compared with 5.5% among European American men (Fujimoto, Leonetti, Kinyoun, Newell-Morris, et al., 1987; Office of Minority Health, 1989), and is about four times that of men in Japan (Tsunehara, Leonetti, & Fujimoto, 1990). An important correlate of this variability in prevalence rates is that dietary patterns of Nisei men are more similar to those of Anglo American men than they are to those of native Japanese men. In addition, among the Nisei, men with diabetes consume more animal protein and fat than nondiabetic men.

Extrapolating from a small sample of 50- to 70-year-old Nisei men ($N = 74$) residing in King County, Washington, who did not self-report having diabetes combined with a sample of 214 men sampled during the first year of the Seattle Diabetes Study, 12.1% of whom reported diabetes when surveyed, Fujimoto and colleagues (1983) estimate that among second-generation Japanese American men, 13.5% have NIDDM and 41.9% IGT (Table 6.4). For comparison, the overall prevalence of diabetes in Japan in 1955 was 0.02% and increased to 0.25% in 1978 (Ohno et al., 1990). In Japan's nationwide surveys of diabetes, among persons aged 40+ years the prevalence of diabetes was 4.1% in 1957-1958, but had increased by 85%, to 7.6%, in 1962 (reviewed in Ohno et al., 1990). In 1982 and 1988, prevalence rates of NIDDM averaged 2.37% and 3.82% in the urban area of Yamagata, Japan, and were not different in men and women (Sekikawa, Tominaga, & Sasaki, 1991). In 1988, these rates increased with cross-sectional age, and were 0.25% at ages 20 to 29, 1.9% at ages 40 to 49, and 9.6% at ages 70 to 79. Taken as a whole these data indicate that a differential of four- to sevenfold may exist between NIDDM prevalence rates in Nisei and native Japanese, however, the possible effects of different age distributions have not been accounted for in these comparisons.

Table 6.4 Prevalence Estimates of NIDDM in Various, Mainly U.S., Adult Populations

Population	Percentage Men	Women	Both	Sample Description (Source)
American Samoan			9-18.8	ages 20+, both sexes (Crews, Bindon, & Ozeran, 1991)
San Francisco Samoan	18.0	9.0		ages 18+ (Pawson & Janes, 1981)
Western Samoan, rural	2.8	6.2		ages 20+ (Zimmet et al., 1981)
Western Samoan, urban	12.6	12.2		ages 20+ (Zimmet et al., 1981)
Native Hawaiian			16.0	ages 40-49, both sexes (Curb et al., 1991)
Native Hawaiian			23.0	ages 50-59, both sexes (Curb et al., 1991)
Hawaii white			0.7	ages 14+ both sexes (Sloan, 1963)
Hawaii Chinese			1.5	ages 14+ both sexes (Sloan, 1963)
Hawaii Filipino			2.2	ages 14+ both sexes (Sloan, 1963)
Hawaii Japanese			2.0	ages 14+ both sexes (Sloan, 1963)
Hawaii Korean			2.0	ages 14+ both sexes (Sloan, 1963)
Japanese American	10-14	—		men aged 40 (Office of Minority Health, 1989)
Japanese American	20.0	—		men aged 46-75 (Fujimoto, Leonetti, Kinyoun, Shuman, et al., 1987)
Japanese American	10.1	5.7		ages 15-39 (Kawate et al., 1980)
Japanese American	19.4	9.8		ages 40-59 (Kawate et al., 1980)
Japanese American	14.3	21.0		ages 60-96 (Kawate et al., 1980)
Japanese American			13.9	age-sex adjusted (Kawate et al., 1980)
Japanese, Hiroshima	8.3	0.0		ages 15-39 (Kawate et al., 1980)
Japanese, Hiroshima	2.9	4.8		ages 40-59 (Kawate et al., 1980)
Japanese, Hiroshima	7.6	10.3		ages 60-96 (Kawate et al., 1980)
Japanese, Hiroshima			6.5	age-sex adjusted (Kawate et al., 1980)
U.S. white	5.5	7.3		ages 20-74 (Harris et al., 1987)
U.S. white	7.7	8.5		ages 45-54 (Harris et al., 1987)
U.S. white	9.1	14.5		ages 55-64 (Harris et al., 1987)
U.S. black	8.6	11.0		ages 20-74 (Harris et al., 1987)
U.S. black	11.1	14.5		ages 45-54 (Harris et al., 1987)
U.S. black	14.4	25.4		ages 55-64 (Harris et al., 1987)
Pima Indian	32.6	37.2		ages 20+ (Knowler et al., 1981)

NOTE: Terms used to describe ethnic groups were used in the original publications.

In an unrelated study, Japanese Americans residing in Hawaii and Los Angeles during 1973-1978 had a 13.9% prevalence rate of

NIDDM, twice that of Japanese living in rural areas around Hiroshima in 1975 to 1978, 6.5%, at ages 15 to 96 (Table 6.4) (Kawate, Yamakido, & Nishimoto, 1980). The greatest difference in prevalence rates was observed among men aged 40 to 59; Japanese Americans showed a 19.4% prevalence rate two-and-a-half-fold that of native Japanese, 7.6%. Overall, men showed greater differentials in NIDDM prevalence than women. Other data show that observed differences are not the result of differences in obesity as estimated from BMI. The Ni-Hon-San study of men living in Nipon, Japan, Honolulu, and San Francisco also reported poorer glucose tolerance in the Hawaii and San Francisco samples (Kagan et al., 1974). Prevalence rates of NIDDM among Filipino, Japanese, Korean, and Chinese Americans residing in Hawaii are about three times the rate in the European Hawaii population (Table 6.4) (Sloan, 1963).

Pacific Islander Americans

Prevalence rates of NIDDM in American Samoans aged 30+ have been estimated at 9% to 18.8%, although the actual rate may be higher (Crews, Bindon, & Ozeran, 1991). Based upon these estimated prevalence rates, and extrapolation of U.S. census figures for 1990 and 1980, my colleagues and I have estimated that among approximately 100,000 Samoan Americans there are as many as 7,000 adults suffering from NIDDM (Crews, Bindon, McCuddin, & Puletasi, 1991). Prevalence rates of NIDDM increase with age among Samoan and Native Hawaiians, as they do in most populations. However, Pacific Islander Americans may suffer a steeper increase in NIDDM prevalence with age than Anglo Americans or African Americans (Table 6.5 and 6.6). For Native Hawaiians NIDDM prevalence rates quadruple between ages 30 to 39 and 40 to 49, an increase from 4% to 16%; between these same ages NIDDM prevalence triples in the NHANES Anglo sample, but only increases from 1% to 3% (Table 6.5) (Curb et al., 1991). Among African Americans in 1976-1980, the estimated prevalence rate of diabetes at ages 45 to 54 was 11.1% in men and 14.5% in women, somewhat below that of Native Hawaiians aged 40 to 49 in 1985, 16.0%; at ages 55 to 64 rates were 14.4% and 25.4% in African American men and women, whereas at ages 50 to 59 rates were 23.9% in Native Hawaiians. These differences indicate that Native Hawaiians are at equal risk for NIDDM in their fifth and sixth decades of life as are African American women (Table 6.6).

Table 6.5 Prevalence of NIDDM in Native Hawaiians and NHANES Anglo Americans in 1985, by Age

| | Age Group | | | |
	20-29	30-39	40-49	50-59
Hawaiian	2.0	4.0	16.0	3.0
Anglo	1.0	1.0	3.0	5.0

SOURCE: Extrapolated from Curb et al. (1991, p. 166).

Non-U.S. Asian Populations

The prevalence and distribution of NIDDM is somewhat better documented among Asian residents and migrants outside the United States than for populations in the United States. Several British research groups have recently documented ethnic variations in the prevalence of diabetes in the United Kingdom. In a sample of 3,193 men and 561 women recruited from among London workers and general practitioners' lists, the prevalence of diabetes was little different across four Asian groups, but was 3.8 to 4.4 times higher than in the comparative European sample (Table 6.7) (McKeigue et al., 1991). In the Southall diabetes survey Asians of undefined ethnicity also showed NIDDM prevalence rates four times those of Europeans at ages 40 to 64 (Mather & Keen, 1985).

Asian Muslims and Hindus in Tanzania show prevalence rates of NIDDM that are only one third to one half the rates among their countrymen in London (Table 6.7) (McLarty, Pollitt, & Swai, 1990). Within the Muslim Indian community in the Dar es Salaam (Tanzania) urban area, prevalence rates of NIDDM are similar to those of

Table 6.6 Estimated Prevalence of NIDDM in U.S. Blacks and Whites, 1976 to 1980

| | Age Group | | | |
	20-44	45-54	55-64	65-74
Black men	2.8	11.1	14.4	29.4
Black women	3.5	14.5	25.4	23.1
White men	1.0	7.7	9.1	18.1
White women	2.2	8.5	14.5	16.1

SOURCE: Adapted from Harris and Hamman (1985, p. IV-12).

Table 6.7 Prevalence Estimates of NIDDM in Various Adult Asian and
non-Asian Populations

Population	Percentage Men	Women	Both	Sample Description (Source)
London European	4.8	2.3		ages 40-69 (McKeigue et al., 1991)
London South Asian	19.6	16.1		ages 40-69 (McKeigue et al., 1991)
London Sikh			20	ages 40-69, divided by language and religion (McKeigue et al., 1991)
London Punjabi Hindu			19	ages 40-69, divided by language and religion (McKeigue et al., 1991)
London Gujarati Hindu			22	ages 40-69, divided by language and religion (McKeigue et al., 1991)
London Muslim			19	ages 40-69, divided by language and religion (McKeigue et al., 1991)
London British			5	ages 40-69, divided by language and religion (McKeigue et al., 1991)
Tanzania Asian Muslim			8.8	both sexes (McLarty et al., 1990)
Tanzania Asian Hindu			8.6	both sexes (McLarty et al., 1990)
Tanzania black			0.9	both sexes (McLarty et al., 1990)
Tanzania Muslim Indian	7.0	7.6		ages 12+ (Swai et al., 1990)
Fiji Indian, rural	12.1	12.9		ages 20+ (Zimmet et al., 1983)
Fiji Indian, urban	11.3	11.0		ages 20+ (Zimmet et al., 1983)
Melanesian, rural	1.1	1.2		ages 20+ (Zimmet et al., 1983)
Melanesian, urban	3.5	7.1		ages 20+ (Zimmet et al., 1983)
South Africa Indian	7.6	13.5		ages 15+ (Omar et al., 1985)
Indian, Eluru	1.9	1.4		all ages combined (Rao et al., 1989)
Indian, Eluru			6.1	both sexes, ages 40+ (Rao et al., 1989)
Indian, Eluru			13.3	both sexes, ages 50-59 (Rao et al., 1989)
Indian, New Delhi			3.1	both sexes, ages 30+ (Verma et al., 1986)
Mauritius Hindu	14.0	10.9		ages 25+ (Dowse et al., 1990)
Mauritius Muslim	12.7	13.8		ages 25+ (Dowse et al., 1990)
Mauritius Chinese	13.5	9.5		ages 25+ (Dowse et al., 1990)
Mauritius Creole	7.7	13.0		ages 25+ (Dowse et al., 1990)
Singapore Indian	13.4	5.1		ages 18+ age-adjusted (Thai et al., 1987)

(continued)

Table 6.7 Prevalence Estimates of NIDDM in Various Adult Asian and non-Asian Populations (Continued)

Population	Percentage Men	Women	Both	Sample Description (Source)
Singapore Malay	9.5	7.3		ages 18+ age-adjusted (Thai et al., 1987)
Singapore Chinese	4.6	4.9		ages 18+ age-adjusted (Thai et al., 1987)
Singapore Indian	13.9	9.9		ages 50-59 (Thai et al., 1987)
Singapore Malay	32.3	19.4		ages 50-59 (Thai et al., 1987)
Singapore Chinese	26.1	25.0		ages 50-59 (Thai et al., 1987)
Indonesian, urban	1.7	1.5		ages 35-44 (Waspadji et al., 1983)
Indonesian, urban	4.0	3.3		ages 45-54 (Waspadji et al., 1983)
Indonesian, urban	11.5	9.2		ages 55-64 (Waspadji et al., 1983)

NOTE: Terms used to describe ethnic groups were used in the original publications.

Tanzania, 7.0% in men and 7.6% in women (Swai et al., 1990). These rates are 8 to 10 times the prevalence rates in native Tanzanian blacks (0.9%) (McLarty et al., 1990) and two to three times prevalence rates among Indians in New Delhi (Verma, Mehta, Madhu, Mather, & Keen, 1986). Similar prevalence rates of NIDDM, for men, 7.6%, but higher rates for women, 13.5%, have been reported for Indians residing in South Africa (Omar, Seedat, Dyer, Rajpu, Motala, & Joubert, 1985), whereas in the Fijian Indian population prevalence rates of NIDDM are 12% in men and 11.0% in women, and 2 to 10 times rates among Fijian Melanesians (Table 6.7) (Zimmet et al., 1983). In Singapore, prevalence rates in men increase from 4.6% in Chinese to 9.5% in Malays to 13.4% in Indians, whereas rates are about equal in Chinese and Indian women but highest in the Malay women (see Table 6.7). Rates of NIDDM increase with cross-sectional age in Chinese, Malay, and Indian residents (Thai et al., 1987). Overall prevalence rates of NIDDM increased by 135% between 1975 and 1985; the largest jumps were seen in Malay men (235%) and women (177%) and Chinese men (153%) and women (157%). On the island of Mauritius, age-standardized NIDDM prevalence rates are generally similar across ethnic groups for Muslim, Hindu, and Chinese men and women (Dowse et al., 1990). However, in all three groups of Asian men prevalence rates of NIDDM were 50% to

100% above those of Creole men, although the Creole women showed rates above those of Hindu and Chinese women (Table 6.7).

It has generally been accepted that overseas Asian Indian populations in locations such as London and Fiji suffer high prevalence rates of NIDDM compared with native resident Indian populations; however, recent data indicate that prevalence rates of NIDDM in India may previously have been underestimated or have risen rapidly during recent decades (Table 6.7) (for a thorough review, see Ramaiya, Kodali, & Alberti, 1990). In a series of studies since 1984, prevalence rates have ranged from 1.8% to 4.7% in Indians aged 10 to 15 years and older and from 2.2% to 9.1% in those aged more than 20 to 30 years (Ramaiya et al., 1990). A recent survey of 9,563 rural Indians from Eluru, India, resulted in a crude prevalence rate for NIDDM of 1.6% (1.9% men; 1.4% women) and rates increased with cross-sectional age (Rao et al., 1989). By ages 50 to 59, 13.3% of persons have NIDDM, and age-adjusted rates are comparable to those from affluent Delhi or Southall, London. In a survey in New Delhi, among those 30+ years of age the overall crude prevalence rate of NIDDM was 3.1% (Verma et al., 1986).

Although prevalence data on NIDDM in Asian populations are in no way complete, surveys carried out among several populations indicate that Chinese migrants experience the lowest and Indian migrants the highest prevalence rates of any Asian groups (King & Zimmet, 1988). In at least one study, individuals of Chinese origin showed higher prevalence of NIDDM, 5.0%, than an Indonesian-origin group, 1.4%, living in the urban area of Jakarta (Waspadji, Ranakusuma, Suyono, Supartondo, & Sukaton, 1983). Furthermore, NIDDM represents a substantial health burden in older urban Chinese, among whom rates as high as 10% have been reported (Woo et al., 1987). In total, available evidence may be interpreted as indicating a "spectrum of underlying genetic susceptibility to NIDDM in Asian populations," with Asian Indian populations possibly exhibiting a greater degree of genetic susceptibility (King & Zimmet, 1988, p. 192). Although no Asian or Pacific Islander group has yet been documented to show NIDDM prevalence rates as high as those among the Pima Indians of the U.S. Southwest, rates ranging from about 50% to 66% of Pima rates have been reported for Japanese American men, American Samoans, Native Hawaiians, and several South Asian groups in London (Table 6.5), whereas most other migrant Asian groups examined attain only about 35% of the Pima rate, about equal that of Anglo Americans.

Estimating the Prevalence of NIDDM in Asian Pacific Americans

In 1980, the Asian American population (excluding Pacific Islander Americans) in the United States numbered 3,466,421 (U.S. Bureau of the Census, 1983). Of these, 716,331 were Japanese Americans (Table 6.8). If the prevalence of NIDDM in this population lies between 2% and 4%, the total number of Japanese Americans affected with NIDDM is 14,000 to 28,000. Estimates of the prevalence of NIDDM are not available for other Asian American populations, such as Chinese, Filipino, Indian, or Korean Americans, but data presented for these populations in other overseas settings indicate that rates may be similarly high and that as many as 69,000 to 140,000 Asian Americans may have been suffering from NIDDM in 1980. In the 1990 census there were 6,908,638 Asian Americans and 365,024 Pacific Islander Americans enumerated in the U.S. total population count (Table 6.8) (ACCIS Program & the Asian American Health Forum, 1991). Using the same estimates of prevalence rates for NIDDM, as many as 138,000 to 276,000 Asian Americans may have suffered from NIDDM in 1990. Using an estimate of 9% to 18% for prevalence rates of NIDDM (Crews, Bindon, & Ozeran, 1991; Pawson & Janes, 1981), there may have been as many as 32,852 to 65,704 Pacific Islander Americans with NIDDM in 1990.

Inherent problems confound all comparisons of prevalence estimates. For one, different criteria have been used to establish the presence of diabetes in the various studies reviewed and, in some cases, rates were age adjusted within the study sample. Therefore, although internally comparable, some rates are not directly comparable across studies. When not age adjusted, some results refer to only specific age groups in the population. In addition, prevalence data such as these depend on two population-specific factors, incidence and survival rates (see King & Zimmet, 1988). Prevalence rates of NIDDM vary across Asian Pacific populations not only because of possible differences in etiological factors but also because of variability in health care access, available treatment modalities, and cultural perceptions. In addition, these population groups are exposed to variable environmental and ecological circumstances. However, recalling these caveats and evaluating the available data as a whole, the conclusion at this time must be that Asian Pacific individuals are at high risk for NIDDM, significantly above that of European and European American samples, when they live an affluent lifestyle such as many adopt in the United States.

Table 6.8 Census Estimates of Asian Pacific American Populations

Population	1970	1980	1990
Chinese	431,583	812,178	1,645,472
Filipino	336,731	781,894	1,406,770
Japanese	588,324	716,331	847,562
Asian Indian	—	387,223	815,447
Korean	68,510	357,393	798,849
Vietnamese	—	245,025	614,547
Laotian	—	47,683	149,014
Thai	—	45,279	147,411
Cambodian	—	16,044	91,274
Pakistani	—	15,792	81,371
Indonesian	—	9,618	29,252
Hmong	—	5,204	90,082
Malaysian	—	—	12,243
Bangladeshi	—	—	11,838
Sri Lankan	—	—	10,970
Burmese	—	—	6,177
Okinawan	—	—	2,247
Other Asian	—	26,757	148,111
Total	1,426,148	3,466,421	6,908,638
Hawaiian	—	—	211,014
Samoan	—	—	62,964
Guamanian	—	—	49,345
Tongan	—	—	17,606
Fijian	—	—	7,036
Palauan	—	—	1,439
North Mariana Islander	—	—	960
Tahitian	—	—	944
Other Pacific Islander	—	—	13,716
Total	—	—	365,024

SOURCES: U.S.Bureau of the Census (1973, 1983), ACCIS Program and the Asian and Pacific Islander American Health Forum (1991).

Diabetes: Mortality

Mortality rates provide an additional representation of cross-cultural variability in the health costs of NIDDM in Asian Pacific Americans. However, there are also inherent errors in estimating denominators for death rates and, among Asian Pacific Americans, numerators may also be underestimated. Differences in diagnostic standards and reporting cause of death across areas and populations influence what causes are listed as underlying. In addition, different ethnic groups may receive differential diagnoses based upon the type of health care to which they have access. Still, the available data allow an estimate of the discordance between Asian Pacific Americans and Anglo Americans in diabetes mortality.

NIDDM mortality rates among Asian Pacific Americans and other groups have been compiled for California for the years 1988 to 1989 (Asian and Pacific Islander American Health Forum, 1991). Unadjusted mortality rates from NIDDM were highest among African Americans. However, Samoan Americans trailed the African Americans by only 17%, with mortality rates that exceeded those of Anglo Americans by 47%. Other Pacific Islander Americans and Japanese Americans showed NIDDM mortality rates of 11.1 and 9.9/100,000, respectively. These almost equaled those of European Americans (10.7) but were slightly above those of Native Hawaiians (8.7) residing in California. Guamanian, other Asian, Fijian, Hispanic, and Chinese Americans all experienced approximately equal NIDDM mortality rates of 6.0 to 7.5/100,000, whereas Korean and Asian Indian Americans showed lower rates, 4.5 and 3.0/100,000, respectively, and all other identified groups were below 2.5/100,000 (Asian and Pacific Islander American Health Forum, 1991). In a separate survey of the 10 leading causes of death, diabetes was ranked seventh in Anglo, Japanese, and Filipino Americans and eighth in Chinese Americans (Yu, Chang, Liu, & Kan, n.d., cited in Office of Minority Health, 1986). In the same nationwide survey, compared with Anglo Americans, age-adjusted mortality ratios for diabetes mellitus were 0.81 for Chinese, 0.64 for Japanese, and 0.49 for Filipino Americans. These results suggest that the differentials observed in the California crude mortality rates may be slightly attenuated with age adjustment and a nationwide database.

Additional support for the hypothesis that Asian Pacific Americans experience an elevated risk of mortality from NIDDM comes from Hawaii, where Filipino, Japanese, Korean, and Chinese Americans experience prevalence and mortality rates that exceed by two- to threefold rates reported among the Anglo American population (Fujimoto, 1985; Office of Minority Health, 1989). Furthermore, mortality rates are higher among Hawaiian-born Asians than among Asians who were born in their native countries. During 1986, the mortality rate from diabetes in Hawaii was 29/100,000, whereas on the U.S. mainland it was 9.8/100,000 for the entire population (Martin, 1990). In American Samoa between 1962 and 1974 the age-adjusted mortality rate from diabetes was 32.2/100,000, more than double the age-adjusted rate in the United States during 1957-1959, 13.4/100,000. As early as 1975, diabetes ranked as the fifth leading cause of death among both men and women in American Samoa (Crews, 1988b).

Correlates and Outcomes

Correlates

As addressed earlier, two of the closest correlates of NIDDM are obesity and age. Unfortunately, among men, U.S.- and Hawaiian-born Asians show greater adiposity than do their counterparts in their native homelands and greater adiposity among the more educated (Klatsky & Armstrong, 1991). A major correlate of increased obesity and diabetes among Asian Pacific American groups appears to be *in situ* and migration-related modernization. Of the many changes encompassed by the terms *modernization* and *acculturation*, the most important for NIDDM are generally believed to include (a) dietary changes, particularly ingestion of more animal protein and fat and simple sugars along with a lower intake of dietary fiber; (b) decreased physical activity at both work and leisure; (c) new patterns of psychosocial stress for which traditional culturally sanctioned responses may not be available; and (d) the aging or graying of the population as life expectancy extends into the sixth and seventh decades of life. The combined effects of these changes likely expose underlying genetic propensities toward obesity and diabetes in rapidly modernizing Asian Pacific Americans, as they do in other populations.

Studies of familial aggregation and concordance among twins have confirmed the strong genetic basis of NIDDM. Included in these data are studies of diabetic Japanese twins, for whom concordance rates of NIDDM were 83% among monozygotic twins and 40% among dizygotic twins, and their families, among whom diabetes is more frequent than might be expected by chance (Japan Diabetes Society, 1988). However, as reviewed earlier, no major gene for NIDDM has yet been identified, although several specific genes and restriction fragment length polymorphisms may be associated with NIDDM in specific populations.

Dietary and activity changes with modernization contribute to the general increase in population obesity among Asian Pacific Islanders, and obese individuals tend to show hyperinsulinemia, an independent risk factor for future NIDDM and hypertension (Dowse et al., 1991; Helmrich, Ragland, Leung, & Paffenbarger, 1991; McKeigue et al., 1991). Of interest in this regard is insulin's effect not only on NIDDM but also on blood pressure and obesity. For example, Asian Indians tend to show higher basal and challenged insulin levels (during glucose tolerance tests) than do Europeans, whether they are nondiabetic normals or diabetic patients (Mohan et al., 1986). This is true even though Europeans in the sample showed higher average BMI and slightly greater average age.

Among a sample of Nisei American men examined in Seattle, Washington, those with IGT had greater mid-thigh fat deposits, whereas diabetic men had larger subscapular and biceps fat deposits than the nondiabetic men (Newell-Morris et al., 1989). In addition, men with IGT were significantly fatter than normal men on 5 of 10 measurements of fat, and diabetic men were fatter on 4 of 10. Furthermore, Japanese American men with diabetes and IGT show significantly higher BMIs, 25.9 and 26.0 kg/m^2, respectively, than do normoglycemic Japanese American men, 24 kg/m^2. Similarly, Chinese men in Hong Kong with diabetes have higher average BMI than do nondiabetic Chinese men residing in the same community (Woo et al., 1987).

The effects of diet and activity changes may be accelerated or enhanced by a particular type of psychosocial stress, status incongruity (see Bindon, Crews, & Dressler, 1991; Dressler, 1991), which tends to increase when the socioeconomic pattern of life moves toward dependency on mass media, a market economy, and adoption of a suite of behaviors and attitudes that have been labeled *Western*. The increase in prevalence of NIDDM in Japan in association with socioeconomic change and improved diagnostic techniques illustrates this pattern (Ohno et al., 1990). After World War II the amount of energy in the Japanese diet increased, carbohydrate intake decreased, the intake of protein and fat increased, and consumption of dairy products (milk, eggs) increased, as physical activity decreased with development of a mechanized economy. During this period obesity also increased such that in 1976, 30% of women aged 50+ were obese; furthermore, diabetes rose in prevalence as its primary age of incidence decreased (Ohno et al., 1990).

A similar process is apparently affecting Asian Pacific American groups as they experience *in situ* modernization on their home islands (Samoa, Hawaii, Guam) and migration-related acculturation in the United States (Samoans, Native Hawaiians, Asian Indians, Japanese, Chinese, Koreans, Vietnamese, Laotians, Filipinos, Cambodians, Thais, Guamanians). Although increases in particular chronic diseases, including diabetes, occur with modernization (Crews & Gerber, 1993; McGarvey, Bindon, Crews, & Schendel, 1989), an additional correlate of modernization is population aging—that is, an increase in the proportion of older individuals—which is among the strongest predictors of degenerative diseases, glucose tolerance, and NIDDM (see Andres, 1971; Crews, 1990). This clear association of NIDDM with modernization prompted one group of researchers to conclude, "Throughout the Asia-Pacific countries, economic progress and urbanisation have a uniformly deleterious effect on diabetes" (Cheah, Wang, & Sum, 1990, p. 501). However, there are still few epidemiological data on obesity, diabetes, diet, physical activity, aging, and glucose and insulin levels from most Asian Pacific American groups.

Outcomes

Included in the major pathological outcomes associated with diabetes are hypertension (high blood pressure), cardiovascular diseases (CVD) and microvascular complications, nephropathy (kidney dysfunction associated with loss of protein in the urine that may progress to renal failure), neuropathy (alterations in the nerve tissue that lead to decreased ability to conduct signals), and retinopathy (progressive proliferative degenerative changes in the eye that may progress to blindness). Data have accumulated from throughout the world confirming that CVD is the leading cause of morbidity and mortality among NIDDM patients (Grabauskas, 1988; Klaff & Palmer, 1986; West, 1978; Yano, Kagan, McGee, & Rhoads, 1982). NIDDM is consistently associated with lipoprotein, triglyceride, and cholesterol levels that are predictive of CVD, and blood pressure is commonly elevated in NIDDM patients (see Curb et al., 1991; Grabauskas, 1988).

In a sample of Asian Indian NIDDM patients from Southall, England, the microalbuminuria/creatinine ratio (a measure used to assess nephropathy) was significantly above the mean among European NIDDM patients (Allawi et al., 1988). In addition, hypertension was highly correlated with the microalbuminuria/creatinine ratio in the Indian but not the European diabetics. These results may indicate that nephropathy and hypertension will be more frequent outcomes of NIDDM among Indian patients than among Europeans, particularly because NIDDM has a higher prevalence and earlier age of onset in the Indian population. Allawi and colleagues (1988) suggest that the kidneys of Indians may be more vulnerable to the effects of raised blood pressure, diabetes, or both. If such a vulnerability exists, Samoans may also suffer from its consequences, because end-stage renal disease is already a frequent underlying cause of death among NIDDM patients in American Samoa (Crews, unpublished data). The degree to which the unavailability of biomedical technology and Western-style treatment modalities influence such outcomes in these settings also remains to be documented.

The primary correlate of these various pathological outcomes and the amount and degree of morbidity among diabetics is the degree to which blood glucose is elevated and, unfortunately, poor control is common among Asian Pacific Americans with diabetes. For example, among American Samoans with diabetes examined in 1989, blood sugar was not controlled and averaged 295.2 mg/dl, whereas glycated hemoglobin, an additional measure of glucose control, averaged 15.7%, more than twice the maximum expected in normoglycemic individuals (Crews, Bindon, & Ozeran, 1991). Diabetic complications indicative of poor glucose tolerance are frequent in Nisei with diabetes residing in Seattle, Washington. Among diabetic men, 11.5% show retinopathy, 46.2% show evidence of peripheral neuropathy, 53.8% have hypertension, 29.5% have ischemic heart disease, and 24.4% show atherosclerosis of the lower leg vessels, compared with 0.0%, 4.0%, 29.1%, 6.3%, and 8.9%, respectively, of men with glucose tolerance values below the diabetic range (Fujimoto et al., 1987b).

Barriers to Care

Barriers to care among Asian Pacific Americans with NIDDM are numerous, in continuous flux, and vary across language/ethnic groups. At any time and place these include at minimum language differences, overt discrimination, and lack of health insurance. To the degree such barriers influence access to the health care system, limit knowledge of the U.S. health care system, increase reliance on traditional health practices, and generate mistrust of the biomedical model of health that is operational in clinical and hospital settings, they lead to increases in late diagnoses of NIDDM and earlier onset of complications and undesirable outcomes (blindness, amputation). Further complicating health care related to obesity and diabetes in some Asian Pacific Americans are traditional body images and cultural beliefs that produce situations, activities, and expectations that may be contrary to health promotion and disease prevention. Culture-specific manifestations of illness and concepts of the organization of the universe, world, body, illness, and healing of many Asian Pacific groups often do not meld with the biomedical paradigm (see the preface to this volume).

Among these communities, language differences are overwhelming. Asian Pacific Americans represent more than 43 nationalities who speak more than 100 different languages and dialects (Asian and Pacific Islander American Health Forum, 1991). They are poorly served by a monolingual health care system and health care materials in but one, two, or even several languages. Diagnosis of obesity and NIDDM and other morbid conditions is hampered when adequate medical histories cannot be obtained, and compliance with treatment regimens for NIDDM is difficult when instructions are not understood because of language differences. In a recent survey of 296 households in Oakland, California's Chinatown, only 13% of respondents were fluent in English (Chen, Lew, Okahara, Ko, & Hirota, 1990). Discrimination in health care, like discrimination in hiring and education, is a pervasive and perverse fact of life for almost all minority populations. For Asian Pacific Americans such discrimination works two ways. First, there is overt racism when these individuals are treated differently by health providers—that is, refused service or given cursory or low-quality service—because providers are unable to understand their health complaints owing to language differences. Second, there is the perception that certain Asian Pacific Americans are healthier than other groups and that, with the large numbers of Asian Pacific physicians, health care among this population is already above average (this factor is documented in the preface to this volume and need not be addressed further here).

Access to health insurance is a primary determinant of health care usage and early diagnosis of problems. In many Asian Pacific communities a large proportion of individuals are not covered by any health insurance plan. For example, in a sample of Korean American residents of Los Angeles County, Han (1990) found that 50% of those under 65 years of age had health insurance; among those aged 65 and older 55% had health insurance, but 91% of these senior citizens had public, rather than private, insurance. Among those who had been residents of the United States for more than 10 years, insurance coverage rates were double those of shorter-term residents. In a similar study conducted in the Chinatown area of Oakland, California, 35% of the respondents from 296 households reported that they did not have health insurance coverage (Chen et al., 1990). Given that the percentage insured was slightly above that observed in Korean residents of Los Angeles, it would be interesting to know whether these Chinese Americans were longer-term residents of the United States than the Los Angeles Koreans. Without health insurance, presentation of persons with obesity and diabetes for medical care is delayed, secondary pathology is more severe, and the ultimate outcome is less promising.

Health Promotion and Disease Prevention Strategies

Health education in relation to obesity and NIDDM among Asian Pacific Americans needs to stress at least four factors: early detection of hyperglycemia, control of body weight, proper diet, and culturally appropriate exercise regimens. After age 25, all Asian Pacific individuals whose weight is more than 20% above ideal or who have a BMI ≥ 27 kg/m^2 need to have their urine tested for glucose with the use of a simple inexpensive dip stick. Those obtaining a positive result need to participate in an oral glucose tolerance test, and their family members need to be tested for urinary glucose. Educational materials, based on culturally appropriate terminology and concepts, need to be developed for these Asian Pacific American patients to aid them in identifying symptoms of both NIDDM (excess weight, blurred vision, numbness in feet and hands, skin infections, slow healing of wounds) and IDDM (frequent urination, excessive thirst, hunger, rapid weight loss, fatigue and weakness). Furthermore, these materials should be graphically informative regarding pathological outcomes of uncontrolled diabetes—retinopathy, nephropathy, neuropathy, and amputation of limbs—to help these patients make informed decisions and comply with treatments.

Health educators must learn to stress diet/food guidelines and patterns of physical activity that are congruent with Asian Pacific Americans' cultural expectations and experiences. Only if appropriate cultural dietary practices are reinforced along culturally acceptable lines, rather than taught through Western concepts and ways, will such guidelines be accepted and followed by any significant proportion of ethnic minority groups. Many members of Asian Pacific ethnic groups residing in the United States today came from areas where subsistence agriculture is an integral aspect of daily life, where a village market is the source for daily purchase and/or exchange of fresh meats, fish, vegetables, and fruits to supplement homegrown foods; refrigerators and freezers are recent innovations; and a person's day may include high levels of physical activity, such as gardening, chopping, and walking. Health educators who stress culturally inappropriate diet or activity patterns are not going to see compliance. For many Asian Pacific Americans, food choices and the preparation and consumption of food are culturally significant events, and the offering of food and drink to friends and other guests is considered a requirement rather than a nicety of social interaction. However, switching from high-fiber, low-calorie food staples such as taro, banana, yam, and breadfruit to low-fiber, high-calorie foods such as cake, pie, meat, chips and other snack items, and alcohol as socially appropriate foods increases calorie consumption while decreasing nutrition, and may significantly influence weight and obesity patterns in people adopting a sedentary lifestyle. Similarly, a switch from group social activities such as dancing, fishing, and hunting to TV watching, video game playing, and other sedentary behaviors reduces caloric expenditures and adversely influences physical fitness.

Among Korean Americans, Han (1990) reports that only 17% of adults exercise regularly, with twice as many men (23%) as women (11.5%) reporting regular exercise. These figures are only one third and one fifth the proportions, respectively, of Anglo American men and women who report regular exercise. Han also reports that the consumption of American-style foods increases with duration of residence in the United States. In particular, the intake of rice decreases and intakes of fruit, beef, pork, poultry, dairy, and vegetables increase. It would also be interesting to know the degree to which frying, particularly in saturated oils, increases in these populations and what types of vegetables and fruits are being eaten.

In the Wai'anae Diet Program a culturally appropriate diet including only pre-Western-contact traditional Hawaiian foods was developed for 20 obese Native Hawaiians (Shintani, Hughes, Beckman, & O'Conner, 1991). One aspect of the program was that participants could eat as much as they desired of traditional Native Hawaiian foods, with limitation only on the amount of fish eaten daily. Over a period of 21 days on this diet, with calories distributed as 7% fat, 78% complex carbohydrates, and 15% protein, all measured chronic disease risk factors decreased and weight loss averaged 7.8 kg (17.2 lb.), about 0.4 kg (0.8 lb.) per day.

Obesity in Asian Pacific Americans likely begins in childhood, as it does in most populations. For instance, among Japanese boys and girls studied at birth and ages 3, 6, 11, 14, and 17 years, obesity at age 17 was related to body habitus at birth in girls and at age 3 in boys (Muramatsu, Sato, Miyao, Muramatsu, & Ito, 1990). Such data indicate that strategies to prevent obesity in Asian Pacific Americans should begin early in life and that adult education needs to stress that parents are responsible for proper diet and physical fitness among their children.

Asian Pacific Americans need special health promotion programs and funding for research projects to study obesity and diabetes in their communities. One "myth" that needs to be either challenged or refuted is that Asian Pacific Americans have greater extended family support available to them than do similar African, Anglo, and Hispanic Americans. It is highly possible that although Asian Pacific Americans do have more support within extended families, the support may become impotent within the Western socioeconomic context. Private organizations may need first to document the need for special health programs through directed research before the federal government will be convinced of the health problems posed by obesity and diabetes in these groups. Health maintenance in Asian Pacific Americans is a legitimate societal concern and should involve cooperation between traditional and biomedical healers, organization of local health offices, and development of Asian Pacific health maintenance organizations. At present, health care for Asian Pacific Americans is fragmented, thus it is difficult to determine the extent of health problems. The need for integrated health care services and reporting of morbid conditions for documentation of the extent of obesity and diabetes cannot be overemphasized; however, without additional pressure on state and local governments to count their Asian Pacific populations, even these activities will not ensure adequate data. Development of integrated health care would allow greater emphasis on culturally appropriate strategies, provide linguistically appropriate services, and link policy decisions and objectives for health to the development of primary prevention strategies in the various Asian Pacific American communities. In addition, these activities would stimulate expansion of research activities as data are centralized and provide better information to policy makers.

Future Research

Health research among Asian Pacific American communities has not proceeded to the extent that it has among the white, black, Hispanic, and Native American communities. There are likely several interacting factors that have led to this lack. Many health administrators are not aware that Asian Pacific Americans have major health disadvantages. This makes it necessary for those concerned with the health of the population to conceive and design research projects to document the extent of obesity and diabetes in these communities. One strategy could be collaborative research projects between university-based investigators and community-based advocacy organizations to gather preliminary data.

Another reason health research among Asian Pacific Americans has not proceeded as rapidly as some might like is the pace at which federal bureaucracies react to emerging problems. Many research priorities of the National Institutes of Health were developed before the recent large immigrations of Asians and Pacific Islanders to the United States, and after scarce research dollars were allocated to long-term health research among Anglo Americans, African Americans, Alaskan Natives, American Indians, and Hispanic Americans. In addition, there are few U.S.-based Asian Pacific health researchers working on these problems in their own communities, and therefore the preliminary data to establish clearly that a health problem exists have heretofore not been compiled in a readily available format.

It is past time to begin well-designed studies of the prevalence and incidence of obesity and diabetes in as many Asian Pacific American populations as possible. Such studies are necessary to establish the need for a long-term commitment to the joint problems of diet, exercise, obesity, and diabetes in the community. Once present and future estimates of the extent of obesity and diabetes in these groups and their associations with lifestyle are available, long-term surveillance and intervention funding should become available to establish cross-sectional and longitudinal risk factors and to determine whether there are unique determinants of obesity and diabetes in these populations.

Summary

Although the material presented here does not represent a complete and exhaustive review of the available literature on obesity and diabetes on all Asian Pacific groups, the data reviewed do illustrate several salient points regarding the prevalence of these health problems in Asian Pacific Americans. Asian Pacific individuals appear to be at high risk for both obesity and NIDDM when they migrate to "Westernized" areas, whether in the United States or elsewhere, or take on the lifestyle associated with "Westernization" in their native lands. Whether in Eluru, India, or in England, Fiji, Tanzania, or Singapore, Asian Indians show prevalence rates of NIDDM that are very similar to those of African American men aged 45 and older but still less than rates among African American women aged 55 to 64 (Tables 6.4 and 6.7). In addition, every migrant Asian Indian population shows rates of diabetes that exceed those of the native populations alongside whom they reside (Table 6.7). Data to make similar comparisons with Asian Indians in the United States are lacking. However, it is clear that Japanese Americans, Korean Americans, Samoan Americans, and Native Hawaiians, at ages 40+, 40+, 30+, and 40+ years, respectively, show prevalence rates of NIDDM that approach those of U.S. blacks of similar age (Table 6.2). Indeed, at ages 50 to 59, Native Hawaiians show prevalence rates that are double those of U.S. whites at ages 55 to 64, approximate those of African American women at ages 55 to 64, and are 65% of the rates observed among Pima Indians aged 20 years and older (Table 6.4). Japanese American men and women also show rates of NIDDM at ages 40 to 59 (19.4 and 9.8) that exceed those of Anglo Americans at ages 45 to 59 years (7.7 and 8.5) and that are twice rates among native Japanese. Although data on the prevalence of obesity in Asian Pacific Americans remain scarce, obesity has been documented as a major problem among Pacific Islanders. More than 60% of Samoan and Native Hawaiian men and women are defined as obese according to commonly accepted criteria, and NIDDM is a major health problem in both groups. Similar data are needed on other Asian Pacific groups, particularly given that in both London and Singapore Asian residents show rates of obesity that equal or exceed those among Anglo Americans (Table 6.2).

In order to determine the extent of the dual problems of obesity and diabetes in Asian Pacific Americans, researchers need to take several steps as soon as possible. The most immediate need, aside from treatment to save lives, is for cross-sectional surveys of representative samples of as many of the Asian Pacific American groups listed in Table 6.8 as possible using standard protocols to determine weight, height, skinfolds, percentage body fat, fat distribution, fasting and challenged serum glucose and insulin, and blood pressure, so that the extent of obesity and diabetes and their sequelae may be documented. The second need is for the establishment of longitudinal studies of relationships among obesity and NIDDM and cultural practices, diet, exercise, access to health care, and health practices, along with testing of treatment modalities and their applications, within several Asian Pacific American communities. A third need is for the establishment of federally funded ethnically based health consulting agencies in each community to help persons at high risk to access needed health care and obtain ethnically appropriate treatment and lifestyle (diet, exercise) advice. Finally, integration of health care services in Asian Pacific American communities is needed to document and report the extent of obesity and NIDDM in each ethnic group.

In closing, it seems appropriate not only to echo Klatsky and Armstrong's (1991) recent call for efforts focused on weight control in Asian men, but also to urge that such efforts be extended to include Asian women along with Pacific Islander American men and women. To recommend a return to a more "natural" or "traditional" diet may seem trite and overly simplistic, but results among Native Hawaiians and Native Americans indicate that such practical modifications work to reduce obesity. Furthermore, regenerating traditional native foodways can be a source of self-esteem and cultural pride in such communities. Our national government has an opportunity to take the lead in these areas by supporting activities that encourage reduced consumption of refined and highly processed foods, while promoting consumption of more natural foods, and that encourage increased physical activity of all Americans.

References

ACCIS Program & the Asian and Pacific Islander American Health Forum. (1991). U.S. Bureau of the Census, STF1A-1991, Magnetic Media.
Allawi, J., Rao, P. V., Gilbert, R., Scott, G., Jarrett, R. J., Keen, H., Viberti, G. C., & Mather, H. M. (1988). Microalbuminuria in non-insulin dependent diabetes: Its

prevalence in Indians compared with Europid patients. *British Medical Journal (Clinical Research), 296,* 462-464.

Aluli, N. E. (1991). Prevalence of diabetes in a Native Hawaiian population. *American Journal of Clinical Nutrition, 53*(Suppl. 6), 1556S-1560S.

Andres, R. (1971). Aging and diabetes. *Medical Clinics of North America, 55,* 835-845.

Asian and Pacific Islander American Health Forum. (1991). *AAHF policy papers: Dispelling the myth of a healthy minority.* San Francisco: Author.

Baker, P. T. (1984). Migrations, genetics, and the degenerative diseases of South Pacific Islanders. In A. Boyce (Ed.), *Migration and mobility* (pp. 209-239). London: Taylor & Francis.

Baker, P. T., & Crews, D. E. (1986). Mortality patterns and some biological predictors. In P. T. Baker, J. M. Hanna, & T. S. Baker (Eds.), *The changing Samoans: Behavior and health in transition* (pp. 93-122). New York: Oxford University Press.

Bindon, J. R., Crews, D. E., & Dressler, W. W. (1991). Life style, blood pressure, and blood glucose interrelations in American Samoan men. *American Journal of Physical Anthropology, 73*(Suppl. 12), 51. (Abstract)

Bouchard, C. (1991). Current understanding of the etiology of obesity: Genetic and nongenetic factors. *American Journal of Clinical Nutrition, 53*(Suppl. 6), 1561S-1565S.

Bunnag, S. C., Sitthi-Amorn, C., & Chandraprasert, S. (1990). The prevalence of obesity, risk factors and associated diseases in Klong Toey slum and Klong Toey government apartment houses. *Diabetes Research and Clinical Practice, 10*(Suppl. 1), S81-S87.

Cheah, J. S., Wang, K. W., & Sum, C. F. (1990). Epidemiology of diabetes mellitus in the Asia-Pacific region. *Annals of the Academy of Medicine, 19,* 501-505.

Chen, A., Lew, R., Okahara, L., Ko, K., & Hirota, S. (1990, November 15-17). *Identification of high risk Asian Pacific American subgroups in a population-based survey.* Paper presented at the Third Biennial Forum of the Asian and Pacific Islander American Health Forum, "Asian Pacific: Dispelling the Myth of a Healthy Minority," Bethesda, MD. (Abstract)

Cox, N. J., Epstein, P. A., & Spielman, R. S. (1989). Linkage studies on NIDDM and the insulin and insulin-receptor genes. *Diabetes, 38,* 653-658.

Crews, D. E. (1988a). Body weight, blood pressure and the risk of total and cardiovascular mortality in an obese population. *Human Biology, 60,* 417-433.

Crews, D. E. (1988b). Multiple causes of death and the epidemiological transition in American Samoa. *Social Biology, 35,* 198-213.

Crews, D. E. (1990). Anthropological issues in biological gerontology. In R. L. Rubinstein (Ed.), *Anthropology and aging: Comprehensive reviews* (pp. 11-38). Boston: Kluwer Academic.

Crews, D. E., Bindon, J. R., McCuddin, C. R., & Puletasi, A. (1991). Health promotion and disease prevention in Samoan populations [Abstract]. In *Towards the Pacific century: The challenge of change* (Proceedings of the XVII Pacific Science Congress) (p. 23). Honolulu: East-West Center.

Crews, D. E., Bindon, J. R., & Ozeran, J. E. S. (1991). Associations of body habitus with diabetes, glucose, and glycated hemoglobin in American Samoans. *Diabetes, 40*(Suppl. 1), 433A. (Abstract)

Crews, D. E., & Gerber, L. M. (1993). Aging and chronic degenerative diseases. In D. E. Crew & R. M. Garruto (Eds.), *Biological anthropology and aging: Perspectives on human variation over the life span* (pp. 154-181). New York: Oxford University Press.

Crews, D. E., & MacKeen, P. C. (1982). Mortality related to cardiovascular diseases and diabetes mellitus in a modernizing population. *Social Science and Medicine, 16,* 175-181.

Curb, J. D., Aluli, N. E., Kautz, J. A., Petrovitch, H., Knutsen, S. F., Knutsen, R., O'Conner, H. K., & O'Conner, W. E. (1991). Cardiovascular risk factor levels in ethnic Hawaiians. *American Journal of Public Health, 81,* 164-167.

Curb, J. D., & Marcus, E. B. (1991a). Body fat and obesity in Japanese men. *American Journal of Clinical Nutrition, 53*(Suppl. 6), 1552S-1555S.

Curb, J. D., & Marcus, E. B. (1991b). Body fat, coronary heart disease, and stroke in Japanese men. *American Journal of Clinical Nutrition, 53*(Suppl. 6), 1612S-1615S.

Davidson, J. K. (1986). The effective approach and management of diabetes in black and other minority groups. In *Report of the Secretary's Task Force on Black and Minority Health: Vol. 7. Chemical dependency and diabetes.* Washington, DC: U.S. Department of Health and Human Services (vol. VII, pp. 297-355).

Dowse, G. K., Gareeboo, H., Zimmet, P., Alberti, K. G. M. M., Tuomilehto, J., Fareed, D., Brissonnette, L. G., & Finch, C. F. (1990). High prevalence of NIDDM and impaired glucose tolerance in Indian, Creole, and Chinese Mauritians. *Diabetes, 39,* 390-396.

Dowse, G. K., Zimmet, P., Gareeboo, H., Alberti, K. G. M. M., Tuomilehto, J., Finch, C. F., Chitson, P., & Tulsidas, H. (1991). Abdominal obesity and physical inactivity as risk factors for NIDDM and impaired glucose tolerance in Indian, Creole, and Chinese Mauritians. *Diabetes Care, 14,* 271-282.

Dressler, W. A. (1991). Social class, skin color, and arterial blood pressure in two societies. *Ethnicity and Disease, 1,* 60-77.

Foster, D. W. (1989). Diabetes mellitus. In C. R. Scriver, A. L. Beaudet, W. S. Sly, S. D. Valle (Eds.), *The metabolic basis of inherited disease* (6th ed., pp. 375-397). New York: McGraw-Hill.

Fujimoto, W. Y. (1985). Diabetes in Asian Americans. In M. Harris & R. F. Hamman (Eds.), *Diabetes in America: Diabetes data compiled 1984* (National Diabetes Data Group, Publication No. NIH 85-1468) (pp. X1-X12). Washington, DC: Government Printing Office.

Fujimoto, W. Y., Hershon, K., Kinyoun, J., Stolov, W. C., Weinberg, C., Ishiwata, K., Kahinuma, H., Kanazawa, N., & Kuzuya, N. (1983). Type II diabetes in Seattle and Tokyo. *Tohoku Journal of Experimental Medicine, 141*(Suppl.), 133-139.

Fujimoto, W. Y., Leonetti, D. L., Kinyoun, J. L., Newell-Morris, L., Shuman, W. P., Stolov, W. C., & Wahl, P. W. (1987a). Prevalence of diabetes mellitus and impaired glucose tolerance among second-generation Japanese-American men. *Diabetes, 36,* 721-729.

Fujimoto, W. Y., Leonetti, D. L., Kinyoun, J. L., Shuman, W. P., Stolov, W. C., & Wahl, P. W. (1987b). Prevalence of complications among second-generation Japanese-American men: Diabetes, impaired glucose tolerance, or normal glucose tolerance. *Diabetes, 36,* 730-739.

Garn, S. M. (1993). Fat, lipid and blood pressure changes in adult years. In D. E. Crews & R. M. Garruto (Eds.), *Biological anthropology and aging: Perspectives on human variation over the life span* (pp. 301-320). New York: Oxford University Press.

Garn, S. M., Bailey, S. M., & Block, W. D. (1979). Relationship between fatness and lipid levels in adults. *American Journal of Clinical Nutrition, 32,* 733-735.

Garn, S. M., Sullivan, T. V., & Hawthorne, V. M. (1989). The education of one spouse and the fatness of the other spouse. *American Journal of Human Biology, 1,* 223-238.

Grabauskas, V. J. (1988). Glucose intolerance as contributor to noncommunicable disease morbidity and mortality: WHO integrated program for community health in noncommunicable diseases. *Diabetes Care, 11,* 253-257.

Han, E. (1990, November 15-17). *Korean health survey in Southern California: A preliminary report on health status and health care needs of Korean immigrants.* Paper presented at the Third Biennial Forum of the Asian and Pacific Islander American Health Forum, "Asian Pacific: Dispelling the Myth of a Healthy Minority," Bethesda, MD. (Abstract)

Harris, M., & Hamman, R. F. (Eds.). (1985). *Diabetes in America: Diabetes data compiled 1984* (National Diabetes Data Group, Publication No. NIH 85-1468). Washington, DC: Government Printing Office.

Harris, M. I., Hadden, W. C., Knowler, W. C., & Bennett, P. H. (1987). Prevalence of diabetes and impaired glucose tolerance and plasma glucose levels in U.S. population aged 20-74 years. *Diabetes, 36,* 523-534.

Helmrich, S. P., Ragland, D. R., Leung, R. W., & Paffenbarger, R. S. (1991). Physical activity and reduced occurrence of non-insulin-dependent diabetes mellitus. *New England Journal of Medicine, 325,* 147-152.

Hughes, K., Yeo, P. P., Lun, K. C., Thai, A. C., Wang, K. W., & Cheah, J. S. (1990). Obesity and body mass indices in Chinese, Malays, and Indians in Singapore. *Annals of the Academy of Medicine, Singapore, 19,* 333-338.

Japan Diabetes Society, Committee on Diabetic Twins. (1988). Diabetes mellitus in twins: A cooperative study in Japan. *Diabetes Research and Clinical Practice, 5,* 271-280.

Kagan, A., Harris, B. R., Winkelstein, W., Jr., Johnson, K. G., Kata, H., Syme, S. L., Rhoads, H. H., Gay, M. L., Nichaman, M. Z., Hamilton, H. B., & Tillotson, J. (1974). Epidemiologic studies of coronary heart disease and stroke in Japanese men living in Japan, Hawaii, and California: Demographic, physical, dietary, and biochemical characteristics. *Journal of Chronic Disease, 27,* 345-364.

Kawate, R., Yamakido, M., & Nishimoto, Y. (1980). Migrant studies among the Japanese in Hiroshima and Hawaii. In W. K. Waldhausel (Ed.), *Diabetes 1970: Proceedings of the 10th Congress of the International Diabetes Federation* (pp. 526-531). Amsterdam: Excerpta Medica.

King, H., & Zimmet, P. (1988). Trends in the prevalence and incidence of diabetes: Non-insulin-dependent diabetes mellitus. *World Health Statistical Quarterly, 41,* 190-196.

Kissebah, A. H., Peiris, A., & Evans, D. J. (1988). Mechanisms associating body fat distribution to glucose intolerance and diabetes mellitus. In C. Bouchard & F. E. Johnson (Eds.), *Fat distribution during growth and later health outcomes* (pp. 203-229). New York: Alan R. Liss.

Klaff, L. J., & Palmer, J. P. (1986). Risks for glucose intolerance. *Cardiology Clinics, 4,* 67-73.

Klatsky, A. L., & Armstrong, M. A. (1991). Cardiovascular risk factors among Asian Americans living in Northern California. *American Journal of Public Health, 81,* 1423-1428.

Knowler, W. C., Pettit, D. J., Savage, P. J., & Bennett, P. F. (1981). Diabetes incidence in Pima Indians: Contributions of obesity and parental diabetes. *American Journal of Epidemiology, 113,* 144-156.

Lipton, R. B., & LaPorte, R. E. (1989). Epidemiology of islet cell antibodies. *Epidemiologic Reviews, 11,* 182-203.

Martin, B. (1990, August 28-29). *Obesity, hypertension, and diabetes mellitus in Native Hawaiians.* Paper presented at the NIH-NHLBI sponsored conference, "Obesity and Cardiovascular Disease in Minority Populations," Bethesda, MD. (Abstract)

Mather, H. M., & Keen, H. (1985). The Southall diabetes survey: Prevalence of known diabetes in Asians and Europeans. *British Medical Journal, 291,* 1081-1084.

McGarvey, S. T., Bindon, J. R., Crews, D. E., & Schendel, D. E. (1989). Modernization and adiposity: Causes and consequences. In M. A. Little & J. D. Hass (Eds.), *Human population biology: A transdisciplinary science* (pp. 263-279). New York: Oxford University Press.

McKeigue, P. M., Shah, B., & Marmot, M. G. (1991). Relation of central obesity and insulin resistance with high diabetes prevalence and cardiovascular risk in South Asians. *Lancet, 337,* 382-386.

McLarty, D. G., Pollitt, C., & Swai, A. B. M. (1990). Diabetes in Africa. *Diabetic Medicine, 7,* 670-684.

Mohan, V., Sharp, P. S., Cloke, H. R., Burrin, J. M., Schumer, B., & Kohner, E. M. (1986). Serum immunoreactive insulin responses to a glucose load in Asian Indians and European Type 2 (non-insulin dependent) diabetic patients and control subjects. *Diabetologia, 24,* 235-237.

Muramatsu, S., Sato, Y., Miyao, M., Muramatsu, T., & Ito, A. (1990). A longitudinal study of obesity in Japan: Relationship of body habitus between at birth and at age 17. *International Journal of Obesity, 14,* 39-45.

Najjar, M. F., & Rowland, M. (1987). *Anthropometric reference data and prevalence of overweight: United States, 1976-1980* (National Center for Health Statistics, Vital and Health Statistics, Series 11, No. 238, DHHS Publication No. PHS 87-1688). Washington, DC: Government Printing Office.

Newell-Morris, L., Treder, R. P., Shuman, W. P., & Fujimoto, W. Y. (1989). Fatness, fat distribution and glucose tolerance in second-generation Japanese-American (Nisei) men. *American Journal of Clinical Nutrition, 50,* 9-18.

Newman, B., Selby, J. V., King, M.-C., Siemenda, C., Fabsitz, R., & Friedman, G. D. (1987). Concordance for type 2 (non-insulin-dependent) diabetes mellitus in male twins. *Diabetologia, 30,* 763-768.

Nomura, M., Iwama, N., Mukai, M., Saito, Y., Kawamori, R., Shichiri, M., & Kamada, T. (1986). High frequency of class 3 allele in the human insulin gene in Japanese type 2 (non-insulin dependent) diabetic patients with a family history of diabetes. *Diabetologia, 29,* 402-404.

Office of Minority Health. (1986). Black and minority health: Report of the Subcommittee on Diabetes. In *Report of the Secretary's Task Force on Black and Minority Health: Vol. 7. Chemical dependency and diabetes* (pp. 191-293). Washington, DC: U.S. Department of Health and Human Services.

Office of Minority Health, Resource Center. (1989). *Closing the gap.* Washington, DC: Author.

Ohno, M., Ikeda, Y., & Abe, M. (1990). Role of obesity in the development of NIDDM. In J. Köbberling (Ed.), *Proceedings of the First Congress on the Clinico-Genetics Genesis of Diabetes Mellitus* (pp. 324-333). Göttingen.

Omar, M. A. K., Seedat, M. A., Dyer, R. B., Rajpu, M. C., Motala, A. A., & Joubert, S. M. (1985). The prevalence of diabetes mellitus in a large group of South African Indians. *South African Medical Journal, 67,* 924-926.

Osei, K. (1990). Predicting Type II diabetes in persons at risk. *Annals of Internal Medicine, 113,* 905-906.

Pawson, I. G. (1986). The morphological characteristics of Samoan adults. In P. T. Baker, J. M. Hanna, & T. S. Baker (Eds.), *The changing Samoans: Behavior and health in transition* (pp. 254-274). New York: Oxford University Press.

Pawson, I. G., & Janes, C. (1981). Massive obesity in a migrant Samoan population. *American Journal of Public Health, 71,* 508-513.

Pi-Sunyer, F. X. (1990). Obesity and diabetes in blacks. *Diabetes Care, 13*(Suppl. 4), 1144-1149.

Ramaiya, K. L., Kodali, V. R., & Alberti, K. G. (1990). Epidemiology of diabetes in Asians of the Indian subcontinent. *Diabetes/Metabolism Reviews, 6,* 125-146.

Rao, P. V., Ushabala, P., Seshiah, V., Ahuja, M. M., & Mather, H. M. (1989). The Eluru survey: Prevalence of known diabetes in a rural Indian population. *Diabetes Research and Clinical Practice, 7,* 29-31.

Rewers, M., LaPorte, R. E., King, H., & Tuomilehto, J. (1988). Trends in the prevalence and incidence of diabetes: Insulin-dependent diabetes mellitus in childhood. *World Health Statistical Quarterly, 41,* 179-189.

Sekikawa, A., Tominaga, M., & Sasaki, H. (1991). Prevalence of diabetes mellitus in Oguni Town Yamagata, Japan. *Diabetes, 40*(Suppl. 1), 433A. (Abstract)

Selby, J. V., Newman, B., Queensbury, C. P., Jr., Fabsitz, R. R., King, M.-C., & Meaney, F. J. (1989). Evidence of genetic influence of central body fat in middle-aged twins. *Human Biology, 61,* 179-193.

Shintani, T. T., Hughes, C. K., Beckman, S., & O'Conner, H. K. (1991). Obesity and cardiovascular risk intervention through the ad libitum feeding of traditional Hawaiian diet. *American Journal of Clinical Nutrition, 53*(Suppl. 6), 1647S-1651S.

Sloan, N. R. (1963). Ethnic distribution of diabetes mellitus in Hawaii. *Journal of the American Medical Association, 183,* 419-442.

Swai, A. B. M., McLarty, D. G., Sherrif, F., Chuwa, L. M., Maro, E., Lukmanji, Z., Kermali, W., Mekene, W., & Alberti, G. M. M. (1990). Diabetes and impaired glucose tolerance in an Asian community in Tanzania. *Diabetes Research and Clinical Practice, 8,* 227-234.

Takeda, J., Seino, Y., Fukumoto, H., Koh, G., Otsuka, A., Ikeda, M., Kuno, S., Yawata, M., Moridera, K., Morita, T., & Imura, H. (1986). The polymorphism linked to the human insulin gene: Its lack of association with either IDDM or NIDDM in Japanese. *Acta Endrocrinol* (Copenhagen), *113,* 268-271.

Temple, R. C., Carrington, C. A., Luzio, S. D., Owens, D. R., Schneider, A. E., Sobey, W. J., & Hales, C. N. (1989, February). Insulin deficiency in non-insulin-dependent diabetes. *Lancet, 11,* 293-295.

Thai, A. C., Yeo, P. P. B., Lun, K. C., Hughes, K., Wang, K. W., Sothy, S. P., Lui, K. F., Ng, W. Y., Cheah, J. S., Phoon, W. O., & Lim, P. (1987). Changing prevalence of diabetes mellitus in Singapore over a ten-year period. In *Epidemiology of diabetes mellitus: Proceedings of the International Symposium on Epidemiology of Diabetes Mellitus* (pp. 63-67). Bangkok: Crystal House.

Tsunehara, C. H., Leonetti, D. L., & Fujimoto, W. Y. (1990). Diet of second- generation Japanese-American men with and without non-insulin dependent diabetes. *American Journal of Clinical Nutrition, 52,* 731-738.

U.S. Bureau of the Census. (1973). *1970 census of population: Vol. 1. Characteristics of the population.* Washington, DC: Government Printing Office.

U.S. Bureau of the Census. (1983). *1980 census of population: Vol. 1. Characteristics of the population.* Washington, DC: Government Printing Office.

Vague, J. (1956). The degree of masculine differentiation of obesities: A factor determining predisposition to diabetes, atherosclerosis, gout, and uric acid calculous disease. *American Journal of Clinical Nutrition, 4,* 20-34.

Vague, J., Björntrop, P., Guy-Grand, B., Rebuffe-Scrive, M., & Vague, P. (Eds.). (1985). *Metabolic complications of human obesities.* Amsterdam: Excerpta Medica.

Verma, N. P. S., Mehta, S. P., Madhu, S., Mather, H. M., & Keen, H. (1986). Prevalence of known diabetes in an urban Indian environment: The Darya Ganj diabetes survey. *British Medical Journal, 293,* 423-424.

Waspadji, S., Ranakusuma, A. B., Suyono, S., Supartondo, S., & Sukaton, U. (1983). Diabetes mellitus in an urban population in Jakarta, Indonesia. *Tohuku Journal of Experimental Medicine, 141*(Suppl.), 219-228.

West, K. (1978). *Epidemiology of diabetes and its vascular lesions.* New York: Elsevier.

Woo, J., Swaminathan, R., Cockram, C., Pang, C. P., Au, S. Y., & Vallance-Owen, J. (1987). The prevalence of diabetes mellitus and an assessment of methods of detection among a community of elderly Chinese in Hong Kong. *Diabetologia, 30,* 863-868.

World Health Organization. (1985). *Diabetes mellitus: Report of a WHO study group* (Tech. Rep. Series 727). Geneva: Author.

Xiang, K. S., Cox, N. J., Sanz, N., Haung, P., Karam, J. H., & Bell, G. I. (1989). Insulin-receptor and apolipoprotein genes contribute to development of NIDDM in Chinese Americans. *Diabetes, 38,* 17-23.

Yano, K., Kagan, A., McGee, D., & Rhoads, G. G. (1982). Glucose intolerance and nine-year mortality in Japanese men in Hawaii. *American Journal of Medicine, 72,* 71-80.

Yu, F., Chang, C. F., Liu, W., & Kan, S. (n.d.). *Asian-white mortality differentials.* Unpublished manuscript, commissioned by the Subcommittee on Diabetes of the Task Force on Black and Minority Health.

Zimmet, P. (1979). Epidemiology of diabetes and its macrovascular manifestations in Pacific populations: The medical effects of social progress. *Diabetes Care, 2,* 144-153.

Zimmet, P., Faaisu, S., Ainuu, J., Whitehouse, S., Milne, B., & DeBoer, W. (1981). The prevalence of diabetes in the rural and urban populations of Western Samoa. *Diabetes, 30,* 45-51.

Zimmet, P., Taylor, R., Ram, P., King, H., Sloman, G., Raper, L. R., & Hunt, R. (1983). Prevalence of diabetes and impaired glucose tolerance in the biracial (Melanesian and Indian) community of Fiji: A rural-urban comparison. *American Journal of Epidemiology, 118,* 673-688.

7

Hypertension and
Other Cardiovascular Risk Factors

AYALA TAMIR
SHIRLEY CACHOLA

There has been a dramatic decline in the death rate owing to cardiovascular disease (diseases of the heart and the blood vessels) during the past 15 years, but this disease is still the main cause of death in the United States. The mortality rate for cardiovascular disease (primarily consisting of coronary heart disease and stroke cases) is nearly the same as the combined rate of all other diseases (National Center for Health Statistics, 1990a). Diseases of the heart are the leading cause of death among Asian Pacific Americans in California. According to California vital statistics data from 1989, Japanese have the highest death rate from diseases of the heart, and Filipinos have the highest numbers of death from this cause. Rate of death from diseases of the heart is higher among Asian Pacific Americans (82 cases per 100,000) than among Hispanic (63 cases per 100,000) Americans, although lower than that for white and African Americans. Table 7.1 and Figure 7.1 describe the prevalence of diseases of the heart among Asian Pacific populations in California in 1989.

There is common agreement that a large proportion of coronary deaths can be prevented through the application of existing knowledge concerning risk factors, but there is still debate over what is the best approach. Those who favor the *population approach* suggest

Table 7.1 Diseases of the Heart: Primary Leading Cause of Death Among
Asian Pacific Americans in California, 1989

Race or Ethnicity	Number of Deaths From Diseases of the Heart	1990 Population in California[a]	Rate of Death From Diseases of the Heart per 100,000 of the Population C/D × 100,000
Japanese	447	312,989	143
Other Pacific Islander	22	19,176	115
Filipino	758	731,685	104
Samoan	32	31,917	100
Chinese	694	704,850	98
Hawaiian	27	34,447	78
Guamanian	14	25,059	56
Asian specified[b]	30	58,058	52
Cambodian	19	68,190	28
Vietnamese	60	280,223	21
Thai	5	32,064	16
Asian and Pacific Islander	2,335	2,845,659	82
Other	215	4,181,234	5
Hispanic	4,875	7,687,938	63
African American	5,267	2,208,801	238
White	56,765	20,524,327	277
Total	69,457	29,760,021	

NOTES: a. U.S. Census population data for 1990 were used as a denominator, as no 1989
population data estimates were available.
b. Includes Laotians and others presumed to be Laotians.

providing health education to the general population, whereas
proponents of the *high-risk approach* would selectively focus on
individuals at particular risk. The population approach can be
successfully applied among populations who are not aware of their
existing risks, such as recent Southeast Asians immigrants to the
United States. The high-risk approach can be applied in more
clinically based settings. In applying this approach, the focus is less
on risk factors that cannot be modified, such as age, gender, and
heredity, and more on risk factors that can be reduced through
changes in lifestyle and personal habits, such as cigarette smoking,
hypercholesterolemia, and hypertension. Development in statistical measurement, analysis, and evaluation has made possible the

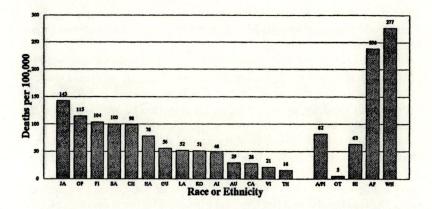

Figure 7.1. Diseases of the Heart: Primary Leading Cause of Death Among Asians and Pacific Islanders in California

SOURCES: California Department of Health Services and U.S. Bureau of the Census. Copyright 1992 Asian and Pacific Islander American Health Forum, Inc. Reprinted by permission.

assessment of separate and combined influences of different risk factors. However, because the causes of heart disease are complex and incompletely understood, it is difficult to distinguish between the direct and indirect risk factors that affect the prevalence of cardiovascular disease. To some extent, all risk factors are linked and influence each other. The purpose of this chapter is to examine each of the major risk factors for cardiovascular disease—namely, hypertension, smoking, hypercholesterolemia, high alcohol consumption, and lack of physical activity—as each relates to the Asian Pacific American populations in the United States.

Hypertension

Hypertension, an elevation in normal blood pressure, is a leading cause of stroke, renal disease, and cardiac disease for all populations in the United States. Most medical studies define hypertension as a condition in which the systolic blood pressure is equal to or exceeds 140 mmHg and the diastolic blood pressure is equal to or more than 90 mmHg. Also, a person taking antihypertensive medications is defined as hypertensive. According to this definition, approximately

30% of the adults in the United States have high blood pressure (National Heart, Lung and Blood Institute, 1985). Hypertension is the most frequent medical disorder for which physician visits are generated and prescriptions written. It is also one of the major modifiable risk factors in prevention of cardiovascular disease mortality. Thus hypertension is one of the most serious public health problems in the developed world, and it is treated or avoided by both pharmacological and nonpharmacological treatment.

Studies of hypertension in the general population have shown that there is a tendency for blood pressure to rise with age and that it is more common in lower socioeconomic groups. Males tend to have a higher prevalence of hypertension in younger age groups, whereas females have a higher prevalence of hypertension in older age groups. Hypertension tends to run in families, suggesting a genetic influence. However, environmental factors have also been shown to play a significant, although controversial, role in the genesis of hypertension, particularly in the areas of excessive calorie and salt intake.

The rapid growth of Asian Pacific ethnic populations in the United States over the past two decades represents a great need for more research in this area. This review of hypertension among Asian Pacific American populations will include recent data on the biological and environmental factors involved in hypertension. For Asian Pacific Americans, hypertension is influenced by changes in acculturation, psychosocial, demographic and other factors. Most of the current information available has been drawn from studies done in Hawaii, California, and New York. These studies address the three major Asian American subgroups: Chinese, Japanese, and Filipino. There are also data available about Southeast Asian Americans (Bates, Hill, & Barrett-Connor, 1989; Centers for Disease Control, 1992). Variables such as age, gender, relative body weight, alcohol consumption, ethnicity, place of birth, level of education, and psychological contributors have been identified as having an impact on blood pressure level.

Age and Gender

Angel, Armstrong, and Klatsky (1989) indicate that in both sexes, increased age is significantly related to hypertension. This strong positive age-hypertension link was also found by Stavig, Igra, and Leonard (1984), who noted that it was particularly dominant among females in their sample. In Stavig et al.'s investigation, subjects who were one standard deviation above the mean of the variable age (54.7 years) had a 30.9% likelihood of being hypertensive, as opposed to 5.7% when the person is one standard deviation below the mean age (24.4 years). Generally, men had higher rates of hypertension than women, but when the effects of confounding variables were removed, gender was not found to have a significant effect.

A positive correlation between age and blood pressure levels was found across all of the various Asian Pacific populations. The American Heart Association (1991) reports on a study in which overall blood pressure levels among Japanese Americans were found to be lower than in Caucasians. However, depending on socioeconomic and demographic factors, the comparative rates of hypertension among Japanese men varied. For example, in the 18 to 49 age group, Japanese men in California had a higher prevalence rate of hypertension (19%) than did Caucasian men (15%), whereas in the 50+ age group it was lower (29% and 39%, respectively). Japanese women had a lower prevalence than Caucasian women in these two age groups.

Among 349 elderly (ages 60 to 96 years) Chinese immigrants in Boston, blood pressure levels were correlated with age and gender (Choi et al., 1990). The prevalence rate of hypertension was 30% among males and 34% among females. In addition, age correlated negatively with diastolic blood pressure in men and positively with systolic blood pressure in women. The prevalence of hypertension in this sample was 28%, similar to that of the elderly population in urban Mainland China (Wu, Lu, Gao, Yu, & Liu, 1982). This prevalence rate is much lower than the rate (39%) of elderly white Americans (Roberts & Maurer, 1977).

Similar relationships are reported by Bates et al. (1989), who examined blood pressure levels among Southeast Asians, a seldom-studied population among the various Asian Pacific American groups. The sample consisted of 55 men and 62 women, of whom 23 were Hmong, 44 Laotian, 45 Vietnamese, and 5 Cambodian. Moderate risk was defined as blood pressure ≥140/90 mmHg, and high risk was defined as blood pressure ≥165/95 mmHg. Mean systolic and diastolic blood pressure was significantly correlated with age. When analyzing the cardiovascular risk factor prevalence among these subjects at two categorically predetermined risk factors levels (moderate-high and high), the researchers found that hypertension was the most commonly defined risk factor among the sampled population:

27% had moderate-high risk and 14% had high risk. Lower prevalence rates for those two categories were found for hypercholesterolemia, cigarette smoking, and body mass index. Another study sampled 397 Southeast Asians in central Ohio (Chen, Kuun, Guthrie, Wen, & Zaharlick, 1991); 84% of the subjects were 49 years old or younger, and 45% overall were on Medicaid. Compared with 22% of the general population in Ohio who had high blood pressure ($\geq$140/90 mmHg), only 17% of the studied population was found to have hypertension. The reason for this comparably low prevalence might be the younger age group of the subjects in this study.

Relative Body Weight

Like age, elevation in body mass has been found to be significantly related to hypertension in both sexes (Angel et al., 1989). Stavig et al. (1984) found that a person whose body mass index was one standard deviation above the mean was estimated to have a 25.2% prevalence rate of uncontrolled hypertension as opposed to 11.4% when the person's body mass index was one standard deviation below the average. In this study, both Filipinos and "other Asians and Pacific Islanders" (those Asian Pacifics who are not Chinese, Japanese, or Filipino) had significantly higher rates of uncontrolled hypertension than did Chinese and Japanese Americans.

There is disagreement among researchers about the causes for hypertension among Asian Pacific populations. For example, comparatively low blood pressure was found among Filipinos in the Philippines, and some have argued that environmental rather than genetic factors contribute to the high rate of hypertension among Filipinos in California (Cabral, Gusman, & Estrada, 1981). However, in another study, hypertension was not found to be more prevalent among U.S.-born Filipinos (Angel et al., 1989), suggesting a nonenvironmental factor. Other research has suggested that the reason for high blood pressure among the Filipino population is partly connected to the proposed sodium-load handling hypothesis examined by Woods, West, Weissberg, and Beevers (1981). These researchers compared the level of activity of the red cell sodium pump among normotensive and hypertensive blacks and whites and found that white hypertensives had an increased level of activity of this pump compared with white normotensives. This difference was not observed between black normotensives and hypertensives.

These findings suggest that there are racial differences in sodium handling and in the pathophysiology of essential hypertension between whites and blacks.

Support for biological factors as the main contributors to high blood pressure has been provided by Reed, McGee, and Katsuhiko (1982). More than 8,000 Japanese men living in Hawaii were studied during a 6-year interval. The age-specific blood pressure of the Japanese in the Hawaiian cohort, when adjusted for relative weight, was similar to the Hiroshima-Nagasaki cohort, although the Japanese men from Hawaii were larger and ate more animal fat and protein (Kagan et al., 1974; Winkelstein, Kagan, Kato, & Sacks, 1975). Even 40 years after migration, the Japanese in the Hawaiian cohort had very similar blood pressure levels to those persons in the areas from which they emigrated. The findings of this study suggest that psychosocial variables have less influence on increasing blood pressure compared with biological determinants. As described previously, other studies have found that environmental factors affect levels of blood pressure (Cabral et al., 1981; Cassel, 1975; Shekelle, 1979), but Reed et al. (1982) claim these studies did not control for body weight.

Alcohol Consumption

Alcohol consumption has also been found to be positively correlated with elevated blood pressure levels, especially among the Filipino American population. One study indicated that alcohol intake that was one standard deviation above the average amount of alcohol consumption resulted in an estimated 22.6% prevalence rate of hypertension as opposed to 14% prevalence rate among persons with alcohol intake one standard deviation below the average (Stavig et al., 1984). Filipinos in that study averaged 1.62 alcoholic drinks per sitting, which is 0.33 above the Asian Pacific average. In another study it was found that for Filipino men, heavy alcohol intake (≥3 drinks/day) was also related to hypertension (Angel et al., 1989).

Ethnicity

Studies about hypertension that have surveyed the Filipino population in the United States indicate that this population has a higher prevalence for hypertension compared with the other Asian Pacific groups (Angel et al., 1989; Klatsky & Armstrong, 1991; Stavig et al., 1984). The study by Angel et al. (1989) included 11,684 Asian Pacific Americans who had health examinations offered by a Northern California prepaid health care program from 1978 to 1985. The ethnic groups in this study were 2,496 Chinese, 1,519 Filipino, 619 Japanese, and 498 other Asians. According to the definition used in this study for hypertension (systolic blood pressure ≥ 140 mmHg and diastolic blood pressure ≥ 90 mmHg), 580 men and 546 women were hypertensive. Filipinos had significantly higher adjusted mean systolic and diastolic blood pressure than each of the other Asian Pacific groups, except that Filipino men did not have higher diastolic blood pressure than Chinese men (75.5 ± 0.3 mmHg in both groups).

These data are similar to those found in an earlier study by Stavig et al. (1984) that examined hypertension among 8,353 adults in California in a statewide random probability household survey conducted in 1979. The primary goal was to obtain baseline estimates of the prevalence, awareness, and degree of control of hypertension in the total adult population of California and among four major racial-ethnic groups: whites (3,396), blacks (1,436), Asians and Pacifics (1,757), and Hispanics (1,764). The proportion with elevated blood pressure among Asian Pacific Americans was 18.3%, compared with 19.8% for the entire adult population. Among the specific Asian Pacific ethnic groups, Filipinos showed the highest rates of elevated blood pressure (24.5%), followed by "other Asians and Pacific Islanders" (20.1%), Chinese (15.7%), and Japanese (12.5%).

In a recent study of cardiovascular risk factors in Northern California, Klatsky and Armstrong (1991) collected data from 13,031 Asian Pacific respondents, resulting in a sample size that is perhaps the largest ever reported in the literature. The subjects were classified as 5,951 Chinese, 4,211 Filipinos, 1,703 Japanese, and 1,166 other Asians. As in most other research, hypertensives were classified as having blood pressure over 140/90 mmHg or on antihypertensive treatment. The adjusted mean systolic (124.4 ± 0.4 mmHg) and diastolic (75.5 ± 0.2 mmHg) blood pressure readings of Filipino males were significantly higher compared with all other Asian Pacific ethnic groups, except that Chinese males were found to have the same diastolic blood pressure as Filipino males. A similar pattern of results was also found for Filipino females (119.2 ± 0.3 and 72.9 ± 0.2 mmHg, respectively).

Most of the studies about Asian Pacific Americans and hypertension have been conducted on the Chinese, Filipino, and Japanese ethnic groups. However, there have been a few studies of other populations, such as the Vietnamese (Centers for Disease Control, 1992) and ethnic Hawaiians (Curb et al., 1991). Vietnamese Americans are one of the most rapidly increasing Asian Pacific populations in the United States and the third largest Asian ethnic group in California after Chinese Americans and Filipino Americans (Fawcett & Carino, 1987). Out of more than 600,000 Vietnamese in the United States, almost 46% reside in California (U.S. Bureau of the Census, 1990). In a recent survey among the Vietnamese population, 10% out of 550 Vietnamese males and 9% out of 443 Vietnamese females were told they had high blood pressure on ≥ 2 occasions, compared with 13% ($n = 1,253$) of males and 16% ($n = 1,448$) of females in the general population (Centers for Disease Control, 1992). The data suggest a lower rate of hypertension among Vietnamese in this study compared with the general population in California. Curb et al. (1991) surveyed 257 Native Hawaiians, ages 20 to 59 years, living on the island of Molokai in Hawaii. The prevalence of hypertension or of taking antihypertensive medications was 24% in females and 26% in males, and these rates were similar to those of whites in the same age group.

A nonrandom survey of Koreans in Southern California in 1988 indicated a 15.9% prevalence rate of hypertension among 32,786 Korean workers employed in industry (Lee, 1988). Other information reported about the prevalence of hypertension among Korean Americans is derived from surveys conducted in 1978 in Orange County, California (Asian and Pacific Islander American Health Forum, 1988). Hypertension has been found to be much more prevalent among Korean males (22.4%) than among Korean females (3.2%), and the overall prevalence rate of hypertension among Korean Americans is lower than that of the general American population. No correlation has been reported between hypertension and dietary factors, such as alcohol, spicy foods, and salt intake. Family history has been found to be the major risk factor among this population. The mortality rate from coronary heart disease is much lower than the rate for leading cause of death among this population, stomach malignancy. Table 7.2 summarizes the findings about hypertension among Asian Pacific populations in the United States.

Table 7.2 Estimated Prevalence of Hypertension Among Asian Pacific Islander Ethnic Groups in the United States

Source	Place and Years	Age Group	Sex	Filipino N	Filipino %HT	Chinese N	Chinese %HT	Japanese N	Japanese %HT	Other Asian N	Other Asian %HT	Hawaiian N	Hawaiian %HT	Indo-chinese N	Indo-chinese %HT	Vietnamese N	Vietnamese %HT	Comments
Angel et al (1989)	Northern California, 1978-1985	18 years old and older	males	1,729	12.2	2,754	10.5	688	12.9	543	6.2							
			females	2,482	9.6	3,197	7.8	1,015	8.8	623	5.4							
Stavig et al (1988)	California, 1979	18 years old and older	males	111	30.5	197	13.3	123	19.8	110	28.5							
			females	160	6.7	195	7.1	147	0.8	87	3.2							
Reed et al (1982)	Hawaii I, 1965-1968	45-49 years old	males (I)					8,006	17									percentage related only to those with
	II, 1974	50 years old and older	males (II)					6,858	23									definite hypertension
Choi et al (1990)	Boston, 1981-1983	60 years old and older	males			127	29.7											elderly Chinese
			females			217	33.5											
Curb et al (1991)	Hawaii, 1985	20-59 years old	males									123	26					
			females									134	24					
Bates et al (1989)	San Diego, CA, 1986	18-75 years old	males and females											117	27			included Hmong, Laotians, Cambodians, and Vietnamese
Centers for Disease Control (1992)	California, 1991	18 years old and older	males													606	15	included self-reported hypertensives and those under treatment
			females													481	14	

NOTE: Hypertension is defined as having systolic blood pressure 140 mmHg and diastolic blood pressure 90 mmHg or taking antihypertensive medications. HT = hypertensives.

Place of Birth

Research into the effect of the country of birth on hypertension has been equivocal. Stavig et al. (1984) found that the prevalence of hypertension was higher among foreign-born (19.4%) than among American-born (15.7%) Asian Pacific individuals in their sample, but this difference was not statistically significant. By contrast, Angel et al. (1989) report finding nativity to be significantly related to hypertension, but only among Chinese men.

Educational Level and Psychological Factors

Among the Asian Pacific population overall, educational level has been negatively correlated with hypertension: Stavig et al. (1984) report that in their sample 15.5% with an educational attainment of one standard deviation above the mean experienced hypertension, compared with 21.1% with one standard deviation below. However, among Filipino men college education has been positively correlated with hypertension (Angel et al., 1989). Psychological factors have also been examined for their link to the prevalence of hypertension. Angel et al. (1989) found that feelings of boredom during the past two weeks and depression or unhappiness were related to a higher rate of hypertension. In addition, it has been suggested that the more social support a person gets from close friends, spouse, and external involvement in the society, the lower the prevalence of hypertension (Stavig et al., 1984).

Knowledge and Awareness

The most striking finding in the central Ohio study concerns the level of knowledge and awareness of the Southeast Asian population with regard to heart health (Chen et al., 1991). In that study, 94% of the subjects did not know what blood pressure is, and 85% did not know what can be done to prevent heart disease. Stavig, Igra, and Leonard (1988) found that Filipinos, who had the highest rates of elevated blood pressure compared with other Asian Pacific groups, were the most likely to be aware of the outcomes of high blood pressure levels (63%) compared with the overall Asian Pacific sample (54%) and the general population (56%) sample. This finding suggests that awareness alone does not mitigate risk factors related to high blood pressure. Compared with the general population, the Asian

Pacific individuals in Stavig et al.'s study had less frequent measurements of their blood pressure (11.6% versus 18.1%) and visited physicians less often (69.3% versus 78.3%). In addition, the Asian Pacifics were less knowledgeable about hypertension.

Treatment and Compliance

Stavig et al. (1988) defined a "controlled hypertensive" as a person with systolic blood pressure below 140 mmHg and diastolic blood pressure below 90 mmHg and taking antihypertensive medications. Those in the Filipino population were found most likely to be under antihypertensive treatment (49%), compared with the Asian and Pacific population (36%) as a whole and the general population (40%). However, their hypertension was poorly controlled by medication, as only 8% of the Filipino patients who took antihypertensive drugs could control their blood pressure levels. The poor level of control also existed for Japanese (8%) and "other Pacific Islanders" (4%). The level of control among the overall Asian and Pacific sample in this study was 9%, compared with 16% among the overall hypertensive population.

In a pilot study among Southeast Asian populations (Bates et al., 1989), more than 50% of those who were categorized as high risk and 40% of those in the moderate-high risk category were under antihypertensive treatment. However, the level of control was poor, as only one-third of the treated patients were successful in lowering their blood pressure levels. Unlike their findings reported above, Chen et al. (1991) found that for Southeast Asians in the Ohio study only 2% of the hypertensive patients reported taking antihypertensive drugs, whereas 17% of those in this sample were defined as being hypertensive.

Implications for Health Care

The linkage between ethnic groups and high blood pressure levels has been studied in several investigations. These studies have discussed the tailoring of hypertensive medications to special patient groups based on age, ethnicity (especially black Americans), and associated medical condition, such as the existence of other cardiovascular risk factors or chronic diseases (Applegate, 1989; Christlieb, 1990; Lund-Johansen, 1987; Zweig, 1990). A review of the existing data about hypertension among Asian Pacific Americans demonstrates that information exists in terms of the prevalence of hypertension in the three major Asian Pacific ethnic groups, but that even within these groups, rates vary by sex and age. We have little or no information on the prevalence of hypertension for other Asian Pacific subgroups that have grown tremendously in the past decade, especially Asian Indians, Koreans, and Southeast Asian groups. Furthermore, the existing studies do not uniformly delineate differences between native-born and foreign-born Asians and Pacific Islanders, which can affect the outcome and interpretation of results.

The independent variables that affect blood pressure levels can be categorized into two general groups: biological variables and sociocultural variables. A family history of hypertension can be derived from both genetic and environmental factors, and culture can affect diet and lifestyle, the influences of which can be determined through biological measures. As in most of the research about hypertension, age, gender, relative body weight, type of diet, and alcohol consumption belong to a set of predictor variables that relates to blood pressure levels.

Women are currently immigrating to the United States at a higher rate than men, for all four ethnic groups in the United States (Urban Associates, 1974). Japanese women outnumber Japanese men in the United States, because there is a higher immigration of Japanese women to the United States and also because women tend to live longer than men. It has been found that the positive link between age and hypertension is dominant among females (Urban Associates, 1974). Therefore, there must be a consideration for increasing health awareness, knowledge, and control of hypertension among females, as it is common to think this problem is unique to males.

Immigration into a new country presents a need for acculturation among the new immigrants. Part of this acculturation includes changes in diet. Although the typical Asian diet includes primarily rice, vegetables, and noodles, the major ingredients of the American diet are animal protein, fats, and sugar. This shift in diet results in an elevation of relative body weight. Chinese and Japanese Americans have tended to preserve their original diets and therefore have historically had lower rates of uncontrolled hypertension. On the other hand, the general Asian diet is not obviously more "healthy"; it contains higher amounts of salt, which by itself could lead to higher risk of hypertension. That can partly explain why Filipino Americans have higher relative body weight and higher levels of hypertension. Some studies indicate that there might be a genetic factor involved (Angel et al., 1989). Higher alcohol consumption has also been found among Filipino Americans, but with its strong correlation to the prevalence of hypertension, there might be a difference between immediate and long-term consumption of alcohol (Shah, 1967).

Ethnicity has been found to be correlated with blood pressure levels. Among the Asian Pacific populations, Filipino Americans have the highest tendency toward hypertension, for reasons that may be biological, sociocultural, or both. It is difficult to determine how each of the factors, such as place of birth, years in the United States, and education, affects blood pressure. Although foreign-born Asian Pacifics might be in more stressful conditions because of the demands of acculturation, U.S.-born Asian Pacifics might have other risk factors that have not been studied or have not been available for study. Studies that investigate the possible correlates affecting outcomes can provide beneficial information to reduce mortality.

In addition, studies that evaluate the health attitudes and practices of the different Asian Pacific ethnic groups can identify important factors that can affect compliance for blood pressure control. Such data can be useful to those attempting to design effective educational and outreach programs to promote the understanding of hypertension and its long-term effects, and in determining which factors, both genetic and environmental, place specific subgroups at higher risk.

Smoking

The major cause of coronary heart diseases (CHD) in the United States, for both sexes, is cigarette smoking. More than one of every six U.S. deaths is a result of tobacco use (U.S. Department of Health and Human Services, 1989). Cigarette smoking increases premature coronary atherosclerosis (Strong & Richards, 1976) and affects blood coagulation (Kannel, Wolf, Castelli, & D'Agostino, 1987) as well as the sympathetic nervous system (Winniford et al., 1986). The combined effects of these factors may contribute to the increased risk of CHD. Cigarette smoking is not determined genetically, whereas other risk factors are determined by both genetic and lifestyle factors. A 1983 report from the U.S. surgeon general indicates that the number of cigarettes smoked daily, the total number of years spent smoking, the degree of smoke inhalation, and the early age of beginning to smoke are all positively correlated with the risk of developing CHD.

In 1958, Hammond and Horn (1958a, 1958b) claimed that smokers had a 70% greater risk of dying from CHD than nonsmokers, and that CHD mortality rates among heavy smokers are two and a half times greater than among nonsmokers. Another finding was that the higher the number of cigarettes smoked per day, the higher the risk of developing CHD. This finding appeared in later studies done with British physicians, in whom the researchers claim stopping smoking significantly reduced the mortality rate from CHD compared with continuing smoking (Doll & Hill, 1964). Daly, Mulcahy, Graham, and Hickey's (1983) study about patients who had unstable angina or myocardial infarction found that the rate of mortality was significantly higher among patients who continued to smoke after their cardiac episodes (82.1%) compared with patients who stopped smoking (36.9%).

One of the findings reported by the U.S. surgeon general is that premenopausal women have lower rates for CHD than men because women both tend to smoke less than men and have smoking habits that are different from those of men (e.g., women smoke fewer cigarettes per day and inhale less deeply than do men). Thus if women had smoking patterns similar to those of men, they would have similar CHD death rates resulting specifically from smoking (U.S. Department of Health and Human Services, 1983). Women who smoke and also use oral contraceptives have been found to have a 10-fold increased risk of a myocardial infarction compared with women who neither smoke nor take oral contraceptives.

Prevalence

The prevalence of smoking among Asians Pacific Americans has been examined by several researchers. Rates of smoking among different Asian Pacific ethnic groups are influenced by age, gender, place of birth, level of education, level of acculturation, and other sociocultural factors. In the following, we discuss the influence of these factors on smoking and propose the development and implementation of smoking prevention and cessation programs.

Among adults in California, the prevalence of smoking is 22.2% (25.5% among males and 19.1% among females). Among Asian

Pacific males, the prevalence of smoking is 23.5%; among females, it is 8.9% (Burns & Pierce, 1992). Across age groups there is a significant difference in the prevalence of smoking between Asian Pacific males and females in California. Whereas among males the highest prevalence (27%) is found in the 25 to 44 age group and a lower prevalence between the ages of 18 and 24 (18%), among females there is almost the same prevalence of smoking (about 10%) for these two age groups.

Klatsky and Armstrong (1991) found that Chinese men and women were less likely to smoke any amount of cigarettes or to smoke heavily compared with other Asian Pacific groups. In their sample, Filipino American men were most likely to smoke (32.9%), followed by "other Asians" (30.9%), Japanese (22.7%), and Chinese (16.2%). Among females, Japanese American women were most likely to smoke, followed by "other Asians" (12.6%), Filipinos (11.4%), and Chinese (7.3%). In addition, Asian Pacifics were lighter smokers than were white smokers in California (with "light smoking" defined as smoking 1 to 14 cigarettes per day). Japanese American males and females were most likely to be heavier smokers (8.2% and 4.6%, respectively), relative to other Asian Pacific subgroups. In the category of heavy smokers, Asian Pacific women born in the United States were more likely to smoke and to be heavier smokers (smoking more than one pack of cigarettes per day) than were women born in Asia. However, the opposite pattern was found for Japanese women. Choi et al. (1990) found smoking to be more common in elderly Chinese American males (39%), compared with the known rate of elderly white American males (20%) (National Institutes of Health, 1980).

A 1991 telephone survey of 1,318 Filipinos in California found that 20% of Filipino men and 6.7% of Filipino women were smokers (Asian and Pacific Islander American Health Forum, 1991). These rates are much lower than those found in Klatsky and Armstrong's (1991) survey of 4,211 Filipinos in Northern California during the years 1978 to 1985, but higher than the rates reported by Burns and Pierce (1992), who conducted a study during the same period and sampled the overall Asian Pacific population in California. Burns and Pierce also found that Asian Pacific females tend to be less heavy smokers (when "heavy smoking" is defined as smoking more than 25 cigarettes per day) than males, but both groups have the same tendency to be occasional smokers, compared with non-Hispanic whites in California.

Some studies have examined the prevalence of smoking among Southeast Asian populations. One study indicated that Southeast Asian women rarely smoke cigarettes, but that men were as likely to smoke as white Americans and twice as likely to be smokers in the youngest and the oldest age groups (National Institutes of Health, 1980). A recent National Health Interview Survey of the Vietnamese population in California compared the prevalence of smoking among Vietnamese to those of the general population (Centers for Disease Control, 1992). The study indicates that 35% of 557 Vietnamese male subjects and less than 1% of 454 Vietnamese females are current smokers, compared with 22% of males and 19% of females among the general population. Levin (1987) analyzed 195 responses to a questionnaire about smoking habits among Laotian refugee males and found that 72% of Laotian males in the sample were current smokers, and that 99% of them had started smoking while still in Laos. The data also indicated that 82% of the subjects started smoking before the age of 20 and 55% of those before the age of 15. Of the 195 Laotian refugees who smoked, 46% smoked 20 cigarettes per day.

A study of Native Hawaiians reveals that 34% of females and 42% of males in that population are smokers (Curb et al., 1991). The highest prevalence of smoking is found among males in the age group 20-29 (48%). The prevalence rate for past smoking is 26% among Hawaiian males and 15% for females. In terms of smoking patterns, 49% smoke less than one pack a day, 44% smoke one to two packs, and 5% smoke more than two packs a day. The 1987 Hawaii Behavioral Risk Factor Survey indicated that 27% of the 305 Hawaiian adults (18 years old and over) were current cigarette smokers. This smoking rate was the highest among all the ethnic groups in Hawaii.

Prevalence of Smoking Among Asians Living in Asia

The smoking rates among Asian populations in Asia are some of the highest in the world. For example, both Japanese males (61%) and South Korean males (75%) report high rates. In China, the consumption of cigarettes is 30% of worldwide consumption (Goldstein, 1990). Generally, men born in Asia are more likely to smoke than are men born in the United States. Li, Jin-Hua, Manlan, and Jiabao (1988) examined behavioral aspects of cigarette smoking among 7,665 students and staff in industrial colleges at Shanghai, China.

The prevalence of smoking among men was 50.5%, compared with 0.33% among women. In this survey, 70% of the male smokers had fewer than 10 cigarettes per day (Li et al., 1988). Another study estimated smoking prevalence in more than half a million Chinese living in China, ages 15 and above (Weng, Hong, & Chen, 1987). The data showed a smoking rate of 33.88%, with rates of 61% among males and 7% among females.

Some studies have analyzed smoking rates relative to age groups. One of these studies, on teenagers in Beijing, China, revealed that as early as ages 10 to 11, 8.2% of the boys were smoking (Ye & Lin, 1982). This rate gradually increased to 34% among the ages of 18 to 19. Among the girls, the prevalence rate was very low; the highest rate found was 1.1% in the age group of 16 to 17. Another study of Chinese individuals aged 15 and over conducted in Shanghai found that the highest percentages of smoking existed among males in the age groups of 50 to 59 (57.5%) and 60 to 69 (58.9%) (Parker, Gong, Shan, Huang, & Hinman, 1982). Among females, the rate of smoking was less than 2% until the age of 49 and reached the highest level of 11.6% in the 60 to 69 age group. Tables 7.3 and 7.4 summarize the prevalence rates of smoking among Asian Pacific populations in the United States and in Asian countries.

Related Factors

Smoking rates have been found to be higher among Asians Pacifics who recently came to the United States, owing to their smoking habits in their countries of origin. Smoking prevalence rates declined with the individuals' acculturation levels, parallel to the reduction of the smoking rate among the overall population in the United States during the past 30 years (U.S. Department of Health and Human Services, 1990).

A variety of factors may influence smoking prevalence among different ethnic groups. In a survey conducted by the Asian and Pacific Islander American Health Forum (1991), Filipino subjects who were apt to speak or think in Filipino dialect(s) more than in English were more likely to smoke. This survey shows that 44% of smokers felt they had to smoke when they were with friends who were smoking. This response is typical of the Filipino cultural traits of hospitality (offering a cigarette) and politeness (accepting what is offered). In comparison, only 21.2% of quitters and 8.3% of nonsmokers felt they should smoke when they were with friends.

Table 7.3 Smoking Prevalence Among Asian Americans

Source	Place and Years	Age Group	Ethnicity	Sex	N	% SM
Klatsky & Armstrong (1991)	Northern California, 1978 to 1985	18 years old and older	Filipino	males	1,729	32.9
				females	2,482	11.4
			Chinese	males	2,754	16.2
				females	3,197	7.3
			Japanese	males	688	22.7
				females	1,015	18.6
			Other Asians	males	543	30.9
				females	623	12.6
Asian American Health Forum (1991)	California, 1991	12 years old and older	Filipino	males	665	20
				females	647	6.7
Hawaii State Department of Health (1991)	Hawaii, 1989	18 years old and older	Hawaiian	males	884	24.5
				females	976	20.2
Choi et al. (1990)	Boston, 1981 to 1983	60 years old and older	Elderly Chinese	males	129	39
				females	217	5
Bates et al. (1989)	San Diego, CA, 1986	18 to 75 years old	Indochinese	males	55	98
Centers for Disease Control (1992)	California, 1991	18 years old and older	Vietnamese	males	557	35
				females	454	<1
Levin (1987)	Cook County, IL, 1988	18 to 57 years old	Laotian	males	195	72

NOTE: SM = smokers.

This survey also found that among Filipinos, the more education individuals had, the less likely they were to smoke. Klatsky and Armstrong (1991) found that among both Asian Pacific females and males, college graduation is negatively correlated with smoking. This correlation has also been found among Chinese living in China (Weng et al., 1987). Alcohol consumption is positively correlated with cigarette smoking, and marriage is positively related to smoking among men (Klatsky & Armstrong, 1991). In another study about Chinese students and staff in Shanghai, men indicated that they began smoking when they started to work (Li et al., 1988).

Table 7.4 Smoking Prevalence Among Asians Living in Asia

Source	Place and Years	Age Group	Ethnicity	Sex	N	% SM
Goldstein (1990)			Japan	males		61
			South Korea	males		75+
Weng et al. (1987)	China, 1984	15 years old and older	China	males	258,422	61
				females	261,178	7
Li et al. (1988)	Shanghai, 1986	15-64 years old	China	males	4,899	50.5
				females	2,440	0.33
World Health Organization (data for 1985)	Santo Tomas, Philippines, 1981	4th-year medical students	Philippines	males	332	44
				females	308	16.2
	Seoul, Korea, 1981	18-29 years old	Korea	males	728	68.5
				males and females		7.4
	Hong Kong, 1982-1984	15 years old and older	Hong Kong	males		32.8
				females		4.1
	Thailand, 1981	10 years old and older	Thailand	males	711	51.2
				males and females		4.4
National Statistics Office, U.S. (data for 1981)		10 years old and older	Thailand	males		92
			Laos	males		98
				females		2.4

NOTE: SM = smokers.

Cessation

In 1987, the smoking rate for males in the United States was 32%; for females it was 27%. The overall smoking rate in 1965 in the United States was 40%, and this was reduced to 29% by 1987. Still, the objective of U.S. health providers is to reduce this rate to 15% by the year 2000. Some investigators claim that the goal of 15% is too challenging and suggest that 22% is a more realistic target. The decline in the rate of smoking since 1965 was achieved despite the addictive nature of tobacco and the aggressive promotion of its use. The highest documented prevalence of smoking was found among Southeast Asian men (55%) in the United States in the years 1984 to 1988, and the objective for the year 2000 is to reduce this rate to 20%.

The implementation of the tobacco control program by the state of California and increased taxes on tobacco purchases might be part of the reason for the sharp decline in smoking (Burns & Pierce, 1992). The readiness to quit smoking and the knowledge that smoking is harmful to one's health have been found to be similar among Asians Pacifics and non-Hispanic whites in California. However, there is a difference between the readiness to quit smoking and actual quit attempt rates when these two ethnic groups are compared. In 1992, 53.6% of male Asian Pacific smokers and 49.2% of female Asian Pacific smokers in California made actual attempts to quit smoking; these rates are slightly higher than the rate of quit attempts among non-Hispanic whites. Asian Pacific males were more successful in their attempts to quit smoking compared with whites, but this differential success rate was not found for females.

In a study conducted in China, the quit rate for smoking was as low as 4.2% among males and 9.7% among females (Weng et al., 1987). Another study examined 7,665 respondents in China and found that individuals perceived themselves as poorly controlled in their ability to abstain from smoking. However, when compared with U.S. adults, they were more successful in giving up their smoking for the short term as well as the long term (Li et al., 1988).

Knowledge and Awareness

The high prevalence of smoking among Vietnamese men and young Southeast Asian men prompted some investigators to examine the knowledge and awareness to the impact of health risks associated with cigarette smoking among these ethnic groups. An unpublished pilot survey of 79 adult Vietnamese refugees in San Diego showed that 72% did not think that smoking was bad for their health (T. Trinh, personal communication). In a study among the Laotian population, almost all of the subjects, who were interviewers and community leaders, claimed there was little or no connection between smoking and associated diseases.

Among the Filipino population in California, 31% of smokers tended to approve of smoking among teenagers if they could afford to buy cigarettes; approval was lower among quitters (21.1%) and nonsmokers (14.1%).

Cigarette smoking during pregnancy accounts for 20% to 30% of low birth weight babies (Kleinman & Madans, 1985), up to 14% of preterm deliveries, and about 10% of all infant deaths (U.S. Department of

Health and Human Services, 1989). Data about pregnant women and smoking show that of more than 5,300 women interviewed, 16.1% smoked before their last pregnancies, whereas among Asian Pacific women, only 4.1% smoked before pregnancy. Among women who were pregnant in the last five years of this research, the Asian Pacific women were more aware of the risks of smoking during pregnancy (97.7%) than were whites (75%) and other ethnic groups. Therefore, among Asian Pacific women, high awareness of the risks associated with smoking during pregnancy might be a crucial factor influencing the low rate of smoking among these women during pregnancy.

Implications for Health Care

Given that smoking is recognized as a major risk factor that can be changed regardless of changes in other risk factors for CHD, smoking prevention alone should result in reduced prevalence rates for CHD. Feinleib (1984) found that a 20% decline in the amount of cigarette smoking produced a 10% decline in CHD mortality rates. Smoking prevention programs must focus on preventing young people from smoking and on increasing the numbers of people who quit. The main thing about cessation programs is that they must provide not only information about the risks of smoking but also long-term assistance.

Furthermore, given that the risk of smoking is strongly attributed to CHD in young women (Rosenberg et al., 1983), more specific educational programs should be geared toward Asian Pacific females, whose prevalence among smokers in the younger ages is increasing. Although Asian Pacific females are less likely to smoke when they become more educated, they tend to have diminished cultural prohibitions against smoking in the United States compared with their home countries, and thus their smoking habits increase. Specific prevention programs must be planned for young females, not only to prevent the elevation of their smoking rates but, more important, to reduce it. These programs must attempt to lower the harmful effects of smoking on Asian Pacific women's health and the health of their children, in the pregnancy period as well as afterward, when the children are at risk of becoming passive smokers.

Hypercholesterolemia

High serum cholesterol is another known risk factor for cardio-vascular disease. It is defined as serum cholesterol equal to or more than 240 mg/dl (Centers for Disease Control, 1987). Cholesterol levels are considered as borderline-high if they are between 200 and 239 mg/dl and desirable if they are less than 200 mg/dl. Morbidity and mortality of CHD increase with increases in blood cholesterol levels. An estimated 60 million American adults require medical advice and treatment to lower their blood cholesterol levels. Current studies indicate that a 1% decline in serum cholesterol results in a 2% decline in the risk of getting cardiovascular disease. Awareness of the risks involved in having high serum blood cholesterol is growing. Compared with the 1960 to 1962 average serum cholesterol levels of 217 mg/dl among men and 223 mg/dl among women in the United States, data from the years 1976 to 1980 show declining levels, with 211 mg/dl among men and 215 mg/dl among women (U.S. Department of Health and Human Services, 1990). During 1976 to 1980, 29% of women and 25% of men in the United States had serum cholesterol levels greater than 240 mg/dl.

The most interesting and most thoroughly investigated issue among the various lipoprotein fractions is the high-density lipoprotein cholesterol (HDL-C), mainly because high levels of HDL-C in the body exert protective effects against CHD (Castelli et al., 1986; Gordon, 1985; Watkins, Neaton, & Kuller, 1985). It has been reported that HDL-C carries cholesterol from peripheral cells to the liver for disposal (Betteridge, 1989), but there might be a more complex mechanism involved. Measurements of the HDL-C, in addition to total cholesterol and triglycerides, can provide a better description of the lipid profile.

Prevalence

A limited number of studies have examined the serum cholesterol levels of Asians Pacific populations in the United States. Klatsky and Armstrong (1991) found that for both men and women, the adjusted mean cholesterol levels were lowest in "other Asians" and highest in Japanese men and women compared with other Asian Pacific ethnic groups. Most studies have found that mean total cholesterol and low-density lipoprotein (LDL) cholesterol levels are lower in Asian countries than in Western countries (Bates et al., 1989; Kesteloot et al., 1985; Nitiyanant, Ploybutr, Harntong, Wasuwat, & Tandhanand, 1987; Shieh, Shen, Fuh, Chen, & Reaven, 1987; Simons, 1986; Szatrowski et al., 1984; Tung, Chen, Liang, Pan, & Xue, 1984; Yao et al., 1988). However, Klatsky and Armstrong (1991) report that, independent of body mass indices differences, they found no difference between the cholesterol levels of U.S.-born Asians and foreign-born Asians (except for Chinese women born in Hong Kong).

Among Native Hawaiians, males and females have been shown to have prevalence rates of 50% and 45%, respectively, for serum cholesterol levels of 5.2 mmol/L (200 mg/dl) or higher. For serum cholesterol levels of 6.2 mmol/L (240 mg/dl) or greater, the prevalence rate for the age group of 50 to 59 has been as high as 40%. When compared with whites, the age-adjusted mean HDL levels are significantly lower among Hawaiian males and especially among females. These results point to high cardiovascular risk for Hawaiians (Curb et al., 1991; Heiss et al., 1980; Lipid Research Clinics Program Epidemiology Committee, 1979).

In another study of the cardiovascular risk factors among Southeast Asians, the levels of total cholesterol were examined for 23 Hmong, 44 Laotians, 45 Vietnamese, and 5 Cambodians, all ages 18 to 75 years old (Bates et al., 1989). The Hmong tended to be older and heavier than those in the other groups, but their average total cholesterol level was significantly below those of the others. The Vietnamese were the leanest and had a higher mean total cholesterol level. Compared with white American women, younger Southeast Asian women had lower cholesterol levels (Kato, Tillotson, Nichaman, Rhoads, & Hamilton, 1973). A behavioral risk factor survey of Vietnamese in California in 1991 estimated that hypercholesterolemia was 38% among Vietnamese males (n = 243) and 32% among Vietnamese females (n = 203) (Centers for Disease Control, 1992). By comparison, among the overall U.S. population, rates of hypercholesterolemia were 29% among males and 28% among females.

A study of the diet of 346 elderly Chinese in Boston indicated that more than 50% of the dietary energy of these subjects was derived from carbohydrates and less than 30% was from fat (Choi et al., 1990). The mean level of HDL-C and LDL-C in this study was relatively low compared with that of whites, and this result has not been described before. Additional information is derived from the Lipid Research Clinics Prevalence Study (Ernst et al., 1980; Schaefer,

Table 7.5 Estimated Prevalence of Hypercholesterolemia Among Asian and Pacific Islander Ethnic Groups in the United States

Ethnicity	% of Hypercholesterolemia Males	Females	Place and Years	Age Group	Source
Filipino	29.8	20.6	Northern California, 1978-1985	18 years old and older	Klatsky & Armstrong (1991)
Chinese	26.6	20.2	Northern California, 1978-1985	18 years old and older	Klatsky & Armstrong (1991)
Japanese	36.6	30.3	Northern California, 1978-1985	18 years old and older	Klatsky & Armstrong (1991)
Other Asian	20.4	13.5	Northern California, 1978-1985	18 years old and older	Klatsky & Armstrong (1991)
Japanese	23.6 (males and females)		Hawaii, 1965-1968	45-69 years old	Reed et al. (1982)
Serum cholesterol (mmol/L)					
Hawaiians	5.28	5.25		20-59 years old	Curb et al. (1991)

Levy, Ernst, Sant, & Brewer, 1981), which found that HDL-C levels correlate negatively with high intake of starch (e.g., rice); this finding might explain the low level of HDL-C among elderly Chinese. Table 7.5 summarizes the prevalence rates of hypercholesterolemia among Asian Pacific populations, compared with the general population in the United States.

Knowledge and Awareness

In the general U.S. population, 55% of men and 57% of women do not know their own cholesterol levels; 22% of men and 23% of women have their cholesterol checked but never find out what their cholesterol levels are. According to the 1989 annual report of the Hawaii State Department of Health, Japanese living in Hawaii have the highest level of awareness of their own blood cholesterol levels of any Hawaiian ethnic group. Level of awareness was measured in this study by the percentage who had their cholesterol checked, who were told their cholesterol levels, and who knew their cholesterol levels. Filipinos were less likely to be aware; only 5.3% of Filipinos knew their cholesterol levels, compared with 28% among Japanese. There were no significant differences in the awareness levels of men and women.

In another study from Hawaii, 45.5% of Hawaii's adult population reported that they had their blood cholesterol checked; 21% reported that they had been told their blood cholesterol levels in numbers, but only 6% were able to provide values for their cholesterol levels. Filipino (34.5%) and Hawaiian and part-Hawaiian (39%) adults were less likely to check their cholesterol levels, and, as in the previous study, Filipinos and Hawaiians and part Hawaiians represented the lower proportion of adults who were told their cholesterol levels in numbers (10.7% and 11.3%, respectively) (Hawaii State Department of Health, 1988).

A majority of Vietnamese men (56%) and women (55%) were never checked for their cholesterol levels, compared with 41% of men and 35% of women in the U.S. population. Vietnamese men were less likely to have their cholesterol checked but were not told (53%) or did not know their cholesterol levels (59%), compared with Vietnamese women (67% and 76%, respectively) (Centers for Disease Control, 1992).

Implications for Health Care

Although limited data exist concerning the levels of cholesterol among Asian Pacific Americans, generally Japanese, Hawaiian, and Filipino Americans are more likely to have higher levels of serum cholesterol compared with other Asian Pacific ethnic groups. Higher mean cholesterol levels among ethnic Japanese men living in Hawaii and California, compared with Japanese living in Japan, are believed to be caused by the higher proportion of fat in the Western diet (Nichaman et al., 1975). As mentioned previously, some investigators have found no differences in serum cholesterol levels between Asian Pacific individuals born in the United States and their counterparts in Asian countries (independent of body weight). These reports also indicate that there has been a rapid increase in the intake of fat and cholesterol in the diets of Asians living in Asian countries (Bates et al., 1989; Chew, Mah, Tan, & Cheong, 1988; Hughes et al., 1989; Nichaman et al., 1975; Nitiyanant et al., 1987; Shieh et al., 1987; Tung et al., 1984; Yao et al., 1988).

Lack of knowledge and awareness is especially typical of Hawaiian and Filipino Americans and among those in Southeast Asian ethnic groups. There is a great need to establish prevention and education programs and/or to emphasize the role of cholesterol in existing cardiovascular heart disease prevention and treatment programs. The objectives of the U.S. Public Health Service are "to reduce the mean serum cholesterol levels among adults to no more than 200 mg/dl" and "to reduce the prevalence of blood cholesterol levels of 240 mg/dl or greater to no more than 20% among adults" (U.S. Department of Health and Human Services, 1990, pp. 400-401). It is estimated that a 5 mg/dl drop in mean cholesterol level will produce a 4.3% drop in mortality rate. Another objective concerning the awareness level is "to increase to at least 60% the proportion of adults with high blood cholesterol who are aware of their condition and are taking action to reduce their blood cholesterol to recommended levels" (p. 402).

Other Risk Factors

There is a growing recognition of the importance of physical activity in preventing cardiovascular disease. Increased physical activity improves the efficiency of heart muscle activity by increasing the pumping capability of the heart and increasing oxygen delivery to the tissues, both at rest and during exercise. Both resting heart rate and heart rate at submaximal exercise decrease progressively with training, and that reduces the load being put on the heart muscle for a given condition. When a malcardiac situation occurs, strong and efficient heart muscle can perform better and thus significantly reduce the damage to the cardiovascular system. Less than 10% of the U.S. adult population exercises at the level recommended by the 1990 objectives: "exercise which involves large muscle groups in dynamic movements for periods of 20 minutes or longer, three or more days per week, and which is performed in an intensity of 60% or greater of an individual's cardiorespiratory capacity" (Caspersen, Christenson, & Pollard, 1986, p. 588). Independent of intensity or type of movement, less than 50% of the adult population in the United States exercises three or more days per week for 20 minutes or longer. The objectives are to increase this percentage to at least 30%.

Differing definitions of *physical activity* have been used in research that has tried to measure and evaluate this factor, so it is difficult to compare studies. A recent study about risk behavior among the Vietnamese population in California defined *sedentary lifestyle* as no physical activity outside of work during the past month of the research. The findings of this study indicate that 40% (n = 556) of Vietnamese males and 50% (n = 453) of Vietnamese females were not exercising, compared with 24% of men and 28% of women in the U.S. population (Centers for Disease Control, 1992). A study of elderly Chinese in Boston defined *active persons* as those who are gainfully employed, exercise regularly, and participate in outdoor activities. Although among elderly Chinese males the proportion of those exercising regularly increased from 34% in the 60 to 69 age group to 44% in the 80+ age group, among elderly Chinese females the rates for the same age groups decreased from 29% to 21% (Choi et al., 1990).

It has been reported that 51.7% of adult Hawaiians have sedentary lifestyles. Only 10% of adult Hawaiians participate regularly in appropriate physical exercise. The 1990 objectives for Hawaiians are to increase this proportion to 60%. Walking, gardening, jogging/running, swimming, and aerobics are the top five physical activities preferred by Hawaiians (Hawaii State Department of Health, 1988). The 1989 Hawaii Department of Health report provides more information about the sedentary lifestyle, which it defines as no physical activity or physical activity fewer than three times per week or less than 20 minutes per occasion. By this definition, Filipinos were most likely to have sedentary lifestyles (76.3%), followed by Japanese (57.1%), and Hawaiians and part-Hawaiians (54.7%). Other factors associated with a lack of physical activity are lower levels of education (about 70%), lower household income (about 64%), and being in the age group of 35 to 54 years (about 61%). Persons over 65 years old, retired persons, and those who are live apart from their spouses are less likely to have sedentary lifestyles (46.4%, 40.8%, and 41.5%, respectively), although these percentages are still high.

In summary, lack of appropriate physical activity is a problem not only among Asian Pacific Americans but also among the overall U.S. population. Although Asian Pacific Americans generally engage in less physical activity compared with the U.S. population, elderly Asian Pacific individuals tend to increase participation in physical activities. Still, because of the different definitions used in the different studies that have been conducted concerning physical activities among the elderly, compared with younger age groups, it is hard to decide if this tendency really exists. In any case, there is an obvious need to consider physical education as an important part of prevention/rehabilitation programs. This can also lead to better acculturation of recent Asian Pacific immigrants, because it might operate in the direction of more emphasis on fitness, which continues to grow in popularity in the United States.

There is a clear relationship between alcohol consumption and blood pressure elevation. Alcohol is a distinct risk factor in prevalence of hypertension and also influences the effectiveness of drug therapy (Beilin & Puddey, 1992). Light or moderate drinkers have lower cardiovascular mortality rates than do abstainers and heavier drinkers. One of the explanations offered for this paradox is selection: Factors that make individuals nondrinkers also increase their risk of cardiovascular diseases. Two studies have addressed this hypothesis (Klatsky, Armstrong, & Friedman, 1990; Thorogood, Mann, & McPherson, 1993). In general, alcohol consumption increases the risk of mortality from hypertension, hemorrhagic stroke, and cardiomyopathy but reduces the risk of coronary artery disease, occlusive stroke, and other cardiovascular conditions. (An extensive review of substance abuse patterns among Asian Pacific Americans is presented in Chapter 12 of this volume.)

Obesity, type of diet, high glucose levels in the blood, diabetes mellitus, and family history are among the other risk factors that can lead to cardiovascular diseases. Some of these factors, such as obesity and diabetes, are described in other related chapters in this book; for other factors there are only very limited or nonexistent data.

Discussion

This review has revealed that among some Asian Pacific groups there is high prevalence of heart disease risk factors, and that these factors vary among ethnic groups. This situation provides justification for targeted disease prevention and health promotion programs and bases for future investigations among these subgroups. Application of "promotion-prevention" strategies can significantly reduce disease dysfunction and premature deaths. However, these strategies have not received enough recognition within U.S. society, and the result has been relatively slow progress in health promotion and disease prevention programs and utilization for Asian Pacific Americans.

As concerns cardiovascular risk factors, Chinese Americans have lower coronary risk compared with Filipino Americans and Japanese Americans, who have the highest risk prevalence among the Asian Pacific ethnic groups. However, Chinese Americans have high stroke risk, so there might be unidentified stroke risk factors that are prevalent in Chinese but not in whites (Choi et al., 1990). Women appear to be at lower risk than men across all the Asian Pacific groups.

In most of the surveys that have examined the Filipino American population, Filipino Americans have been found to have higher prevalence of hypertension or high blood pressure compared with other Asian Pacific Americans, as well as a greater prevalence of excess weight. One of the main reasons for this high proportion of risk factors is Filipino Americans' common use of meat, salted red eggs, and sauces high in salt in their diet (Picache, 1992). Hawaiians are another ethnic group with high risk of premature coronary heart disease and stroke because of high proportions of obesity, hypertension, hypercholesterolemia, smoking, and diabetes mellitus, and low levels of LDL.

Foreign-born immigrants, particularly recent immigrants, usually have lower levels of acculturation. Studies that have considered different risk factors, and especially hypertension, have found that those in this group of Asian Pacific Americans are less aware of hypertension and use more traditional medications. This is not surprising, given that often recent immigrants cannot access health care providers who speak the same languages or dialects, have the same cultural backgrounds, or deliver services in close proximity to the immigrants' residences.

Increasing acculturation to the U.S. lifestyle and in particular the U.S. diet might be associated with elevated risk for cardiovascular disease among Asian Pacific Americans (U.S. Department of Health and Human Services, 1986). In many cases, Asian Pacific Americans are going through an acculturation process that results in their eating more animal protein, fats, and refined sugar, and at the same time keeping their traditional foods (e.g., salted and pickled vegetables, soy and other high-sodium sauces) (Chen et al., 1991). This bicultural diet combination is harmful for individuals trying to prevent hypertension.

Conclusions and Recommendations

The most recent and inclusive research on Asian Pacific Americans was in California conducted by Klatsky and Armstrong (1991). In their conclusions, these researchers present four main topics for the focus of future studies among this population:

- Weight control in Asian Pacific men
- Cigarette smoking control among Asian Pacific women
- Diagnosis and treatment of hypertension among Filipino American men and women
- Control of hypercholesterolemia in all Asian Pacific Americans

The American Health Association's (1991) recent medical/scientific statement defines goals and objectives for future research on hypertension among minorities in the United States. These recommendations might be applied also to other risk factors. The AHA says that future research must put greater emphasis on identifying and correcting environmental factors, including the access and utilization of health services relevant to the prevention/treatment of cardiovascular risk factors. When examining the nature of the prevalence of CHD risk factors, investigators need to define the characteristics of the disease/risk factor in the original environment of the ethnic subgroup and to find out what created the different prevalence rates among the ethnic subgroups. That is, are the differences in prevalence inherent or related to immigration to the United States?

The question of access to diagnosis and treatment, and how access affects incidence, morbidity, and mortality from cardiovascular disease, is crucial, and there is a great need to characterize this access among Asian Pacific Americans compared with other minorities. In addition, follow-up and compliance must also be investigated, considering the influences of a variety of cultural and ethnic factors, such as health care beliefs, folk remedies, and traditional medicine.

If we can come to a better understanding of these issues, we will be able to obtain more information about the determinants of cardiovascular diseases among Asian Pacific Americans and about the epidemiology and pathophysiology of specific risk factors, especially the etiology of hypertension and genetic-environmental interactions. Eventually we might be able to reduce the prevalence of different risk factors for the different ethnic subgroups and to concentrate outreach and services to those most at risk.

Prevention and Treatment Programs

A growing number of prevention and treatment programs for Asian Pacific Americans have been developed and implemented all over the United States, especially in the states that have high concentrations of these populations, such as California, New York, Texas, and Illinois. The following steps are recommended for designers attempting to establish cardiovascular prevention/ treatment programs for these ethnic groups (American Health Association, 1991):

- Establish baseline information about the health status for each minority group.
- Compare the incidence, prevalence, treatment, and pathophysiological measurements of the different ethnic groups to those of their countries of origin.
- Analyze the access and use of health services by these groups. Define how the lack of medical insurance influences the lower numbers of coronary angiogram and coronary artery bypass among minorities.
- Create educational campaigns and outreach programs to encourage hypertensive persons to seek services in detection, diagnosis, and treatment.

In 1987 the Office on Minority Health published a report on prevention in minority communities. That agency's list of the characteristics that affect health care access and services for Asian Pacific communities includes the following: acculturation, acupuncture, communication with community leaders and religious leaders, educational levels, family structure/influence, folk medicine/ remedies, health awareness and health beliefs, health care delivery system, herbalists, knowledge of health care services, language, mass-media use, stress, and urban/rural location. Any approach to the issue of health care access and services must consider all these factors. For example, Chinatown in San Francisco is one of the areas of greatest concentration of Chinese Americans in the United States. In 1985, the American Health Association founded the Chinese Community Cardiac Council, which provides innovative heart-health education to meet the special needs of youth and monolingual Chinese adults. The council sponsors several projects on education for risk factor prevention, including bilingual, culturally sensitive heart-health education material and educational conferences and other events that provide heart-health information, free blood pressure screening, and nutritional education (Lew, 1992). Recently, the American Health Association approved the establishment of the Filipino Community Heart Council (FCHC), the first of its kind for the Filipino community in the Bay Area in California. The FCHC has developed and applied new health and prevention programs for the Filipino community. Outreach programs have been implemented in churches, schools, and professional and regulatory organizations in order to reach a substantial segment of the Filipino community (Picache, 1992).

As mentioned previously, programs must be adjusted to the characteristics of each ethnic group, depending on their prevalence for each risk factor and their access to health care providers and services as well as to the media. For example, for Southeast Asians in the United States, Chen et al. (1991) recommend one-to-one counseling (based on a Red Cross course), cooking classes (based on the American Heart Association Culinary Hearts Kitchens course adapted for Southeast Asian foods), and attractive calendars in Southeast Asian languages that include educational material about heart health. Like the Filipino population in California, 98% of Southeast Asian Americans in Franklin County, Ohio, have access to VCRs. Popular Southeast Asian movies combined with information about hypertension screening are offered for loan to members of this ethnic group without charge. Because there is a relatively low level of knowledge and awareness about cardiovascular risk within this population, the aim of the program is to increase knowledge about cardiovascular health.

Asian Pacific Americans are the fastest-growing minority in the United States. Despite their growing numbers and their increased distribution across the nation, knowledge about their health risks and morbidity patterns has been based upon a few epidemiological studies conducted in Hawaii and California. Recently, more studies have been conducted in Ohio because of the growing immigration of Southeast Asians to that state. In each region a variety of factors—such as place of birth, years in the United States, level of acculturation, barriers to health care services, and education—might differentially influence levels of blood pressure. To obtain more accurate information about the cardiovascular risk factors among Asian Pacific groups, it is necessary to analyze each risk factor with respect to the diverse sociocultural and demographic factors within each ethnic group. This method had been partially applied in recent research, such as the study by Klatsky and Armstrong (1991). Clearly, more research efforts similar to that one in scope and sophistication are needed to address the influence of cardiovascular risk factors among the various Asian Pacific populations.

References

American Heart Association. (1991). Cardiovascular diseases and stroke in African Americans and other racial minorities in the United States: Special report. *Circulation, 83,* 1463-1480.

Angel, A., Armstrong, M. A., & Klatsky, A. L. (1989). Blood pressure among Asian Americans living in Northern California. *American Journal of Cardiology, 64,* 237-240.

Applegate, W. B. (1989). Hypertension in elderly patients. *Annals of Internal Medicine, 110,* 901-915.

Asian and Pacific Islander American Health Forum. (1988). Asian and Pacific Islander American Health Forum national agenda for Asian and Pacific Islander health. In *Proceedings of the Second Asian and Pacific Islander American Health Forum.* San Francisco: Author.

Asian and Pacific Islander American Health Forum. (1991). *Filipino smoking prevalence survey.* Unpublished manuscript.

Bates, S. R., Hill, L., & Barrett-Connor, E. (1989). Cardiovascular disease risk factors in an Indochinese population. *American Journal of Preventive Medicine, 5*(1), 15-25.

Beilin, L. J., & Puddey, I. B. (1992). Alcohol and hypertension. *Clinical and Experimental Hypertension, Part A. Theory and Practice, 14*(1-2), 119-138.

Betteridge, D. J. (1989). High density lipoprotein and coronary heart disease. *British Medical Journal, 298,* 974-975.

Burns, D., & Pierce, J. P. (1992). *Tobacco use in California 1990-1991.* Sacramento: California Department of Health Services.

Cabral, E. L., Gusman, S. V., & Estrada, J. (1981). Prevalence and severity of hypertension in individuals aged fifty years or over from urban and rural communities in the Philippines. In G. Onesti & K. E. Kim (Eds.), *Hypertension in the young and the old* (pp. 299-305). New York: Grune & Stratton.

Caspersen, C. J., Christenson, G. M., & Pollard, R. A. (1986). Status of the 1990 physical fitness and exercise objectives: Evidence from NHIS 1985. *Public Health Reports, 101,* 587-592.

Cassel, C. (1975). Studies of hypertension in migrants. In O. Paul (Ed.), *Epidemiology and control of hypertension* (pp. 41-62). New York: Stratton Intercontinental Medical.

Castelli, W. P., Garrison, R. J., Wilson, P. W. F., Abbott, R. D., Kalousdian, S., & Kannel, W. B. (1986). Incidence of coronary heart disease and lipoprotein cholesterol levels: The Framingham study. *Journal of the American Medical Association, 256,* 2835-2838.

Centers for Disease Control. (1987). Cholesterol awareness in selected states: Behavioral risk factor surveillance. *Morbidity and Mortality Weekly Report, 27*(16).

Centers for Disease Control. (1992). Behavioral risk factor survey of Vietnamese: California, 1991. *Morbidity and Mortality Weekly Report, 41*(5), 69-72.

Chen, M. S., Kuun, P., Guthrie, R., Wen, L., & Zaharlick, A. (1991). Promoting heart health for Southeast Asians: A database for planning interventions. *Public Health Reports, 106,* 304-309.

Chew, W. L. S., Mah, P. K., Tan, Y. T., & Cheong, C. K. (1988). A comparison of the levels of total serum cholesterol (1974-1984) and its relations to ischemic heart disease in Singapore and the United States of America. *Singapore Medical Journal, 29,* 6-10.

Choi, E. S. K., McGandy, R. B., Dallal, G. E., Russell, R. M., Jacob, R., Schaefer, E. J., & Sadowski, J. A. (1990). The prevalence of cardiovascular risk factors among elderly Chinese Americans. *Archives of Internal Medicine, 150,* 413-418.

Christlieb, A. R. (1990). Treatment selection considerations for the hypertensive diabetic patient. *Archives of Internal Medicine, 150,* 1167-1174.

Curb, D. J., Emmett, A. N., Kautz, J. A., Petrovitch, H., Knutsen, S. F., Knutsen, R., O'Conner, H. K., & O'Conner, W. E. (1991). Cardiovascular risk factor levels in ethnic Hawaiians. *American Journal of Public Health, 81,* 164-167.

Daly, L. E., Mulcahy, R., Graham, I. M., & Hickey, N. (1983). Long-term effect on mortality of stopping smoking after unstable angina and myocardial infarction. *British Medical Journal, Clinical Research Edition, 287,* 324-326.

Doll, R., & Hill, A. B. (1964). Mortality in relation to smoking: Ten years' observations of British doctors. *British Medical Journal, Clinical Research Edition, 1,* 1460.

Ernst, N., Fisher, M., Smith, W., Gordon, T., Ritkind, B. M., Little, J. A., Mishkel, M. A., & Williams, O. D. (1980). The association of plasma high-density cholesterol with dietary intake and alcohol consumption: The Lipid Research Clinics Prevalence Study. *Circulation, 62*(4), 41-52.

Fawcett, J. T., & Carino, B. V. (Eds.). (1987). *Pacific bridges: The new immigration from Asia and the Pacific Islands.* Staten Island, NY: Center for Migration Studies.

Feinleib, M. (1984). Changes in cardiovascular epidemiology since 1950. *Bulletin of the New York Academy of Medicine, 60,* 449-464.

Goldstein, C. (1990, March 29). Drags to riches. *Far Eastern Economic Review,* pp. 62-63.

Gordon, D. J. (1985). Plasma high-density lipoprotein cholesterol and coronary heart disease in hypercholesterolemic men. *Circulation, 72,* 111-185.

Hammond, E. C., & Horn, D. (1958a). Smoking and death rates: Report on forty four months of follow-up of 187,783 men: I. Total mortality. *Journal of the American Medical Association, 166,* 1159.

Hammond, E. C., & Horn, D. (1958b). Smoking and death rates: Report on forty four months of follow-up of 187,783 men: II. Death rates by cause. *Journal of the American Medical Association, 166,* 1294.

Hawaii State Department of Health, Health Promotion and Education Office. (1988). *Hawaiians' health risk behaviors, 1987.* Honolulu: Author.

Hawaii State Department of Health. (1991). *Annual report: Statistical supplement 1989.* Honolulu: Author.

Heiss, G., Tamir, I., Davis, C. E., Tyroler, H. A., Ritkand, B. M., Schonfeld, G., Jacobs, D., & Frantz, I. D., Jr. (1980). Lipoprotein-cholesterol distributions in selected North American population: The Lipid Research Clinics Program Prevalence Study. *Circulation, 61,* 302-315.

Hughes, K., Yeo, P. P. B., Lun, K. C., Sothy, S. P., Thai, A. C., Wang, K. W., & Cheah, J. S. (1989). Ischemic heart disease and its risk factors in Singapore in comparison with other countries. *Annals of the Academy of Medicine in Singapore, 18,* 245-249.

Kagan, A., Harris, B., Winkelstein. W., Johnson, K., Kato, H., Syme, S., Rhodes, G., Gay, M., Nichaman, M., Hamilton, H., & Tillotson, J. (1974). Epidemiologic studies of coronary heart disease and stroke in Japanese men living in Hawaii and California: Demographic, physical, dietary and biochemical characteristics. *Journal of Chronic Disease, 27,* 34-35.

Kannel, W. B., Wolf, P. A., Castelli, W. P., & D'Agostino, R. B. (1987). Fibrinogen and risk of cardiovascular disease: The Framingham study. *Journal of the American Medical Association, 258,* 1183-1186.

Kato, H., Tillotson, J., Nichaman, M., Rhoads, G. G., & Hamilton, H. B. (1973). Epidemiologic studies of coronary heart disease and stroke in Japanese men living in Japan, Hawaii and California. *American Journal of Epidemiology, 97,* 372-385.

Kesteloot, H., Huang, D. X., Yang, X. S., Claes, J., Rosseneu, M., Geboers, J., & Joossens, J. V. (1985). Serum lipids in the People's Republic of China: Comparison of Western and Eastern populations. *Arteriosclerosis, 5,* 427-433.

Klatsky, A. L., & Armstrong, M. A. (1991). Cardiovascular risk factors among Asian Americans living in Northern California. *American Journal of Public Health, 81,* 1423-1428.

Klatsky, A. L., Armstrong M. A., & Friedman, G. D. (1990). Risk of cardiovascular mortality in alcohol drinkers, ex-drinkers and nondrinkers. *American Journal of Cardiology, 66,* 1237-1242.

Kleinman, J. C., & Madans, J. H. (1985). The effect of maternal smoking, physical stature, and educational attainment on the incidence of low birthweight. *American Journal of Epidemiology, 121,* 843-855.

Lee, D. (1988, May). *Epidemiology study of hypertension among Koreans.* Paper presented at a symposium of the Asian and Pacific Islander American Health Forum, San Francisco.

Levin, B. L. (1987). *Cigarette smoking habits and characteristics in the Laotian refugees: A perspective pre- and postresettlement.* Unpublished manuscript.

Lew, D. R. (1992). *Overview of Chinese Community Cardiac Council.* San Francisco: American Heart Association.

Li, V. C., Jin-Hua, H., Manlan, Z., & Jiabao, Z. (1988). Behavioral aspects of cigarette smoking among industrial college men of Shanghai, China. *American Journal of Public Health, 78,* 1550-1553.

Lipid Research Clinics Program Epidemiology Committee. (1979). Plasma lipid distributions in selected North American populations: The Lipid Research Clinics Program Prevalence Study. *Circulation, 60,* 427-439.

Lund-Johansen, P. (1987). Treatment of essential hypertension today: The role of beta-blockers, calcium antagonists and ACE inhibitors. *Medical Clinics of North America, 71,* 947-957.

National Center for Health Statistics. (1990a). *Health, United States, 1989* (DHHS Publication No. PHS 90-1232). Hyattsville, MD: U.S. Department of Health and Human Services.

National Center for Health Statistics. (1990b). *1987 National Health Interview Survey* (CD-ROM Series 10, No. 1). Hyattsville, MD: U.S. Department of Health and Human Services.

National Heart, Lung and Blood Institute. (1985). Hypertension prevalence and the status of awareness, treatment and control in the United States: Final report of the Subcommittee on Definition and Prevalence of the 1984 Joint National Committee. *Hypertension, 7,* 457-468.

National Institutes of Health. (1980). *The Lipid Research Clinics Prevalence Study (North America): Population studies data book* (DHEW Publication No. 80-1527). Bethesda, MD: U.S. Department of Health, Education and Welfare.

Nichaman, M. Z., Hamilton, H. B., Kagan, A., Grier, T., Sacks, T., & Syme, S. L. (1975). Epidemiologic studies of coronary heart disease and stroke in Japanese men living in Japan, Hawaii and California: Distribution of biochemical risk factors. *American Journal of Epidemiology, 102,* 491-501.

Nitiyanant, W., Ploybutr, S., Harntong, S., Wasuwat, S., & Tandhanand, S. (1987). Lipid and lipoprotein contents in normal Thai subjects. *Journal of the Medical Association of Thailand, 70,* 20-23.

Office on Minority Health. (1987). *The literature on prevention in minority communities: Some lessons to be learned.* College Park: University of Maryland, Minority Health Research Laboratory.

Parker, R. L., Gong, Y.-L., Shan, L.-G., Huang, D.-Y., & Hinman, A. R. (1982). The sample household health interview survey. *American Journal of Public Health, 72,* 65-70.

Picache, B. R. (1992). Healthier diet needed in Filipino community. *Asian Week, 13*(31).

Reed, D., McGee, D., & Katsuhiko, Y. (1982). Biological and social correlates of blood pressure among Japanese men in Hawaii. *Hypertension, 4,* 406-414.

Roberts, J., & Maurer, K. (1977). *Blood pressure levels of persons 6-74 years: United States, 1971-1974* (Vital and Health Statistics, Series 11, No. 203; DHEW Publication No. HRA 78-1648). Washington DC: Health Resources Administration.

Rosenberg, L., Miller, D. R., Kaufman, D. W., Helmrich, S. P., Van de Carr, S., Stolley, P. D., & Shapiro, S. (1983). Myocardial infarction in women under 50 years of age. *Journal of the American Medical Association, 250,* 2801-2806.

Schaefer, E. J., Levy, R. I., Ernst, N. D., Sant, F., & Brewer, B. (1981). The effects of low cholesterol high polyunsaturated fat, and low fat diets on plasma lipid and lipoprotein cholesterol levels in normal and hypocholesterolemic subjects. *American Journal of Clinical Nutrition, 34,* 1758-1763.

Shah, V. V. (1967). Environmental factors and hypertension with particular reference to prevalence of hypertension in alcohol addicts and teetotalers. In J. Stamler, R. Stamler, & T. N. Pullman (Eds.), *The epidemiology of hypertension* (pp. 204-217). New York: Grune & Stratton.

Shekelle, R. (1979). Psychosocial factors and high blood pressure. *Cardiovascular Medicine, 4,* 1249.

Shieh, S.-M., Shen, M., Fuh, M. M.-T., Chen, Y.-D. I., & Reaven, G. M. (1987). Plasma lipid and lipoprotein concentrations in Chinese males with coronary artery disease, with and without hypertension. *Atherosclerosis, 67,* 49-55.

Simons, L. A. (1986). Interrelations of lipids and lipoproteins with coronary artery disease mortality in 19 countries. *American Journal of Cardiology, 57,* 5G-10G.

Stavig, G. R., Igra, A., & Leonard, A. R. (1984). Hypertension among Asians and Pacific Islanders in California. *American Journal of Epidemiology, 119,* 677-691.

Stavig, G. R., Igra, A., & Leonard, A. R. (1988). Hypertension and related health issues among Asians and Pacific Islanders in California. *Public Health Reports, 103,* 28-37.

Strong, J. P., & Richards, M. L. (1976). Cigarette smoking and atherosclerosis in autopsied men. *Atherosclerosis, 23,* 451-475.

Szatrowski, T. P., Peterson, A. V., Jr., Shimizu, Y., Prentice, R. L., Mason, M. W., Fukunaga, Y., & Kato, H. (1984). Serum cholesterol, other risk factors, and cardiovascular disease in a Japanese cohort. *Journal of Chronic Disease, 27,* 569-584.

Thorogood, M., Mann, J., & McPherson, K. (1993). Alcohol intake and the U-shaped curve: Do non-drinkers have a higher prevalence of cardiovascular-related disease? *Journal of Public Health Medicine, 15,* 245-249.

Tung, C.-L., Chen, W.-C., Liang, S.-P., Pan, S.-R., & Xue, W. (1984). A reappraisal of the changing proportion of the various types of heart diseases in Shanghai and its relationship to serum cholesterol levels. *Chinese Medical Journal, 97,* 171-174.

Urban Associates. (1974). *A study of selected socioeconomic characteristics of ethnic minorities based on the 1970 census: Vol. 2. Asian Americans.* Washington, DC: U.S. Department of Health, Education and Welfare.

U.S. Bureau of the Census. (1990). *1990 U.S. population census: Summary tape file IA.* Washington, DC: Government Printing Office.

U.S. Department of Health and Human Services, Office on Smoking and Health. (1983). *The health consequences of smoking: Cardiovascular disease* (DHHS Publication No. PHS 84-50204). Rockville, MD: Author.

U.S. Department of Health and Human Services, Office on Smoking and Health. (1989). *Reducing the health consequences of smoking: 25 years of progress* (DHHS Publication No. CDC 89-84-11). Washington, DC: Author.

U.S. Department of Health and Human Services, Public Health Service. (1990). *Healthy People 2000: National health promotion and disease prevention objectives* (DHHS Publication No. PHS 91-50212). Washington, DC: Government Printing Office.

U.S. Department of Health and Human Services, Secretary's Task Force on Black and Minority Health. (1986). *Cardiovascular and cerebrovascular diseases* (Vol. 4, pt. 2). Washington, DC: Government Printing Office.

Watkins, L. O., Neaton, J. D., & Kuller, L. H. (1985). High-density lipoprotein cholesterol and coronary heart disease incidence in black and white MRFIT usual care men. *Circulation, 71,* 417A.

Weng, X.-Z., Hong, Z. G., & Chen, D.-Y. (1987). Smoking prevalence in Chinese aged 15 and above. *Chinese Medical Journal, 100,* 886-892.

Winkelstein, W., Kagan, A., Kato, H., & Sacks, S. (1975). Epidemiologic studies of coronary heart disease and stroke in Japanese men living in Japan, Hawaii, and California: Blood pressure distributions. *American Journal of Epidemiology, 102,* 502-513.

Winniford, M. D., Wheelan, K. R., Kramers, M. S., Ugolini, V., Van den Berg, E., Jr., Niggemann, E. H., Jansen, D. E., & Hillis, L. D. (1986). Smoking induced coronary vasoconstriction in patients with atherosclerosic coronary disease: Evidence of adrenergically mediated alterations in coronary artery tone. *Circulation, 72,* 662-667.

Woods, K. L., West, M. J., Weissberg, P. L., & Beevers, D. G. (1981). Studies of red cell transport in white and black essential hypertensives. *Postgraduate Medical Journal, 57,* 769.

Wu, Y. K., Lu, C. Q., Gao, R. C., Yu, J. S., & Liu, G. C. (1982). Nationwide hypertension screening in China during 1979-1980. *Chinese Medical Journal, 95,* 101-108.

Yao, C.-H., Wu, Z.-S., Hong, Z.-G., Xu, X.-M., Zhang, M., Wu, Y.-Y., Yu, S.-E., & Wu, Y.-K. (1988). Risk factors of cardiovascular diseases in Beijing. *Chinese Medical Journal, 101,* 901-905.

Ye, G.-S., & Lin, W.-S. (1982). Cigarette smoking among Beijing high schoolers. *Chinese Medical Journal, 95*(2), 95-100.

Zweig, J. (1990, September). Anti-hypertensive drug therapy tailored to the individual. *Kaiser Permanente Monograph.*

8

Acquired Immunodeficiency Syndrome

TERRY S. GOCK

On June 5, 1981, the *Morbidity and Mortality Weekly Report*, publish-ed by the Centers for Disease Control (CDC), contained a descrip-tion of five cases of an unusual type of pneumonia in young gay men. Although the significance of this publication would not be truly appreciated until a few years later, it nevertheless serves as a milestone to mark the beginning of what would often be referred to as the "AIDS epidemic" in the years to come. It should, however, be mentioned here that, as Shilts (1987) points out, isolated cases of the disease were apparent in this country in the late 1970s despite the lack of any medical term at that time to label the disease syndrome suffered by these patients.

In the early years of this epidemic, the number of reported cases of the disease among Asian Pacific Americans was small when compared with other racial/ethnic groups. This led to a peculiar complacency among our communities that acquired immune defi-ciency syndrome (AIDS) was not a concern for Asian Pacific Ameri-cans. After all, as the rationalization often went, "AIDS is a disease affecting only gay (and generally white) men and drug users, and we don't have that kind of people among us." This was further reinforced by some people in the mainstream scientific community, who, in view of the virtual nonexistence of reported AIDS cases in the Asian Pacific communities, postulated that Asian Pacific Ameri-cans were somehow genetically immune to the retrovirus that causes AIDS (Lee & Fong, 1990).

The above-described synergistic "conspiracy of silence" maintained by both the mainstream and Asian Pacific American communities themselves created a dangerous illusion that we are not affected by this disease. In fact, some Asian Pacific community members to this day still hold on to the belief that they are somehow immune to AIDS. Therefore, the overall objective of this chapter is to summarize the available scientific evidence in an attempt to counteract the strong veil of denial existing both in the mainstream and within Asian Pacific American communities. The bottom line is that Asian Pacific Americans are affected by AIDS just as the other racial and ethnic communities in this country are. As will be shown below, the trend is, in fact, very disturbing, in that Asian Pacific Americans are perhaps suffering from AIDS at a rate *higher* than other racial and ethnic communities.

In the rest of this chapter, I will discuss three general areas that I believe are important for understanding AIDS in Asian Pacific American communities: (a) the clinical aspects of AIDS and human immunodeficiency virus (HIV) infection, (b) the epidemiological aspects of Asian Pacific American AIDS cases, and (c) the actions required to address AIDS in Asian Pacific American communities.

Clinical Aspects of AIDS and HIV Infection

What Is AIDS?

Acquired immunodeficiency syndrome, or AIDS, is a term used to describe a number of diseases or medical conditions resulting from someone's being infected by a retrovirus called the human immunodeficiency virus. In the time since the condition was discovered more than 10 years ago, an impressive body of knowledge has been gathered about the biological aspects of the retrovirus and the infection process. This information has been detailed in a number of highly readable publications (e.g., Douglas & Pinsky, 1991; Gong, 1985), and so it will not be repeated here. However, a brief synopsis is provided below.

For surveillance and monitoring purposes, the term *acquired immunodeficiency syndrome* was initially coined by the CDC in 1982 to define a spectrum of diseases that the retrovirus HIV can cause. Because HIV infection was seen to manifest itself in a variety of ways, AIDS characterized a number of conditions that were the consequences of suffering from significant and severe compromise to the immune system. Since then, modifications have been made to encompass other conditions as the understanding of HIV infection has increased. As of the time of this writing, the most current definition of AIDS includes, among others, a number of opportunistic protozoal and helminthic infections (e.g., *Pneumocystis carinii* pneumonia), fungal infections (e.g., cryptococcosis), bacterial infections (e.g., mycobacterium avium complex), viral infections (e.g., cytomegalovirus), rare forms of cancer (e.g., Kaposi's sarcoma), wasting syndrome, and dementia (Centers for Disease Control, 1991).

The infections mentioned above are called *opportunistic* because although the microorganisms causing the various disease manifestations may be present in the bodies of many healthy people and do not affect their physical well-being, they become health threatening when an individual's immune system has been pervasively damaged by a condition such as HIV infection. As summarized by the Institute of Medicine/National Academy of Sciences (1986): "There have been no recorded cases of prolonged remissions from AIDS. Most patients die within two years of the appearance of the clinical disease; few survive longer than three years" (p. 7). Recent advances in medical treatment, however, may have increased survival limits somewhat. In all, the cumulative case-fatality rate for adolescents and adults with AIDS between 1981 and the end of 1990 was about 63% (Centers for Disease Control, 1991).

The Spectrum of HIV Infection

Several blood tests, generally known as HIV antibody tests (e.g., Western blot), have been available for a few years to detect in a person's blood the presence of antibodies that specifically recognize the retrovirus. This serves as a marker that a person is HIV infected. Such a person, however, may not show any clinical symptoms of AIDS for months or even years. Although some experts believe that all HIV-infected persons will eventually develop AIDS, the disease course of HIV infection is still far from clear at this time. In fact, according to a report by the Institute of Medicine/National Academy of Sciences (1988), an eight-and-a-half-year monitoring of a group of gay men who had previously given blood for hepatitis vaccine research revealed that only slightly more than 40% of the HIV-infected members had developed AIDS. Other HIV-infected persons may either be asymptomatic or develop conditions that have been subsumed under the rubric of *AIDS-related complex*, or ARC.

In general, the term *ARC* has been used to describe a number of conditions that indicate a lesser degree of immune suppression than those diseases associated with AIDS described above. They include such presenting problems as diarrhea, weight loss, swollen lymph nodes, and night sweats that persist for an extended period of time. At present, we do not have a definite answer to the question of whether ARC is a step in the progression toward full-blown AIDS. Furthermore, the utility of having this separate diagnostic category has been seriously questioned. For example, the Institute of Medicine/National Academy of Sciences (1988) recently recommended that HIV infection itself be viewed as a disease and asserted that the term *ARC* is no longer useful from either a clinical or a public health perspective.

Currently, there is no cure for HIV infection, nor is there a vaccine to guard against infection. However, as summarized by Allen (1988), cures and different forms of symptom alleviation are available for a number of the opportunistic diseases and conditions resulting from HIV infection. Furthermore, antiviral drugs such as azidothymidine (AZT) have been shown to be effective in arresting the destructive effects of HIV on the immune system and thus prolonging the health of those infected.

Modes of Transmission

As we shall see later in this chapter, a clear understanding not only of how HIV is transmitted but also of how it is *not* transmitted is particularly important for developing an effective campaign against AIDS and HIV infection in the Asian Pacific American communities. I present here a brief summary of our current state of knowledge about HIV transmission.

Although persons who are HIV infected may not show any clinical symptoms of AIDS or ARC, they can infect others with the retrovirus. This long and often undetected "incubation period" complicates control of the spread of the retrovirus. However, it is now apparent that the route of viral transmission is quite limited. HIV spreads from infected persons through (a) unprotected anal and vaginal intercourse (including mouth-anal contacts), (b) sharing of contaminated intravenous (IV) needles and syringes, (c) transfusion of contaminated blood or blood products (including in the treatment of hemophilia), and (d) in utero transmission from infected mothers to their unborn infants or through breast milk after birth.

Besides our current understanding of the modes of HIV transmission, it is now also clear how HIV is not transmitted. As succinctly summarized by the Institute of Medicine/National Academy of Sciences (1986):

> Studies show no evidence that infection is transmitted by so called casual contact—that is, contact that can be even quite close between persons in the course of daily activities. Thus, there is no evidence that the virus is transmitted in the air, by sneezing, by shaking hands, by sharing a drinking glass, by insect bites, or by living in the same household with [a person with AIDS] or an HIV-infected person. (p. 6)

Along the same lines, touching or hugging an HIV-infected person does not transmit the retrovirus. Similarly, the risk of HIV transmission is nonexistent for someone who is donating blood. Furthermore, because of the blood screening procedures developed in recent years, the risk of receiving contaminated blood or blood products during transfusion for medical purposes has been greatly reduced.

Epidemiological Aspects of Asian Pacific American AIDS Cases

Incidence and Prevalence

The currently available epidemiological data are unequivocal in attesting to the fact that AIDS is no longer a "gay white male disease." Indeed, the disease affects all ethnic, racial, and other socioeconomic strata. For example, ethnic minorities have been described as the "second wave" of the AIDS epidemic in this country (Brickman, 1989). More recently, Taylor (1991) reported that the annual rate of increase of AIDS cases for women in 1990 was higher than that for men.

As pointed out earlier in this chapter, Asian Pacific Americans generally have not been concerned about the AIDS epidemic because

they may have perceived AIDS as a uniquely Western (and therefore culturally foreign) phenomenon. This perception was further
reinforced by the lack of statistical recognition of reported AIDS
cases within the Asian Pacific communities in the United States. In
fact, AIDS cases among Asian Pacific Americans were not identified
separately until June 1987, when, in a footnote, the CDC reported
that buried within the "others" category of its monthly surveillance
reports were 232 cumulative Asian Pacific American AIDS cases. By
that time, the cumulative number of total reported AIDS cases in
the United States was nearly 40,000.

According to the Centers for Disease Control (1991), by the end
of 1990 there was a cumulative total of 997 reported AIDS cases
among Asian Pacific Americans in the United States, out of a total
of 161,073 cases. Asian Pacific Americans thus represent 0.6% of all
reported AIDS cases in this country. Furthermore, the 1990 rate of
AIDS cases per 100,000 population for Asian Pacific Americans
stood at 3.8. This was the lowest rate of AIDS when compared with
other racial/ethnic groups in this country. However, such incidence
and prevalence data ignore some disturbing trends about AIDS in
the Asian Pacific American communities.

As can be seen in Table 8.1, the annual rate of increase in reported
AIDS cases for Asian Pacific Americans nationwide since 1987,
when the Asian Pacific American data became routinely available,
at least parallels that of other racial/ ethnic minority groups combined. Such cursory data, though important enough by themselves,
still do not underscore the problems faced by Asian Pacific Americans
in this area. For example, in a report by the now-defunct National
AIDS Network (1989), the incidence of AIDS in the Asian Pacific
communities was described as doubling about every 10 months. Moreover, in such metropolitan areas as San Francisco and Los Angeles,
where large concentrations of Asian Pacific Americans reside, the
Asian Pacific American group has the highest rate of increase in
reported AIDS cases when compared with other racial/ethnic groups
(Asian Pacific AIDS Education Project, 1990; Toleran, 1991).

Diversity

As we all know, the Asian Pacific American population in the
United States is not a homogeneous entity. There are many ethnic
subgroups under the general category of "Asian Pacific Ameri-

Table 8.1 Comparison of the Annual Rate of Increase in Reported AIDS Cases (Cumulative) Between Asian Pacific Americans and Other Racial/Ethnic Groups, 1987-1990 (in percentages)

| | Racial/Ethnic Group | |
Year	Asian Pacific Americans	Other Racial/ Ethnic Groups
1987-1988	66	65
1988-1989	47	43
1989-1990	39	39

SOURCE: Centers for Disease Control (1991, Table 4).

cans." Although the national surveillance data kept by the CDC do not provide a breakdown of Asian Pacific American AIDS cases by ethnic groups, other statistics do provide some information on this. For example, Table 8.2 shows the Asian Pacific American ethnic breakdown for the reported AIDS cases in Los Angeles County through 1990. Of importance here is not the absolute numbers (because they change monthly), but the fact that all major Asian and

Table 8.2 Reported (Cumulative) AIDS Cases Among Asian Pacific American Ethnic Groups In Los Angeles County (as of December 31, 1990)

Ethnic Group	Total
Cambodian	1
Chinese	21
Filipino	44
Japanese	26
Korean	4
Pacific Islanders	12
Taiwanese	1
Thai	11
Vietnamese	8
Unknown	22
Total	150

SOURCE: Los Angeles County Department of Health Services (1991, Table 2).

Table 8.3   Reported (Cumulative) Adult/Adolescent AIDS Cases by Exposure Category and Race/Ethnicity, Through December 31, 1990 (in percentages)

| | Racial/Ethnic Group | | | | |
Exposure Category	Asian Pacific Americans	Whites	Blacks	Latinos	American Indians
Male homosexual/bisexual contacts	74[a]	76	36	40	54
IV drug use (female and heterosexual male)	4	8	39	40	17
Male homosexual/bisexual and IV drug use	2	7	7	6	13
Hemophilia/coagulation disorder	2	1	0	0	4
Heterosexual contact	4	2	11	6	4
Recipient of blood transfusion and blood products	7	3	1	2	3
Others/undetermined	7	2	5	5	5

SOURCE: Centers for Disease Control (1991, Table 4).
NOTES: Percentages for each racial ethnic category may not add up to 100 because of rounding.
a. Because the number of Asian Pacific American AIDS cases is comparatively small, minor fluctuations can drastically change these percentages. The consistency of these percentages over the past few years, however, suggests that they may be relatively stable.

Pacific Islander subgroups are represented. This phenomenon corroborates that described by Aoki, Ngin, Mo, and Ja (1989) in San Francisco. In other words, not only are Asian Pacific Americans, as a community, no longer able to consider themselves immune, but no single Asian Pacific ethnic subgroup is insusceptible.

Table 8.3 compares figures concerning the reported modes of HIV transmission for Asian Pacific American adolescent and adult AIDS cases nationwide through 1990 with those of other racial/ethnic groups. As is apparent from these figures, Asian Pacific Americans, unlike other ethnic minority groups, are similar to whites in HIV transmission in that they tend to be exposed to the retrovirus through male same-gender sexual contacts (as opposed to IV drug use). This is important to note because it suggests that, like the white community and unlike other ethnic minority communities, the Asian Pacific American community must clearly give priority to developing preventive education efforts and addressing treatment issues that are of relevance to those engaging in high-risk male same-gender sexual behaviors.

Limitations of Epidemiological Data

Despite the valuable information that can be obtained from the analysis of such epidemiological data as those mentioned above, there are certain important limitations that must be kept in mind when reviewing the available surveillance data. For example, the technical notes contained in the CDC (1991) surveillance report acknowledge that the number of reported AIDS cases in this country, in general, represents an underestimation. In addition, it appears that certain cultural and practical factors further work against researchers' ability to obtain an accurate number of AIDS cases in the Asian Pacific American communities. Given these additional factors, it is likely that the number of Asian Pacific American AIDS cases shown in official records (such as those maintained by the CDC) may be lower than the actual number of Asian Pacific Americans with AIDS by more than the usual 5% to 10% estimated underreporting rate for the general population.

Among these cultural factors that may contribute to a disproportional underestimate of Asian Pacific American AIDS cases, shame and loss of face about having contracted such a socially stigmatized disease are likely the front-runners. An indirect indication of such concerns, even among those Asian Pacific Americans who have been diagnosed with AIDS, is evident in Table 8.3. In contrast to other racial/ethnic groups, Asian Pacific Americans reported two to seven times more HIV transmission through receipt of blood and blood component transfusions than other groups. Because there is no apparent reason to believe that Asian Pacific Americans should contract the retrovirus in such disproportional numbers through blood transfusion, an alternative explanation is that it is more culturally and socially acceptable for some Asian Pacific Americans with AIDS to report having contracted the disease through the most "neutral" transmission mode among the known routes.

In addition to the cultural factors described above, there are certain practical factors that tend to limit further the accuracy of the official AIDS surveillance data as far as Asian Pacific American populations are concerned. To understand this, one must first be cognizant of the fact that there is great variability between public and private medical personnel in terms of the completeness and accuracy of their reportage of AIDS cases. As pointed out by the Los Angeles County HIV Planning Council (1990), the reporting of AIDS cases by private practice physicians is more delayed and/or

incomplete than that of their counterparts in public service. Because many Asian Pacific immigrants for linguistic reasons tend to
seek health services from physicians in private practice within their
communities, the accuracy of the reporting of Asian Pacific American AIDS cases may be compromised. Moreover, many immigrants
seek help on medical issues from indigenous folk medicine practitioners for both linguistic and cultural reasons. This practice increases the likelihood that AIDS cases may be either undiagnosed
or misdiagnosed and thereby go unreported to CDC.

Actions in Response to AIDS in the Asian Pacific Communities

Preventive Education

Given that no vaccination against or cure for AIDS is in sight, in
general the best public health action alternative available is still the
development of sound strategies to reduce high-risk behaviors.
Moreover, as the current number of reported AIDS cases among
Asian Pacific Americans is comparatively low, the window of opportunity is still open for preventing any significant increase in the
incidence and prevalence of HIV infection within the Asian Pacific
American populations. However, this opportunity must be seized
immediately. In other words, the development and implementation
of effective preventive education in Asian Pacific American communities are particularly crucial at this time.

The urgency of coordinating an effective education campaign is
underscored by the results of a number of "knowledge, attitudes,
beliefs, and behaviors" (KABB) studies conducted recently in San
Francisco's Chinese, Filipino, and Japanese communities (Gorrez &
Araneta, 1990; Ja, Kitano, & Ebata, 1990a, 1990b). Although the
generalizability of these results beyond San Francisco awaits testing in replication studies, all three studies consistently point to the
lack of accurate information on many salient dimensions of AIDS
and HIV infection within the Asian Pacific American communities,
including how the retrovirus is transmitted and how it is not
transmitted. For example, Ja et al. (1990a, 1990b) found that although Chinese and Japanese respondents were generally accurate
in terms of identifying ways of HIV transmission, significant numbers also incorrectly believed that casual contacts (such as drinking

from the same glass as an AIDS-infected person, mosquito bites, and being close to gay men) were methods of transmission. Gorrez and Araneta (1990) found that their Filipino survey respondents scored low in terms of their knowledge about HIV transmission. Such contacts as via needles used for vaccinations or laboratory tests and donating blood were erroneously viewed as HIV transmission modes by a high number of the community members.

As a result of inaccurate and incomplete information about AIDS, excessive fear of the disease and advocacy of extreme and unreasonable measures to avoid contact with those who are HIV infected were common among survey respondents. For example, a majority of the Chinese respondents actually endorsed the use of quarantine for persons with AIDS. Perhaps of even more concern than the consequences of ignorance described above is the common finding in all three studies that a significant number of respondents with adequate understanding of efficacious preventive measures against HIV infection continued to engage in high-risk behaviors (such as participating in unprotected high-risk sexual activities).

As suggested by Ja et al. (1990a, 1990b), comprehensive and coordinated multimedia campaigns (including, but not limited to, ethnic-specific advertisements, newspaper articles, radio public service announcements, and TV programs) are essential to promote AIDS-related risk-reduction behaviors successfully in the Asian Pacific American communities. These campaigns must offer complete and accurate information in culturally sensitive and linguistically understandable ways in order to combat such high-risk activities as unprotected sexual activities (especially with multiple partners) and IV drug use, as well as to dispel the excessive fear of relating to people with AIDS and HIV infection. In addition, as I have pointed out in previous work, alcohol and drug use in general (not just IV drug use) increases the risk of HIV infection, because the resulting altered state of consciousness tends to reduce an individual's judgment and ability to negotiate for safer sexual practices and/or to refuse the offer of IV drugs (Gock, 1991). The "harm reduction" approach to substance use (Bunning, 1990), which stresses the minimization of HIV infection risk caused by substance use, must therefore also be included as part of the overall preventive education strategy.

Given our understanding of the knowledge level about AIDS in the Asian Pacific American communities described above, a community preventive education approach must, therefore, include efforts to (a) combat unfounded fears about AIDS and those living with HIV infection, (b) increase accurate knowledge about AIDS and HIV infection, and (c) foster communitywide norms for low-risk sexual practices and substance use behaviors.

The Asian Pacific American communities pose some particular problems for the coordination of such a comprehensive prevention campaign that are not experienced by other racial/ethnic groups. Although these problems are not insurmountable, program designers must be aware of and ready to address them if they are to be successful in reducing the risk behaviors associated with HIV transmission in this population. The need for linguistically appropriate and culturally responsive preventive education efforts seems apparent from the KABB studies mentioned above, in that primarily non-English-speaking Asian and Pacific Islander immigrants tend to have the lowest level of accurate AIDS-related information. They, as a group, are therefore of particularly high risk for HIV infection. In fact, an analysis of the reported AIDS cases among Asian Pacific Americans in Los Angeles reveals that more than two thirds are found in first-generation (i.e., foreign-born) Asian Pacific Americans (Los Angeles County Department of Health Services, 1989).

The necessity of having linguistically and culturally sensitive education campaigns seems obvious enough, and the logistical problems of implementing such prevention efforts in the Asian Pacific American communities are equally apparent. For example, in order to reach most Asian Pacific Americans in the United States adequately, such a campaign would require targeting at least 10 Asian Pacific subgroups that use more than 15 languages and dialects. Given current funding shortages, arguing for a coordinated preventive education effort of such a magnitude will be quite a challenge.

In addition to logistical and funding problems, a more fundamental problem is that the Asian Pacific American communities' preventive education efforts are at a more elementary stage than are those of other racial/ethnic and high-risk behavior groups. For example, it seems clear from the KABB studies mentioned previously that the ethnic print and electronic media are important and effective ways of disseminating accurate and crucial HIV-related information to Asian Pacific American community members, especially those with limited English-speaking capabilities. However, such approaches are considered outmoded in the mainstream HIV prevention field by now and thus are generally not looked upon as innovative enough to be worthy of funding. Trying to convince funding sources to make an exception for the Asian Pacific American communities, especially when many of them are not sensitive to or cognizant of the importance of such efforts in the first place, is like going against the tide. Thus strong institutional education and advocacy efforts are required on behalf of Asian Pacific American communities.

Although problematic in terms of the aspects described above, the fact that the Asian Pacific American communities are at a more rudimentary stage in HIV preventive education is not necessarily a disadvantage, because Asian Pacific Americans can profit from the successes, and do not have to repeat the mistakes, of prevention efforts already attempted. For example, what we now know about the interrelationship between alcohol and other substance use, high-risk sexual behaviors, and HIV infection suggests the necessity of tackling all three components of this unholy trinity together. Although some innovative theoretical frameworks and model programs (e.g., "Stop AIDS" in San Francisco and Los Angeles) are now available for those in the mainstream community, the challenge for the Asian Pacific American communities is to create from these some versions that are culturally relevant and linguistically appropriate.

Besides a comprehensive multimedia campaign aimed at the general Asian Pacific American populations, specific targeting of groups at higher risk for HIV infection must also be conducted as an integral part of the overall preventive education strategy. In other words, Asian Pacific Americans who are gay and bisexual men, adolescent and young adult heterosexual women and men, and substance abusers need to be reached with sensitive and relevant subcultural approaches. The urgency of doing so is highlighted by a recent study by Strunin (1991), in which Asian youth were found to be least knowledgeable about HIV transmission risks when compared with adolescents of other ethnic groups. Given the particular concern for privacy in Asian and Pacific Islander cultures, there is no shortcut to the labor-intensive process of (a) identifying appropriate social, community, and religious groups to provide preventive education presentations; (b) conducting small group and/or one-on-one discussions to disseminate HIV-related information and encourage risk-reduction behaviors; and (c) training community gatekeepers (such as community and religious leaders, service providers, and schoolteachers) in HIV risk-reduction strategies so that they can have an impact on those Asian Pacific Americans with whom they come in contact in their various capacities.

Within cultures that are historically reticent to talk about sex and sexuality (not to mention same-gender sexual behaviors and diversity in sexual orientations), to acknowledge the presence of substance abuse among its community members, and to discuss death and dying openly, any attempt to mention any of these three areas, let alone all of them together, is no small feat. Given the number of potential Asian Pacific American lives at stake, efforts to counteract such cultural reluctance are, however, of paramount importance and particularly urgent. In this regard, a number of recent studies have paved the way to addressing such issues as Asian sexuality and HIV infection (e.g., Cochran, Mays, & Leung, 1990), substance abuse (e.g., Sasao, 1991; Zane & Sasao, in press), and substance abuse and AIDS (Gock, 1991) in the Asian Pacific American communities.

Early Intervention and Treatment

Perhaps more than many other illnesses, AIDS and HIV infection have emphasized the myriad of physical, emotional, social service, legal, and spiritual dimensions that must be attended to if we are to provide care for those with the disease. For example, Jue (1987) highlights the special sensitivity practitioners must have if they are to adequately and competently look after the psychosocial needs of racial/ethnic minority clients with AIDS, including those of Asian and Pacific Islander background. In addition, Dornette (1987) and Wood (1988) discuss the complexity of the legal and ethical issues surrounding the treatment of AIDS and HIV infection. Kübler-Ross (1987) explores the spiritual dimension of HIV-related care.

Because the number of reported Asian AIDS cases is relatively small, it is difficult to justify the development of comprehensive treatment programs that are specific to Asian Pacific Americans. This is especially the case if the programs are to include many or all of the dimensions and considerations mentioned above. This state of affairs, however, does not diminish the many problems faced by Asian Pacific Americans living with AIDS as they seek treatment and other services that are responsive to their cultural backgrounds and sensitive to their linguistic requirements.

Given the current limitations described above, the training of a sufficient number of medical and psychosocial personnel who are bilingual and bicultural (and who are housed within existing programs) is therefore advisable, especially in those geographic areas with critical concentrations of Asian Pacific American AIDS cases (such as Hawaii, Los Angeles, New York, and San Francisco). These staff can then directly assist monolingual Asian Pacific American persons living with HIV infection in all aspects of their treatment process, including HIV pre- and posttest counseling. Because the pool of such personnel within any locale is necessarily limited, the sharing of staff resources among agencies must be encouraged, so that Asian Pacific American linguistic and service needs can be adequately covered. In addition, the education of mainstream service providers must also be considered, with emphasis on helping them respond appropriately to the demands of those Asian Pacific Americans they will encounter when offering HIV-related treatment services. Furthermore, a pool of qualified interpreters familiar with HIV-related concerns and issues of particular relevance to the Asian Pacific American communities should be developed to augment the effectiveness of mainstream providers in serving Asian Pacific Americans living with AIDS and HIV infection.

In addition to focusing on treatment for people with AIDS, the past few years have seen an increasing emphasis on early intervention. The advances made in antiviral drugs that delay the course of HIV progression, as well as the development of medications that are more effective in treating the opportunistic diseases associated with HIV infection and AIDS, have encouraged such an approach. In fact, early prophylactic treatments have become hopeful stopgap measures short of any known cure for HIV infection and AIDS. However, like members of other racial/ethnic minority groups (compared with whites), Asian Pacific Americans tend to delay the identification, detection, and treatment of HIV infection. In these days when early detection and intervention offer better chances for a healthier and prolonged lifespan, such delays can be costly, if not deadly.

There are numerous reasons why a significant number of HIV-infected Asian Pacific Americans delay seeking early intervention and other treatment services. Often, when such services are avoided, several nonmedical factors are likely operating. For Asian Pacific Americans, these factors include (a) lack of knowledge about the availability of appropriate treatment resources among many indigenous health care providers with whom primarily monolingual Asian Pacific Americans tend to consult first; (b) the fear of being identified as HIV infected and thus risking the loss of acceptance by significant others, such as family members; and (c) the shame of accepting infection status because it implies that one has engaged in sexual and drug use behaviors that are social and cultural taboos.

In addition to factors that hamper treatment access and compliance, the Asian Pacific American communities have not been mobilized adequately to support HIV-related early intervention and other treatment efforts by reducing the above-described stigma, fear, and shame associated with HIV infection. As mentioned previously, the KABB studies conducted in San Francisco reveal that the Asian Pacific American communities surveyed all tend to be quite inaccurate in terms of knowing how HIV is *not* transmitted (Gorrez & Araneta, 1990; Ja et al., 1990a, 1990b). For example, a significant number of respondents still believed that contact with hospital needles, donating blood, and being close to gay men were methods of transmission. Such misinformation often leads to unreasonable fear, avoidance, and feelings of shame on the part of both community members at large and Asian Pacific Americans living with AIDS and HIV infection. The challenge here is thus to develop strategies that will change the community perceptions of the disease and those infected by it. In other words, we need to fight HIV infection, not the people with the disease, in order to encourage those who are HIV infected to seek proactive treatment instead of suffering health deterioration silently and unnecessarily.

Research Directions

Virtually no currently available medical and social science research studies in the HIV area include Asian Pacific Americans in their samples. For example, in conducting a recent literature search on "AIDS and Asians" in preparation for writing this chapter, I found only 13 references. Even more disturbing is the fact that most of these were not substantive in nature; many were identified only because they contained the word *Asian* in the text (e.g., in such phrases as "Asian old world monkeys" and "non-Asian-born people with tuberculosis").

Given the current state of affairs described above, the research directions in the Asian Pacific AIDS area are wide open. One possible research focus may be that of conducting clinical drug trials that include representative Asian Pacific American samples. Another possible research avenue in the medical arena is that of comparative studies on drug dosages and effectiveness for Asian Pacific Americans versus dosages for other racial/ethnic groups. In addition, the effectiveness of alternative treatment approaches that are indigenous to Asian Pacific communities (such as herbal medicine and acupuncture) may be an interesting and potentially fruitful field of examination. In fact, Zhang and Ziolkowski (1990) describe some of the areas within this general topic that are currently under scientific investigation. More rigorous studies in this area would undoubtedly enrich the knowledge base concerning effective treatment approaches.

As pointed out by Dudley (1990), research questions in the AIDS area have moved away from asking such questions as "How do people get HIV?" to "What are the effects of HIV infection for those infected and for society as a whole?" In other words, social science research studies will likely gain more prominence in the understanding of AIDS and HIV infection in the years to come. Currently, the field is also wide open for examination of social science-related topics as they relate to Asian Pacific American AIDS concerns. Some possible research topics include (a) how to develop culturally sensitive and effective prevention strategies, (b) how to encourage and maintain low-risk behaviors within the Asian and Pacific Islander populations, and (c) how to minimize the effects of the negative cultural sanctions experienced by those Asian Pacific Americans living with AIDS and HIV infection. Obviously, these topics barely scratch the surface of potential possibilities and crucial questions. The only limitation here is our own creativity and commitment.

Conclusion

We are at a juncture in history when our choices in the preventive education, treatment, and research agenda can significantly affect the future course of AIDS and HIV infection in the Asian Pacific American communities. It is my hope that the issues raised in this chapter will help us move in the direction of stopping the spread of HIV through sensitive and effective preventive education, compassionate treatment services, and rigorous knowledge acquisition based on research. The work is indeed ahead of us.

References

Allen, A. (1988). AIDS 201. In T. Eidson (Ed.), *The AIDS caregiver's handbook* (pp. 13-45). New York: St. Martin's.

Aoki, B., Ngin, C. P., Mo, B., & Ja, D. Y. (1989). AIDS prevention models in Asian-American communities. In V. N. Mays, G. W. Albee, & S. F. Schneider (Eds.), *Primary prevention of AIDS: Psychological approaches* (pp. 290-308). Newbury Park, CA: Sage.

Asian Pacific AIDS Education Project. (1990). *Asian Pacific AIDS statistics, August 1990*. (Available from Asian Pacific AIDS Education Project, Asian Pacific Health Care Venture, 1313 W. Eighth Street, Suite 201, Los Angeles, CA 90017)

Brickman, A. (1989). Lessons for antibody test counselors from the AIDS Conference. *Focus: A Guide to AIDS Research and Counseling, 4*(Suppl. 10), 1-2.

Bunning, E. (1990). The role of harm-reduction programmes in curbing the spread of HIV by drug injectors. In J. Strang & G. Stimson (Eds.), *AIDS and drug misuse* (pp. 153-161). New York: Routledge.

Centers for Disease Control. (1991, January). *HIV/AIDS surveillance: Year-end edition*. (Available from Division of HIV/AIDS, Center for Infectious Diseases, Centers for Disease Control, Atlanta, GA 30333)

Cochran, S. D., Mays, V. M., & Leung, L. (1990). *Sexual practices of heterosexual Asian American young adults: Implications for risk of HIV infection*. Unpublished manuscript, University of California, Los Angeles.

Dornette, W. H. L. (1987). *AIDS and the law.* New York: John Wiley.

Douglas, P. H., & Pinsky, L. (1991). *The essential AIDS fact book.* New York: Pocket Books.

Dudley, J. (1990, March). Changes in the protocols: What it means to you. *LAMS Newsletter.* (Available from L.A. Men's Study, UCLA, School of Public Health, 10833 Le Conte Ave., Los Angeles, CA 90024-1772)

Gock, T. S. (1991, April). *AIDS and the Asian Pacific communities: Considerations for substance abuse treatment agenda planning.* Paper presented at the Office of Treatment Improvement meeting, "Treatment Agenda for Asian Pacific Islanders," Honolulu.

Gong, V. (1985). *Understanding AIDS: A comprehensive guide.* New Brunswick, NJ: Rutgers University Press.

Gorrez, L., & Araneta, M. R. G. (1990). *AIDS knowledge, attitudes, beliefs, and behaviors in a household survey of Filipinos in San Francisco: Vol. 1. Findings, summary, and conclusions.* San Francisco: San Francisco City and County Department of Public Health.

Institute of Medicine/National Academy of Sciences. (1986). *Confronting AIDS: Directions for public health, health care, and research.* Washington, DC: National Academy Press.

Institute of Medicine/National Academy of Sciences. (1988). *Confronting AIDS: Update 1988.* Washington, DC: National Academy Press.

Ja, D. Y., Kitano, K. J., & Ebata, A. (1990a). *Report on a survey of AIDS knowledge, attitudes and behaviors in San Francisco's Chinese communities: Executive summary.* San Francisco: San Francisco City and County Department of Public Health.

Ja, D. Y., Kitano, K. J., & Ebata, A. (1990b). *Report on a survey of AIDS knowledge, attitudes and behaviors in San Francisco's Japanese communities: Executive summary.* San Francisco: San Francisco City and County Department of Public Health.

Jue, S. (1987). Identifying and meeting the needs of minority clients with AIDS. In C. Leukfeld & M. Fimbres (Eds.), *Responding to AIDS: Psychosocial initiatives* (pp. 65-79). Washington, DC: National Association of Social Workers Press.

Kübler-Ross, E. (1987). *AIDS: The ultimate challenge.* New York: Macmillan.

Lee, D. A., & Fong, K. (1990, February/March). HIV/AIDS and the Asian and Pacific Islander community. *SIECUS Report,* pp. 16-22.

Los Angeles County Department of Health Services. (1989). *Asian Pacific AIDS cases, Los Angeles County, April 15, 1989.* (Available from Asian Pacific AIDS Education Project, Asian Pacific Health Care Venture, 1313 W. Eighth St., Suite 201, Los Angeles, CA 90017)

Los Angeles County Department of Health Services. (1991, January). *Monthly AIDS report, December 1990.* Los Angeles: Author.

Los Angeles County HIV Planning Council. (1990). *Los Angeles County HIV strategic plan, fiscal years 1990/91-1992/93.* (Available from the AIDS Program Office, Los Angeles County Department of Health Services, 600 S. Commonwealth Ave., 6th Floor, Los Angeles, CA 90005)

National AIDS Network. (1989). The many faces of Asian AIDS. *NAN Multi-Cultural Notes on AIDS Education and Services, 2*(3), 1-2.

Sasao, T. (1991). *Statewide Asian drug service needs assessment in California* (Contract No. D-0008-9). Sacramento: State of California, Department of Alcohol and Drug Programs.

Shilts, R. (1987). *And the band played on.* New York: St. Martin's.

Strunin, L. (1991). Adolescents' perception of risk for HIV infection: Implications for future research. *Social Science and Medicine, 32,* 221-228.

Taylor, C. S. (1991, April 1). Federal health officials say 1990 figures indicate more women are catching AIDS virus than males. *Metropolitan News-Enterprise,* p. 15.

Toleran, D. E. (1991). Pakikisama: Reaching the Filipino community with AIDS prevention. *MIRA, 5*(1), pp. 1, 8-10.

Wood, W. J. (1988). Whether to take experimental drugs: Counseling issues. *Focus: A Guide to AIDS Research, 3*(6), 1-2.

Zane, N. W. S., & Sasao, T. (in press). Research on drug abuse among Asian Pacific Islanders. *Drugs and Society.*

Zhang, Q., & Ziolkowski, H. (1990). Treating HIV disease with Chinese medicine. *Focus: A Guide to AIDS Research and Counseling, 5*(10), 1-2.

9

Mental Health

STANLEY SUE

For decades, a popular belief among the general U.S. public has been that Asian Pacific Americans are extremely well adjusted, as reflected in their low rates of social deviance (e.g., juvenile delinquency and criminality) and divorce as well as high socioeconomic mobility (e.g., educational and occupational attainments) (Sue & Morishima, 1982). Although there is increasing recognition that the popular conception of well-adjusted Asian Pacific Americans is actually a stereotype, little knowledge exists on the mental health problems experienced by members of this community or on strategies to increase the availability and effectiveness of services for this population. The intent of this chapter is to review the available data and literature on mental disorders and intervention programs or services for Asian Pacific Americans.

Prevalence of Mental Disorders

Unlike other ethnic groups, such as African and Hispanic Americans, Asian Pacific Americans have had to confront stereotypes of extraordinary well-being and mental health. In psychological research on Asian Pacific Americans, the critical question is not whether mental health problems exist, because all groups encounter these problems. The meaningful questions involve the extent of mental disorders, the nature of psychopathology, and the particular Asian

Pacific American groups at risk for disorders. I will address these questions in this section by discussing some prevalence, personality, and needs assessment studies.

Prevalence Studies

Prevalence studies attempt to specify the new and ongoing cases of disorders in a particular population over a specified period of time. This is usually accomplished by surveying a population or a representative sample of the population, using a valid measure of psychological disturbance. For example, in the Epidemiologic Catchment Area Study, one of the largest and most rigorous prevalence investigations ever undertaken in the United States, Myers et al. (1984) used the Diagnostic Interview Schedule to ascertain the mental health status of thousands of Americans in different cities across the United States. The investigators found that over a 6-month period, nearly 20% of Americans had experienced or were currently experiencing a mental disorder. The most frequent disorders involved were anxiety and depression.

Unfortunately, in the case of Asian Pacific Americans, no large-scale prevalence studies have been conducted. Thus it is difficult to specify what the rates of mental disorders are within this population, or to compare the various Asian Pacific American groups with each other and with non-Asian Pacific American groups. Because the population of Asian Pacific Americans is relatively small (less than 3% of the U.S. population) and is composed of many different groups, researchers have had difficulty finding adequate and representative samples with which to conduct studies. Furthermore, lack of funding for research on Asian Pacific Americans and problems in finding cross-culturally valid measures of psychopathology have also hindered attempts to study the prevalence of psychiatric disorders among this population. The few available investigations of Asian Pacific Americans have been small-scale studies, often based on selected groups or on selected disorders, and some have not been true prevalence studies. The data that are available, however, provide evidence that suggests the rates of psychopathology among Asian Pacific Americans have been underestimated. Examples of studies with selected groups include the work of Westermeyer, Vang, and Neider (1984), who studied a small group of Laotian Hmong refugees in Minnesota. Using various measures of psychopathology (e.g., the Self-Rating Depression Scale and the Symptom

Checklist-90), these researchers found that the refugees had very high rates of psychiatric disorders. Other studies have also revealed that Southeast Asian refugees are at risk for mental disorders (Berry & Blondel, 1982; Lin, 1986). Investigations by Kuo (1984; Kuo & Tsai, 1986) have examined community samples of four different Asian American groups: Chinese, Japanese, Filipino, and Korean. Using the Center for Epidemiological Studies-Depression Scale, Kuo found that Asian Americans had higher average scores on the measure than did whites. About 19% of the Asian Americans studied were identified as potential cases of depression on the measure.

Finally, in an epidemiological study, Hurh and Kim (1990) examined the correlates of mental health in more than 600 Korean Americans. For male immigrants, being married and being employed in a high-status occupation were related to better subjective mental health. In the case of female immigrants these variables were also important, but less so than in the case of males. The investigators interpreted the findings in terms of Korean gender role ideology.

Personality Surveys

In addition to prevalence studies, personality investigations have provided insight into the mental health problems of Asian Pacific Americans, because they often assess levels of adjustment. Using the Omnibus Personality Inventory (OPI), Sue and his colleagues compared Japanese and Chinese American college students with non-Asian students at the University of California, Berkeley (D. Sue, 1973; Sue & Frank, 1973; Sue & Kirk, 1973). No differences between Chinese and Japanese American students reached significance. However, when race-by-sex comparisons were conducted, significant differences were found. In terms of anxiety level, Chinese American males and females expressed significantly more discomfort than did their control counterparts. On the Personal Integration Scale, Chinese American males and females and Japanese American males expressed more feelings of isolation and loneliness than did their control counterparts. On the Social Extroversion Scale, these three groups also had greater tendency to withdraw from social contacts. Japanese American females did not differ from the control females on any of these scales. Finally, in their responses to the Impulse Expression Scale, Chinese American males and females and Japanese American females were more likely to inhibit the expression of impulses than were control males and females. These results suggest that Chinese American males and females and Japanese American males show more feelings of anxiety, discomfort, loneliness, and isolation than their control counterparts. In addition, they are less socially extroverted and less likely to express impulses than other students. The results are less clear for Japanese American females.

A more recent study using the OPI found similar results between Chinese American students at UCLA and those from the UC Berkeley study that was conducted more than 10 years earlier (Sue & Zane, 1985). Most important, the study revealed that anxiety levels of students were directly related to acculturation: Recent immigrants were more likely to experience anxiety than were immigrants who had been in the United States longer. Interestingly, the academic achievement levels (i.e., academic grades) of the Chinese students exceeded those of the general student body. Thus the fact that Asian Americans perform well in terms of academic achievement should not be used as an indicator of emotional well-being or adjustment.

Needs Surveys

Needs surveys are intended to provide information on the needs that particular groups have. The needs investigated may include economic, housing, legal, employment, and service requirements. These surveys frequently assess mental health needs and provide an understanding of the extent and nature of emotional/adjustment problems of a given community. Two early needs surveys among Asian Pacific Americans are quite revealing. B. L. C. Kim (1978) studied Chinese, Japanese, Korean, and Filipino Americans (immigrants and citizens) in the Chicago area. Kim assessed social, economic, educational, and mental health needs as well as attitudes and beliefs about social service organizations and cultural resources. He found important differences within and between Asian American groups, but one of the more general problems he found was that of language. Not surprisingly, Asian Americans tended to be concerned about English proficiency. The lack of English facility seemed to exacerbate virtually every problem faced by the Asian Americans in Kim's study. Other common problems included cultural differences, insufficient income, employment problems, and experiencing discrimination.

The second revealing needs survey, conducted in Hawaii, provides insight into the public awareness and perception of mental health services (Prizzia & Villanueva-King, 1977). A significant proportion of respondents in this survey were unaware of the availability of local mental health services, although the vast majority considered such services important. About a third of the respondents reported that they would feel some degree of discomfort in using services, particularly Samoan and Filipino Americans; there was less discomfort among whites and Japanese Americans.

These early needs surveys helped to document the kinds of problems faced by Asian Pacific Americans and their attitudes toward services. In view of the rapid increase in Asian and Pacific Islander immigrants and refugees in recent years, a more current appraisal of needs was undertaken by Zane, Fujino, Nakasaki, and Yasuda (1988) in Los Angeles. These researchers held meetings with community leaders and residents and conducted key informant interviews to assess the needs of various Asian Pacific American groups, such as Cambodians, Chinese, Japanese, Koreans, Laotians, Filipinos, Samoans, Thais, Tongans, and South Vietnamese. In general, employment, legal, and English-language needs were of top priority, especially for recent immigrants and refugees. Mental health needs were also considered important, although they were secondary to employment and language needs.

The findings from the available research on prevalence, personality, and needs strongly imply that major mental health problems exist among Asian Pacific Americans. The few prevalence and personality studies demonstrate some of the emotional problems (i.e., anxiety and depression) that are common. Although the validity of measures for ethnic minority groups can always be questioned in the absence of validation studies, the evidence is quite convergent. The needs assessment research reveals that mental health needs are judged to be secondary to language, employment, and legal concerns. However, emotional well-being and adjustment are likely to be strongly related to these concerns. Although it is difficult to specify the prevalence of disorders, the available research findings are contrary to the widespread belief that Asian Pacific Americans are extraordinarily well-adjusted.

Disorders and High-Risk Groups

Given the fact that little is known about the nature and distribution of mental disorders among Asian Pacific Americans, one can only speculate as to the kinds of emotional problems individuals in this population experience. Many Asian Pacific Americans report conflicts involving the family, such as in parent-child interactions. Children often feel that parents maintain traditional role relationships that hinder the children's attempts to be independent. For example, a first-generation father may perceive a second-generation son as being disobedient and no good; in turn, the son may view the father as authoritarian, distant, and old-fashioned. Another common problem among Asian Pacific Americans is extreme shyness and the identity conflicts that can result. Although shyness is not intrinsically negative, many Asian Pacific Americans find this personality pattern disturbing and want to be less shy, especially in a society that values assertiveness and where ethnic minority group individuals encounter stereotypes and discrimination. How these problems are reflected in rates of actual mental disorders is unclear.

We also know that certain groups are at greater risk than others for mental health problems. Recent immigrants, for example, encounter numerous problems involving English-language skills, minority group status, cultural conflicts, and employment that are basic to survival and well-being. The Sue and Zane (1985) study mentioned above demonstrated that recent Chinese immigrants are more likely to report anxiety than are later immigrants or American-born Chinese. Other studies have revealed that Southeast Asian refugees are at particular risk for depression and post-traumatic stress disorder, because of premigration traumas and the postmigration stressors of adapting to and living in a new culture (Gong-Guy, 1987; Westermeyer et al., 1984).

Aside from interest in the distribution of disorders and high-risk groups, researchers have focused attention on somatization among various Asian Pacific American groups. Investigators have argued that certain groups, such as the Chinese, exhibit somatic complaints in their psychiatric symptomatology. For example, researchers have found that many Asians who are treated for mental health problems complain of headaches, back and chest pains, and the like (Kleinman, 1982; Sue & Morishima, 1982). In a study of cultural differences in symptom expression, Kitano (1969) found that Japanese schizophrenics, compared with Caucasian schizophrenics, were more likely to be withdrawn and to exhibit fewer acting-out behaviors. He attributes the differences to cultural factors, such as the tendency for many Japanese to react to stress by becoming more inward (ga-man)—somatizing and suffering without showing overt signs of agitation. Among many Asians there is a belief in unity between the mind and the body, so emotional disturbances are often reflected in somatic symptoms. For example, in a study of the symptoms exhibited by whites, blacks, and Chinese, Chang (1985) found ethnic differences in the patterns of depressive symptomatology. Cognitive concerns characterized the white group, a mixture of affective and somatic complaints was found among blacks, and Chinese were the most likely to exhibit somatic complaints in depressive symptomatology. Similarly, Tung (1985) asserts that in the case of many Southeast Asians, somatic symptoms such as headaches, insomnia, fatigue, loss of memory, and poor appetite are quite common. These complaints may represent more culturally legitimate means of expressing distress, as physical affective symptoms are less stigmatizing than are emotional or psychiatric problems.

The meanings of findings pertaining to somatization have been debated. One view is that somatization actually represents a depressive disorder (Kleinman, 1982). Somatization may be a socially acceptable means of suppressing direct depressive affect while allowing the individual to receive secondary gain—for example, the attention and dependency that comes with the sick role. Another view is that somatization is a function of the lack of available social supports rather than of the suppression of emotions. The lack of social support leads to feelings of hopelessness, which may cause somatization, especially in cultures where the conceptualization and labeling of mental illness is different from Western cultures, where direct "psychologizing" of problems exists (W. H. Kuo, personal communication, 1989). Others have argued that somatization is often under the control of display rules that dictate when, where, and what symptoms are shown (Cheung, 1982). In this view, it is not so much that Chinese suppress or repress affective symptoms as that the context of the situation influences what is presented. Chinese may display somatic symptoms to mental health workers but show depressive symptoms to others. Although these explanations are similar in some respects and are culture based, they differ in emphasis, on whether somatization is viewed as being under the control of intrapsychic or environmental demands. The issues surrounding somatization are important for assessment and treatment. If somatization represents an underlying depressive condition, then the validity of assessment instruments that do not take into account cultural expressions of symptoms may be called into question. If somatization operates under certain display rules, then it is important for a practitioner to understand the rules before rendering a diagnosis. In terms of treatment, confusion over the meaning of somatic symptoms hinders the determination of appropriate forms of treatment and the problems that should be addressed.

Mental Health Services

In the past, utilization of mental health services was used as an indicator of psychopathology in particular populations. The assumption was that if one group had a high prevalence of mental disorders, that group would tend to utilize services more often than would a group with a lower prevalence rate: The *demand* for services was considered to be a reflection of the *need* for services. It is now widely recognized that demand does not indicate need, especially for some groups. Nevertheless, utilization of services must be examined, because it reveals possible cultural differences in defining and approaching mental health problems, provides information about the kinds of problems clients have, indicates the responsiveness of the mental health care system, and yields some insight into how we may better treat or prevent problems. In this section I will examine studies of utilization and then discuss factors that influence help seeking in the service system.

Utilization

Table 9.1 lists a number of studies that have examined utilization among various Asian Pacific American groups. Almost all past studies have demonstrated low rates of utilization among Asian Pacific Americans. Kitano (1969) presented findings on the admission of patients to California state mental hospitals; admission rates for mental disturbance were many times lower for Japanese and Chinese Americans than for Caucasian Americans during each of the years from 1960 to 1965. Data from the state of Hawaii also revealed low Asian and Pacific Islander rates of admission to state hospitals for mental disorders. Chinese, Hawaiian, Japanese, and Filipino Americans all exhibited lower rates of admissions than expected from their proportions in the population.

These and more recent studies consistently demonstrate that Asian Americans tend to be underrepresented in psychiatric clinics and

Table 9.1 Studies Examining Mental Health Service Utilization Among
             Asian Pacific Americans

Study	Population	Measures	Findings
Sue and Sue (1974)	students	MMPI, critical items	underutilization, more disturbed, high dropout
Kitano (1969)	general population/ inpatients	—	underutilization
Hawaii State Department of Health (1970)	general population	—	underutilization
Brown et al. (1973)	general population/ inpatients	ratings	underutilization, more disturbed
S. Sue (1977)	general population	diagnosis	underutilization, more disturbed, high dropout
L.A. County Department of Mental Health (1984)	general population	—	underutilization
Cheung (1989)	general population	—	underutilization
O'Sullivan et al. (1989)	general population	GAS	no underutilization, no greater disturbance, low dropout
Snowden and Cheung (1990)	general population/ inpatient	diagnosis	underutilization, longer stay
Sue et al. (1991)	general population	diagnosis	underutilization, greater disturbance
Matsuoka (1990)	general population	—	underutilization

hospitals compared with their proportions in the larger population
(Brown, Huang, Harris, & Stein, 1973; Cheung, 1989; Los Angeles
County Department of Mental Health, 1984; Snowden & Cheung,
1990; S. Sue, 1977; Sue, Fujino, Hu, Takeuchi, & Zane, 1991). The
underrepresentation occurs whether student or nonstudent populations, inpatients or outpatients, or different Asian Pacific American

groups are considered. In one of the most comprehensive analyses conducted to date, Matsuoka (1990) examined Asian Pacific Americans' use of services at state and county mental hospitals, private psychiatric hospitals, Veterans Administration psychiatric services, residential treatment centers for emotionally disturbed children, nonfederal psychiatric services in general hospitals, outpatient psychiatric clinics, multiservice mental health programs, psychiatric day/night services, and other residential programs in the United States. In general, Matsuoka found that utilization of services by Asian Pacific American populations was low, regardless of their population density in various U.S. states. The only exception to findings of underutilization is found in a study by O'Sullivan, Peterson, Cox, and Kirkeby (1989). Analyzing the community mental health service utilization rates for ethnic groups in the Seattle area, the investigators found that Asian Americans were not underrepresented as users. It is unclear why the results of this study are at variance with all of the others. One potential explanation is that the utilization figures for 1983 were compared with Seattle population data from the 1980 census. If the Asian Pacific American population had marked growth from 1980 to 1983 in Seattle (as it did elsewhere—Asian Pacific Americans represent the fastest-growing ethnic minority in the United States), then this group may indeed be underrepresented as clients. Perhaps the findings are unique to Seattle. In any event, underutilization appears to be the rule rather than the exception.

Severity of Disturbance

The term *underutilization* implies that Asian Pacific Americans are not using services when they need to. Is it possible that this population is relatively better adjusted than other populations, so that greater utilization of services is unnecessary? Every population underutilizes in the sense that not all individuals with psychological disturbance seek help from the mental health system. For example, in the Epidemiologic Catchment Area Study, which compared the prevalence rate of mental disorders with the rate of utilization of mental health care services, the vast majority of afflicted individuals did not seek services (Shapiro et al., 1984). The real issue is whether Asian Pacific Americans with psychiatric disorders have a greater propensity to avoid using services than do other populations. Although this issue cannot be fully addressed in the absence of information on prevalence rates, considerable indirect evidence exists that Asian Pacific Americans are more likely than the general population to underutilize services. As mentioned earlier, the available small-scale prevalence, personality, and needs assessment studies of Asian Pacific Americans suggest that considerable mental health problems exist, and yet utilization is dramatically low. Other lines of evidence, such as severity of disturbance, also point to underutilization.

A study in which I took part in the 1970s analyzed the Asian American (primarily Chinese, Japanese, and Korean) students who utilized the student psychiatric clinic at the University of California, Los Angeles (Sue & Sue, 1974). We obtained information on the number of Asian American student clients, MMPI test scores, and therapists' impressions of these clients. Our findings indicated that Asian American students, who represented 8% of the campus population, constituted only 4% of the clients at the psychiatric clinic— an underrepresentation factor of one half. When we examined the MMPI records, we found that Asian American students exhibited more severe disturbances than other students. Therapists' clinical notes also confirmed that the Asian American students had more serious symptoms than did non-Asian students. The findings revealed that Asian Americans underutilized mental health services and exhibited greater disturbance among the client population. Our inference was that moderately disturbed Asian Americans, unlike Caucasian Americans, are more likely to avoid using services (unless one takes the unusual and unsupported position that Asian Americans have low rates of overall disturbance but high rates of severe mental disorders).

Other studies demonstrate that the phenomena of low utilization and greater severity among Asian Pacific American clients are not confined to students. Brown and his colleagues (1973) investigated Chinese American patients at Resthaven Community Mental Health Center in the Chinatown area of Los Angeles. They examined records of 23 Chinese and 23 Caucasian American patients who were matched on variables such as sex, age, financial status, and legal status (voluntary or involuntary admission). The researchers obtained data from patients' backgrounds, treatment records, and behavioral rating measures. Ratings of patients on the Twelve Psychotic Syndromes Scale revealed that Chinese Americans scored significantly higher than Caucasian Americans on psychomotor retardation, seclusiveness, help needed, and psychotic disorganization.

Brown et al. also found that Chinese Americans underutilized the community mental health center by about half the rate expected on the basis of their proportion of the population in downtown Los Angeles.

In the Seattle Project, I collected records of clients from different Asian American groups, such as Chinese, Japanese, Korean, and Filipino Americans, as well as non-Asian groups, from 17 community mental health centers for a 3-year period (S. Sue, 1977). My intent was to investigate utilization rates, severity of disorders, and demographic characteristics of clients. Relatively few Asian Americans used services: Although they represented about 2.4% of the population served by the centers, only about 100 (or less than 1%) of the 13,000 patients were Asian Americans. To determine whether they were more severely disturbed than whites, I compared Asians with whites in the proportion of functional psychotic diagnoses. A significantly higher percentage of Asian American patients (22%) were diagnosed as psychotic, compared with the 13% figure for white patients. The difference persisted even after I controlled for demographic differences between the two groups in age and educational attainments.

Finally, the National Research Center on Asian American Mental Health at UCLA acquired a large data set on thousands of clients seen in the Los Angeles County mental health system from 1983 to 1988. Preliminary analysis of the data set revealed that Asian Pacific Americans were underrepresented in the outpatient mental health system. They represented 8.7% of the county population, but they constituted only 3.1% of the clients. Latinos were also underrepresented. On the other hand, blacks used services in proportions greater than expected given their relative proportion in the population. When the proportions of clients having psychotic diagnoses were tabulated by ethnic group, Asian Pacific Americans were more likely than whites, blacks, and Latinos to have individuals with psychotic diagnoses in inpatient and outpatient services.

The evidence is quite convergent that few Asian Pacific Americans use the mental health service system. This underutilization is found among all Asian Pacific Americans groups studied, among inpatient and outpatient facilities, and among students and adults. Furthermore, the studies consistently show that on a variety of measures Asian Pacific Americans have greater disturbance levels than do non-Asian clients. The alternative explanation that low utilization of services is caused by the low rate of mental disturbance is weakened by findings that Asian Pacific Americans who seek treatment are more severely disturbed than are Caucasian Americans who do so. These findings suggest that more moderately disturbed Asian Pacific Americans may simply not be using professional mental health services. Lin, Inui, Kleinman, and Womack (1982) found that Asian Americans were more likely than whites to have delays in the recognition of mental health symptoms and in actual participation in a treatment program.

Reasons for Underutilization of Services

A number of factors affect utilization and effectiveness of mental health services, including accessibility (e.g., ease of using services, financial cost of services, location of services), availability (e.g., existence of services), cultural and linguistic appropriateness of services, knowledge of available services, willingness to use services, and existence of alternative and competing services. Further, the nature of an individual's problems also influences utilization. In this section I will focus on culture-based factors such as shame and stigma, conceptions of mental health, and alternative services as factors that affect utilization and appropriateness of mainstream services (i.e., services that are available to the general U.S. population).

For many Asian Pacific American groups, cultural attitudes and beliefs must be considered in the analysis of service utilization. Particularly important is the concept of shame or face. Haji among the Japanese, hiya among the Filipinos, mentz among the Chinese, and chaemyun among the Koreans are terms that reveal concerns over the process of shame or the loss of face (B. L. C. Kim, 1978). The existence of certain problems in the family—such as juvenile delinquency and acting-out behaviors, mental disorders, AIDS, poverty—is considered shameful and likely to bring disgrace on the entire family (Sue & Morishima, 1982). Consequently, many Asian Pacific Americans tend to avoid the juvenile justice or legal system, mental health agencies, health services, and welfare agencies, because the utilization of services for certain problems is a tacit admission of the existence of these problems and may result in public knowledge of familial difficulties. For example, Asian Pacific Americans have been found to differ from white Americans in help-seeking behaviors for emotional difficulties. They are less likely to request outside help for these difficulties, turning first to their families for help and to outside agencies or mainstream services only as a last resort (Tracey, Leong, & Glidden, 1986). Although most Americans are likely to turn to their families as the first resource, and to feel shame or stigma over certain problems, the avoidance of mainstream services is more pronounced among Asian Pacific Americans. That is, there is a differential effect caused by the strong concern over loss of face among Asian Pacific Americans.

Because of shame and stigma, several consequences can be hypothesized. First, those behaviors that create shame and stigma are the ones that are most likely to be denied. For example, the behaviors of children and adolescents are considered a reflection of family upbringing. Therefore, parents may delay using services for their children if such services are needed for problems that would bring shame upon the family. It should be noted that the shame associated with having health and mental health problems may be experienced more acutely by Asian Pacific Americans who reside in immigrant communities. In such communities there are great expectations for doing well in America for the sake of family members both in the United States and back in the country of origin. The personal networks in these communities are often extensive, and information about others is easily shared and disseminated. Within this context, the development of a mental health problem that may compromise a person's productivity or status can generate significant loss of face. Moreover, the need to seek outside help for such a problem only exacerbates the shame. Thus available services tend to be underutilized. Second, as mentioned earlier, the need for services is not equivalent to the demand for services. Asian Pacific Americans may have needs for certain services that are not reflected in their utilization patterns. Third, if services are avoided and used as a last resort, problems may be exacerbated by the delay in finding assistance. Fourth, because Asian Pacific Americans pay taxes for services that they avoid using, they do not receive their fair share of services.

The nature of mental health is strongly influenced by culture. As noted earlier, cultural influences help to shape the symptoms an individual exhibits when emotionally disturbed. Cultural factors also affect interpretations of the causes of disorders and interventions deemed appropriate to overcome health and mental health problems (Leong, 1986). In traditional Chinese culture, for example, many diseases or physical afflictions are attributed to an imbalance of cosmic forces—yin and yang. The task is to restore balance through proper diet, exercise, and psychosocial relationships with others. Essentially, this is a holistic approach to health. Kinzie (1985) notes that many Southeast Asians have a folk tradition in which illness is believed to be caused by physiological factors or supernatural forces (e.g., as the consequence of offending a deity or spirit). Thus they may be unwilling or unable to differentiate among psychological, physiological, and supernatural causes of illness.

Because of the cultural factors that influence symptom expression and conceptions of illness, it is apparent that Asian Pacific Americans are likely to differ from mainstream Americans in the types of interventions used to prevent or treat emotional disturbances and illnesses. The interventions may involve restoration of balance and holistic approaches that are consistent with their cultural beliefs: use of herbal medicine, consultations with folk healers or fortune tellers, acupuncture, certain forms of exercise, and so on. The extent of utilization of these alternatives among different Asian Pacific American groups is unknown, although it is assumed to be highest among recent immigrants or those who are relatively less acculturated to American society. In a study of the utilization of medical care systems among Chinese Americans in Boston, Hessler, Nolan, Ogbu, and New (1975) divided utilization patterns into Chinese medical care only, Western medical care only, predominantly Chinese care, and predominantly Western care. Demographic variables, as well as identification with being Chinese, predicted the type of health care sought. Not surprisingly, Chinese medicine was favored by those subjects less acculturated to American society. Other Asian Pacific American groups also make use of alternative forms of treatment.

The notion that underutilization is, in part, caused by the use of alternative resources is supported by studies of Asians in other countries. For example, Lin, Tardiff, Donetz, and Goresky (1978) found that Chinese resorted to family for support before seeking assistance from medical professionals. Only after a long period of delay did they enter the mental health care system. Although most Americans tend to rely on family and friends before turning to mental health workers (Gourash, 1978; Gurin, Veroff, & Feld, 1960; Lieberman & Glidewell, 1978), there is a marked tendency for Asian Pacific Americans to avoid mental health providers.

These studies suggest that Asian and Caucasian Americans do have different conceptions of mental health and disturbance. Asian

Pacific Americans tend to perceive more organic or somatic involvement in emotional disturbance. They also believe that the exercise of willpower, the avoidance of morbid thoughts, and a focus on pleasant cognitions are means to enhance psychological well-being (Sue & Morishima, 1982). Because professional mental health treatment often stresses insight-oriented approaches that require self-disclosure of morbid (that is, disturbing and embarrassing) thoughts, Asian Americans may avoid Western forms of mental health treatment and seek medical treatment for emotional problems.

Enhancement of Services

Counseling and psychotherapy in the United States generally represent a particular (white, middle-class, Western) worldview. The characteristics of American therapy may conflict with values, styles, and expectations commonly found among Asian Pacific Americans (S. C. Kim, 1985). Thus services may not be culturally consistent with the backgrounds and experiences of Asian Pacific Americans. How can services be organized to respond better to the needs of Asian Pacific Americans? Three directions are discussed below: changes in mental health programs, awareness of interpersonal processes in treatment, and community education.

Organization of Services

In another context I have offered three suggestions for more effectively meeting the mental health needs of Asian Pacific Americans (Uba & Sue, in press). First, in mainstream mental health facilities where there are few Asian Pacific American personnel, service providers can receive training for working with Asian Pacific American clients. Such training would cover assessment, psychotherapy, and case management and would include issues such as cultural values and behaviors and pre- and postmigration experiences. The intent of the training would be to enhance skills and knowledge about Asian Pacific Americans. Special Asian Pacific American consultants should be available to the service providers. Second, mainstream mental health programs should employ more Asian Pacific American personnel who are bilingual and bicultural. Such personnel can be of immense benefit in the effective provision of services. In recent work my colleagues and I have found that when Asian Pacific American clients are matched with therapists who are of the same ethnicity and who speak the clients' language, they stay in treatment longer, tend not to terminate services prematurely, and have better treatment outcomes (Sue et al., 1991). Third, parallel or nonmainstream services should be created. Parallel services are those that may be similar to mainstream ones (e.g., a clinic or hospital) but are specifically designed to serve an ethnic population. For example, a specific ward was created to serve Asian Pacific Americans at San Francisco General Hospital, and in Los Angeles, the Asian Pacific Counseling and Treatment Center was established. Such services typically employ bilingual and bicultural personnel, post notices in English and Asian languages, serve "Asian" foods or drinks, and so on—all in an attempt to respond to the cultural needs of Asian Pacific Americans. Existing parallel services should be strengthened, and new parallel programs should be designed.

Interpersonal Processes

In addition to organizational changes in the service delivery system, therapists must develop skills for working with Asian Pacific Americans. How can clinicians become more effective in working with Asian and Pacific Islander clients? Traditionally, researchers and practitioners have advocated two strategies—one concerning the importance of knowing the culture and background of clients and the other concerning specific techniques to use with ethnic minority clients. Neither strategy has been very effective. Acquiring cultural knowledge is important, but such knowledge has not led directly to an increased understanding of how to conduct psychotherapy. For example, if a practitioner knows that South Vietnamese are family oriented, how should he or she apply this knowledge in therapy? Several other questions can be raised. How much cultural knowledge is necessary? Isn't it impossible to know enough about all the cultures of all the diverse groups in the United States? Does studying the cultural background of a client lead to the danger of stereotyping the client?

The difficulties in addressing these questions have led some investigators to question whether cultural knowledge is a sufficient condition for conducting effective psychotherapy and to offer more concrete suggestions on how to conduct therapy. Some clinicians have attempted to devise what are considered culturally consistent forms of intervention. For example, Asian Pacific Americans tend to prefer psychotherapists who provide structure, guidance, and direction rather than nondirectiveness in interactions (S. C. Kim, 1985), and therapists have been advised to be directive with Asian Pacific Americans. Similar suggestions have been made for other minority group clients. However, these recommendations also raise questions. Is it possible for therapists to change their therapeutic orientations in working with ethnic clients? For instance, a psycho-analytic therapist might find it very difficult to become more directive when working with an Asian client. By using a specific approach—one presumably based on the culture of the client—how does one deal with intragroup variability, given that ethnic minority clients may show many individual differences? Is there a single, culturally consistent form of treatment for each ethnic group? Given the problems in fully answering these questions, Nolan Zane and I have recommended the investigation of therapeutic processes rather than simply argued for cultural knowledge or culture-specific forms of treatment (Sue & Zane, 1987). The two processes we believe to be critical, at least in initial treatment sessions, are credibility and gift giving (i.e., seeing that the client receives a benefit early in the treatment process).

Credibility. Two factors are important in the area of credibility: ascribed status and achieved status. *Ascribed* status is an individual's position or role as it is assigned by others or by cultural norms. For example, in some cultures the young are subordinate to elders, women defer to men, and those who are naive submit to those in authority. Credibility can also be established through *achieved* status. In a clinical context, achieved credibility comes about through the skills and actions of the therapist in treatment, as when the therapist does something that is perceived by the client as being helpful. Ascribed and achieved credibility undoubtedly are related, but they tend to have distinct and different implications for ethnic clients in terms of the psychotherapeutic process. Lack of ascribed credibility seems to relate to clients' willingness to use services, whereas lack of achieved credibility may better explain premature termination and problems related to poor rapport.

Giving. Asian Pacific American clients often wonder how self-disclosure of personal problems to psychotherapists can result in the alleviation of emotional and behavioral distress. Generally, clients need to feel a direct benefit from treatment. I refer to this benefit as a "gift." This gift is essentially a gesture of caring on the part of the therapist. The therapist cannot simply raise the expectations of Asian Pacific American clients about outcomes; he or she must give direct benefits that can be experienced by these clients early in treatment. In this way the therapist can achieve status and, thereby, impart credibility to the therapy. Further, immediate treatment benefits address skepticism about Western forms of treatment on the part of many Asian Pacific Americans.

What kinds of gifts can be offered? Much depends on the particular client and situation, but several gifts can be considered. For example, clients who are depressed or anxious will perceive gains in therapy if they experience an alleviation or reduction of these negative emotional states. The therapist can frequently help clients who are in a state of crisis and confusion to develop cognitive clarity or a means of understanding the chaotic experiences they encounter. Such a technique is often used in crisis intervention. Also, therapists can lead clients through the process of normalization, through which the clients come to realize that their thoughts, feelings, or experiences are common to others as well. This may be a gift to those who do not talk to others and mistakenly believe that others do not have similar problems. Gift giving is intended to provide some type of meaningful gain early in therapy. The process of giving, of course, can be conceptualized as a special case of building rapport or establishing a therapeutic relationship. The main point is that therapists need to focus on gift giving and attempt to offer benefits from treatment as soon as possible for Asian Pacific American clients. Therapists should think of the gifts that they can offer, even in the first session.

Community Education

One of the most valuable strategies to use in addressing the mental health needs of Asian Pacific Americans is community education. Many Asian Pacific Americans are unfamiliar with Western mental health concepts and available services. They may consider mental health problems to be shameful or private and may lack understanding about how services can help. In such situations, education is needed to modify attitudes and to indicate methods by which problems can be addressed. Such educational efforts can be made through schools, mass media (radio, television, ethnic newspapers), community forums, and other institutions, coordinated with mental health agencies.

Several points are important to make in the educational messages aimed at Asian Pacific Americans:

1. *Personal and interpersonal problems are common.* These problems can involve generational conflicts in the family, difficulties in adjusting to American society, anxieties, and depression. Unless the problems are addressed, individuals will continue to feel upset, to have interpersonal problems, and to fail to achieve more. (Examples of common problems should be given.) There is no need to be ashamed of having problems; shame simply hinders one's willingness to find means of overcoming them.

2. *Much can be done to prevent or overcome problems.* Learning how to anticipate or manage problems by oneself and talking with others are often very helpful approaches. (The early identification of potential emotional problems, stress management techniques, and communication skills should be emphasized.)

3. *Individuals should seek services for mental health problems if they find their problems too difficult to manage by themselves.* Although traditional, ethnic folk healing may be helpful, mental health services can be effective and should be considered a viable resource. Clients' problems are kept confidential (in accordance with laws) and therapists are available who can speak the ethnic language of clients. (A description of where services are available and the kinds of services available would be very helpful.)

In other words, educational programs should be designed that will describe accurately the nature of mental health problems and services, will provide some ideas of the means of handling problems, and will make services more accessible and acceptable.

Summary

In this chapter I have discussed the mental health problems among Asian Pacific Americans and some services and strategies for increasing the effectiveness of services to those in that population. The major themes can be readily summarized. First, although there has been little research on this population, Asian Pacific Americans have been shown to experience considerable mental health and adjustment problems. Second, particular groups, such as refugees, are especially at risk for psychopathology. Third, adequate resources for Asian Pacific Americans are lacking, and evidence suggests that individuals in this population underutilize mental health services. Finally, much can be done to improve the delivery of services, such as reorganizing services and hiring appropriate ethnic personnel, training effective psychotherapists, and establishing educational programs.

References

Berry, J. W., & Blondel, T. (1982). Psychological adaptation of Vietnamese refugees in Canada. *Canadian Journal of Community Mental Health, 1*, 81-88.

Brown, T. R., Huang, K., Harris, D. E., & Stein, K. M. (1973). Mental illness and the role of mental health facilities in Chinatown. In S. Sue & N. Wagner (Eds.), *Asian-Americans: Psychological perspectives* (pp. 212-231). Palo Alto, CA: Science and Behavior.

Chang, W. (1985). A cross-cultural study of depressive symptomatology. *Culture, Medicine, and Psychiatry, 9*, 295-317.

Cheung, F. K. (1982). Psychological symptoms among Chinese in urban Hong Kong. *Social Science and Medicine, 16*, 1339-1344.

Cheung, F. K. (1989). *Culture and mental health care for Asian Americans in the United States.* Paper presented at the annual meeting of the American Psychiatric Association, San Francisco.

Gong-Guy, E. (1987). *The California Southeast Asian mental health needs assessment.* Oakland, CA: Asian Community Mental Health Services.

Gourash, N. (1978). Help-seeking: A review of the literature. *American Journal of Community Psychology, 6*, 413-423.

Gurin, G., Veroff, J., & Feld, S. (1960). *Americans view their mental health.* New York: Basic Books.

Hawaii State Department of Health. (1970). *Statistical report of the Department of Health.* Honolulu: Author.

Hessler, R. M., Nolan, M. F., Ogbu, B., & New, P. K. (1975). Intraethnic diversity: Health care of the Chinese-Americans. *Human Organization, 34*, 253-262.

Hurh, W. M., & Kim, K. C. (1990). Correlates of Korean immigrants' mental health. *Journal of Nervous and Mental Disease, 178*, 703-711.

Kim, B. L. C. (1978). *The Asian-Americans: Changing patterns, changing needs.* Montclair, NJ: Association of Korean Christian Scholars in North America.

Kim, S. C. (1985). Family therapy for Asian-Americans: A strategic-structural framework. *Psychotherapy, 22*(Suppl.), 342-348.

Kinzie, J. D. (1985). Overview of clinical issues in the treatment of Southeast Asian refugees. In T. C. Owan (Ed.), *Southeast Asian mental health: Treatment, prevention, services, training, and research* (pp. 113-136). Washington, DC: U.S. Department of Health and Human Services.

Kitano, H. H. (1969). Japanese-American mental illness. In S. C. Plog & R. B. Edgerton (Eds.), *Changing perspectives in mental illness* (pp. 256-284). New York: Holt, Rinehart & Winston.

Kleinman, A. M. (1982). Neurasthenia and depression: A study of somatization and culture in China. *Culture, Medicine, and Psychiatry, 6*, 117-189.

Kuo, W. H. (1984). Prevalence of depression among Asian-Americans. *Journal of Nervous and Mental Disease, 172*, 449-457.

Kuo, W. H., & Tsai, Y. (1986). Social networking hardiness and immigrants' mental health. *Journal of Health and Social Behavior, 27*, 133-149.

Leong, F. T. (1986). Counseling and psychotherapy with Asian-Americans: Review of the literature. *Journal of Counseling Psychology, 33*, 196-206.

Lieberman, M. A., & Glidewell, C. G. (1978). Overview. In The helping process [Special issue]. *American Journal of Community Psychology, 6*, 413-411.

Lin, K. M. (1986). Psychopathology and social disruption in refugees. In C. L. Williams & J. Westermeyer (Eds.), *Refugees and mental health* (pp. 61-73). Washington, DC: Hemisphere.

Lin, K. M., Inui, T. S., Kleinman, A., & Womack, W. (1982). Sociocultural determinants of the help-seeking behavior of patients with mental illness. *Journal of Nervous and Mental Disease, 170*, 78-85.

Lin, T., Tardiff, K., Donetz, G., & Goresky, W. (1978). Ethnicity and patterns of help-seeking. *Culture, Medicine, and Psychiatry, 2*, 3-13.

Los Angeles County Department of Mental Health. (1984). *Report on ethnic utilization of mental health services.* Unpublished manuscript.

Matsuoka, J. (1990). *The utilization of mental health programs and services by Asian/Pacific Islanders: A national study.* Unpublished manuscript.

Myers, J. K., Weissman, M. M., Tischler, G. L., Holzer, C. E., Leaf, P. J., Orvaschel, H., Anthony, J. C., Boyd, J. H., Burke, J. D., Kramer, M., & Stoltzman, R. (1984). Six-month prevalence of psychiatric disorders in three communities. *Archives of General Psychiatry, 41*, 959-967.

O'Sullivan, M. J., Peterson, P. D., Cox, G. B., & Kirkeby, J. (1989). Ethnic populations: Community mental health services ten years later. *American Journal of Community Psychology, 17*, 17-30.

Prizzia, R., & Villanueva-King, O. (1977). *Central Oahu community mental health needs assessment survey (Part III): A survey of the general population.* Honolulu: Management Planning and Administration Consultants.

Shapiro, S., Skinner, E., Kessler, L., Von Korff, M., German, P., Tischler, G., Leaf, P., Benham, L., Cottler, L., & Regier, D. (1984). Utilization of health and mental health services. *Archives of General Psychiatry, 41*, 971-978.

Snowden, L. R., & Cheung, F. K. (1990). Use of inpatient mental health services by members of ethnic minority groups. *American Psychologist, 45*, 347-355.

Sue, D. W. (1973). Ethnic identity: The impact of two cultures on the psychological development of Asians in America. In S. Sue & N. N. Wagner (Eds.), *Asian Americans: Psychological perspectives* (pp. 140-149). Palo Alto, CA: Science and Behavior.

Sue, D. W., & Frank, A. C. (1973). A typological approach to the psychological study of Chinese and Japanese American college males. *Journal of Social Issues, 29*, 129-148.

Sue, D. W., & Kirk, B. A. (1973). Differential characteristics of Japanese-American and Chinese-American college students. *Journal of Counseling Psychology, 20*, 142-148.

288   HEALTH STATUS

Sue, S. (1977). Community mental health services to minority groups: Some opti-
mism, some pessimism. *American Psychologist, 32,* 616-624.
Sue, S., Fujino, D., Hu, L., Takeuchi, D., & Zane, N. (1991). *Community mental health
services for ethnic minority groups: A test of the cultural responsiveness hypothesis.*
Manuscript submitted for publication.
Sue, S., & Morishima, J. (1982). *The mental health of Asian Americans.* San Francisco:
Jossey-Bass.
Sue, S., & Sue, D. W. (1974). MMPI comparisons between Asian- and non-Asian-
American students utilizing a university psychiatric clinic. *Journal of Counseling
Psychology, 21,* 423-427.
Sue, S., & Zane, N. (1985). Academic achievement and socioemotional adjustment
among Chinese university students. *Journal of Counseling Psychology, 32,* 570-579.
Sue, S., & Zane, N. (1987). The role of culture and cultural techniques in psychother-
apy: A critique and reformulation. *American Psychologist, 42,* 37-45.
Tracey, T. J., Leong, F. T. L., & Glidden, C. (1986). Help seeking and problem
perception among Asian Americans. *Journal of Counseling Psychology, 33,* 331-336.
Tung, T. M. (1985). Psychiatric care for Southeast Asians: How different is different?
In T. C. Owan (Ed.), *Southeast Asian mental health: Treatment, prevention, services,
training, and research* (pp. 5-40). Washington, DC: U.S. Department of Health and
Human Services.
Uba, L., & Sue, S. (in press). Nature and scope of multicultural mental health services
for Asian/Pacific Islanders. In N. Mokuau (Ed.), *Handbook of social services for
Asian and Pacific Islanders.* Westport, CT: Greenwood.
Westermeyer, J., Vang, T. F., & Neider, J. (1984). Symptom change over time among
Hmong refugees: Psychiatric patients versus nonpatients. *Psychopathology, 17,*
168-177.
Zane, N., Fujino, D., Nakasaki, G., & Yasuda, K. (1988). *United Way Asian Pacific needs
assessment technical report.* Los Angeles: United Way.

10

Tuberculosis

RICHARD S. HANN

Tuberculosis is a disease that antedates recorded history. There is evidence of spinal tuberculosis in neolithic and pre-Columbian skeletons. Tuberculosis was well known to ancient Greek physicians such as Aristotle and Hippocrates, who used the term *phthisis*, which later translated into "consumption." However, tuberculosis did not become a major problem until the crowded living conditions of the early Industrial Revolution provided a favorable environment for its spread.

Prevalence

It is estimated that in the eighteenth and nineteenth centuries, tuberculosis accounted for one fourth of adult deaths in Europe (Dubos & Dubos, 1952). At the beginning of the twentieth century, tuberculosis was the leading cause of death in the United States; since then, there has been a steady decline in the mortality rate, from 202/100,000 population in 1900 to approximately 3.3/100,000 or 6,500 deaths in 1968.

With the advent of modern treatment there is no longer a high mortality rate for tuberculosis. Thus the new case rate became a more accurate measure of clinical problems. The new case rate has also been steadily declining in recent years. However, with the influx of new immigrants from highly endemic regions of the world,

289

including the Caribbean Islands, Central America, and Indochina, tuberculosis has again become a significant issue. Among Indochinese refugees entering the United States in 1978 to 1979, approximately 2% had Class A (active or suspected active) or Class B (inactive, but requiring further medical attention) tuberculosis. The estimated prevalence of tuberculosis among refugees at the time of their arrival in the United States as of 1981 was 1,138/100,000, and an additional 407/100,000 refugees without evidence of disease upon arrival developed tuberculosis during the ensuing year ("Tuberculosis," 1981).

Southeast Asian Refugees

As many as 550,000 refugees from Vietnam, Laos, and Cambodia have settled in the United States since 1975. About 34% of this population is concentrated in California, 31% settled in seven other states (Texas, Washington, Pennsylvania, Illinois, Minnesota, Virginia, and Oregon), and the remaining one third is scattered across the nation (American Public Welfare Association, 1981).

Overseas Medical Screening

Prior to entry into the United States, all immigrants are screened medically by the Intergovernmental Committee for European Migration according to guidelines formulated by the Centers for Disease Control (CDC) of the U.S. Public Health Service. The purpose of such screening is to identify potential immigrants afflicted with excludable medical conditions, including active tuberculosis, among others. Approximately 4% of Southeast Asians screened abroad have excludable medical conditions (Robinson, 1980).

Medical Processing at U.S. Port of Entry

The vast majority of Indochinese refugees enter the United States through San Francisco. The majority (94%) have been judged "within normal limits" of good health, and 0.1% have required immediate hospitalization. The refugees carry, among other papers, Medical Examination Form OF-157, which contains the results of overseas medical screening and denotes medical conditions requiring follow-up, especially tuberculosis, and chest radiographs. At the same time, state and local health officials are notified of refugees with Class A and Class B tuberculosis who require further medical attention.

Pathogenesis

Tuberculosis is for the most part an airborne infection. It is usually caused by inhalation of *Mycobacterium tuberculosis*. Infections by *Mycobacterium avis* may also present significant problems unique to Asian and Pacific Islander Americans. The disease is confined to the lungs but may spread to almost any organ, including meninges, kidneys, bones, and lymph nodes, causing granulomas. Sensitized T cells participate in the development of delayed hypersensitivity and the formation of caseation of the granulomas; humoral antibodies play a minimal role in the disease. Clinical manifestations of the disease may appear sometime after the infection, most commonly within a year, or may arise after a variable period of dormancy, extending from years to decades, particularly when immunity has been compromised.

The pathogenesis of tuberculosis depends on the social and economic environment. In populations living in primitive and crowded environments, it causes higher infant and child mortality and a second peak in early adult years. In more affluent and/or hygienic environments, the disease becomes more common in older people and in immunologically compromised populations.

Most patients newly infected with tubercle bacilli will have few clinical manifestations of the disease but will show delayed hypersensitivity to tuberculoprotein and thus are designated positive tuberculin reactors. Although they are not symptomatic, the tubercle bacilli survive in the tissues for years and can multiply and spread whenever immunity decreases. Most of these reactivated cases show only pulmonary involvement.

Shortly after the initiation of infection, cellular immunity begins to develop and becomes manifest within 4 to 6 weeks. The interaction of sensitized T cells and macrophages help necrotize the tubercle, resulting in caseation necrosis, which diminishes the risk of dissemination at the cost of irreversible damage to the lung.

Transmission depends on the excretion of large inoculum of viable tubercle bacilli in the sputum. This cavitary pulmonary tuberculosis increases the risk of spread to others and also impairs the prognosis for the patient. For these reasons and many others, early identification and treatment of sputum-positive patients is an important element in the control of tuberculosis.

Diagnosis

The screening test of choice in the United States is the tuberculin skin test with 5 TU of PPD injected intradermally, as described by Charles Mantoux; it is administered to refugees as part of their routine health assessment. Because of technical difficulties in administration and interpretation, this test is not routinely used in refugee screening programs abroad.

As many as 50% to 60% of screened refugees are found to be tuberculin positive. Conversion rates of 20% to 43% after initially negative skin tests have been noted. Possible explanations for this high rate of apparent conversion include (a) technical errors in administering and interpreting tests; (b) the incubation period of tuberculosis at the time of the initial skin test; (c) anergic state owing to tuberculosis, malnutrition, concurrent viral illness, or vaccination with live viral vaccines; (d) booster effect of the first test; and (e) contraction of disease after arrival in the United States. Irrespective of the explanation, a single tuberculin test is not sufficient to exclude tuberculosis reliably in this population; the test should be routinely repeated at least once, 12 to 16 weeks after arrival.

Repeated testing of uninfected persons does not sensitize them to tuberculin (Turkey, Dufour, & Seibert, 1950). However, once delayed hypersensitivity to tuberculin has been established by infection with any species of *Mycobacterium* or by BCG vaccination, it may gradually wane over the years. The reaction to a test several years later may not be significant, but the stimulus of the retest may boost the size of the reaction to the repeat test, sometimes causing an apparent conversion or development of sensitivity. The booster effect can be seen after a second test done as soon as a week after the initial one and can persist for a year or more. For this reason, an initial two-step testing technique has been advocated for use whenever serial tuberculin testing is to be done (Atkinson & Farer, 1979). If the reaction to the first test is classified as not significant, a second test should be given a week later. If the second test result remains below the cutoff point, the reaction is classified as nonsignificant. In such a person a significant reaction to a third test within the next few years with an increase of more than 6 mm is likely to represent the acquisition of infection with *M. tuberculosis* in the interval. If the reaction to the second of the initial two tests is significant, this probably represents a boosted reaction signifying old tuberculosis infection and should be managed accordingly.

Vaccination with BCG in significant numbers of Asians and Pacific Islanders presents a serious problem in interpretation of test results. There is no reliable method of distinguishing tuberculin reactions caused by BCG vaccination from those caused by natural mycobacterial infections. It is prudent, therefore, to consider large reactions in BCG vaccinated persons as indicating infection with *M. tuberculosis*. The cutoff point for defining a significant reaction in BCG-vaccinated persons ideally would vary, depending on the potency of the vaccine used, the recentness of vaccination, and the prevalence of tuberculosis in the patient's past environment. If the cutoff point is set at 10 mm, there is a significant chance of making false-positive diagnosis of tuberculosis. But again, one has to remember that many BCG-vaccinated persons are coming from areas of the world where the prevalence of tuberculosis is high.

Although not recommended by the CDC, BCG is routinely given in some refugee transit camps, including those in Thailand (to newborns) and Hong Kong (to those 12 years of age or younger). This unfortunate practice should be discontinued in the case of refugees who headed for the United States (Minh, Prendergast, & Engle, 1982). Thus it is generally recommended to disregard a history of prior BCG administration when interpreting tuberculin skin test results. Because detection of newly infected persons requires accurate testing and reading, multiple-puncture devices should not be used in surveillance programs (Catanzaro, 1985).

The most reliable tuberculin test is still the intradermal Mantoux test, which is performed by intracutaneous injection of 0.1 ml of PPD containing 5 TU into the volar surface of the forearm with a short, bluntly beveled, 27-gauge needle with a glass or plastic tuberculin syringe. The injection should be made just beneath the surface of the skin, with the needle bevel upward. A discrete, pale elevation of the skin of 6 to 10 mm diameter should be produced when the prescribed amount of fluid (0.1 ml) is injected intracutaneously.

The tablet forms of PPD should be replaced as soon as possible with liquid PPD containing polysorbate (tween) or a product of comparable stability. The PPD tuberculin should be injected immediately after the syringe is loaded (Houk, 1972). Test doses should be removed from the vial under strictly aseptic conditions, and the remaining solution should be kept refrigerated (not frozen) and should never be transferred from one container to another. Tuberculin should be stored in the dark as much as possible, and exposure to strong light should definitely be avoided (Landis & Held, 1975).

Using the Mantoux technique, surveys of patients with tuberculosis conducted throughout the world have shown a remarkable degree of concordance in reactions to S-TU of PPD-S or its equivalent. Catanzaro (1985) conducted a comparative study between multiple puncture skin tests and Mantoux tests among Southeast Asian refugees. He found that PPD tine, OT tine, and Aplitest demonstrated a bimodal distribution in a unimodal population by the Mantoux test. For this reason, he does not recommend multiple puncture tests as a screening tool for Southeast Asians. Thus the Mantoux test remains the preferred skin test, in screening as well as diagnostic situations.

Chest X Rays

The incidence of chest X-ray abnormalities consistent with active or inactive tuberculosis is approximately 5% (Centers for Disease Control, 1975; Waldman, Lege, Oseid, & Carter, 1979) in adults and under 1% in children (Centers for Disease Control, 1975). These figures must be interpreted with caution, because many diseases mimic pulmonary tuberculosis radiographically. These include paragonimiasis, melioidosis, ascariasis, hookworm infestation, and tropical eosinophilia. Among them, paragonimiasis, with its chronic hemoptysis, lung infiltrations, and pleural effusion (American Thoracic Society, 1974; Coleman & Root, 1981; Mayer, 1979; Minh et al., 1981), deserves special attention in differential diagnosis. As the two conditions potentially can coexist, the documentation of one condition cannot rule out the other in a refugee from Southeast Asia.

Extrapulmonary Tuberculosis

Tuberculous adenitis is quite common in Southeast Asia (Barrett-Connor, 1978). The prevalence of atypical mycobacterial infection is uncertain, but *Mycobacterium bovis* is rare, perhaps because milk is not commonly drunk (Barrett-Connor, 1978).

Treatment

In studies of drug resistance done between 1961 and 1973 by both U.S. veterans' hospitals and the Centers for Disease Control, the rate of overall drug resistance was 4% to 8% among mostly non-Hispanic and Asian populations (Banks, 1982). Drug resistance represents a major problem that complicates treatment of Southeast Asian refugees. Several independent surveys reviewing drug-resistant tuberculosis in the Indochinese population were summarized by the Centers for Disease Control in 1981. Approximately one third of isolates of M. tuberculosis from Indochinese refugees were found to be resistant to one or more of the standard antituberculosis agents ("Drug-Resistance," 1981; "Primary Resistance," 1981; "Tuberculosis," 1981). Primary resistance to isoniazid (INH) among the refugee patients with active tuberculosis ranges from 10% to 30% (Centers for Disease Control, 1975, 1979; Coleman & Root, 1981). In Southeast Asia, single-drug therapy, usually with INH that is self-administered, has been virtually the rule. Also, acquired resistance after inadequate duration of therapy or the use of one drug (monotherapy) has been documented (Costello, Caras, & Snider, 1980). After 2 weeks of therapy with INH alone, some resistance has been reported in 23% of positive cultures. Resistance to ethambutol and rifampin is negligible.

Current guidelines for INH chemoprophylaxis were defined jointly by the American Thoracic Society and the Centers for Disease Control regardless of prior vaccination with BCG (American National Tuberculosis and Respiratory Disease Association & Centers for Disease Control, 1971). The rationale for the guidelines is valid; INH chemoprophylaxis is safe when properly monitored, and protection from BCG vaccination is marginal at best (Minh et al., 1982). Rifampin chemoprophylaxis has also been proposed for people exposed to INH-resistant strains (Fairshter, Randazzo, & Garlin, 1975; Glassroth, Robins, & Snider, 1980; Koplan & Farer, 1980).

Active tuberculosis in refugees should be treated with these drugs: isoniazid (10 mg/kg/day up to a maximum of 300 mg/kg/day), rifampin (10-20 mg/kg/day up to 600 mg/kg/day), and ethambutol (15-20 mg/kg/day) (Centers for Disease Control, 1979). However, high-dose treatment with ethambutol (25 mg/kg/day) should be avoided considering the severe optic neuritis observed in many refugees who received such treatment overseas. Streptomycin (20 mg/kg/day intramuscularly) should be substituted for ethambutol when visual acuity cannot be evaluated; this regimen is also recommended for children. Low zinc levels in the blood have been speculated to be the cause of optic neuritis in refugees (Wong & Leopold, 1979).

Despite the conclusions of some workers that two drugs are sufficient in culture-positive cases (Dean, 1979), the third drug is still recommended because of the increased incidence of isoniazid resistance. The British Medical Research Council found the three-drug regimen of isoniazid, rifampin, and pyrazinamide to be quite effective even in patients with isoniazid-resistant strains. The recommended duration of therapy is 12 months for culture-negative patients, or until sputum cultures have been negative for 12 months (Centers for Disease Control, 1979).

Authorities disagree on the choice of agent for "preventive" therapy for the Indochinese refugee with a positive tuberculin skin test in the absence of signs of disease. Some recommend INH alone; others advise a combination of INH and rifampin. Still others would withhold antimicrobial therapy until/unless the patient shows evidence of disease (Centers for Disease Control, 1979).

The American Thoracic Society has issued guidelines on isoniazid preventive therapy in the following six categories:

1. Household members and other close contacts of persons with potentially infectious tuberculosis
2. Newly infected persons, including those who have had a tuberculin skin test conversion within the past 2 years and reactors under the age of 5 years
3. Persons who had tuberculosis in the past but did not receive adequate antituberculosis therapy
4. Persons with tuberculin skin test reactions and abnormal chest roentgenograms
5. Persons with tuberculin skin test reactions who also have silicosis, diabetes mellitus, hematologic or reticuloendothelial disease, acquired immunodeficiency syndrome (AIDS) or antibodies to the AIDS virus, end-stage renal disease, or substantial rapid weight loss or chronic undernutrition, as well as those who are also receiving corticosteroid or immunosuppressive therapy
6. Tuberculin skin test reactors under the age of 35 years

These guidelines for the American public in general are very well applicable to Southeast Asian Americans. However, there has been some concern about the last of the above categories. To apply INH prophylaxis on all tuberculin skin reactors under 35 years of age invites serious risk of causing hepatitis; reactivated pulmonary tuberculosis is a treatable disease, but hepatitis is not. Case-fatality rate from INH-related hepatitis has been shown to be slightly higher than that from tuberculosis itself.

The efficiency of short-term chemoprophylaxis has been examined. Daily INH of 3 months has been found to reduce the reactivation rate by 33%, of 6 months by 65%, and of one year by 75%, compared with untreated controls. Moreover, those patients who carefully adhered to the 12-month treatment experienced an 85% to 90% decrease in reactivation rate. Thus, although short-term prophylaxis was effective, it did not reduce relapse rates as well as did 12 months of prophylaxis.

Nolan, Aitken, Elarth, Anderson, and Miller (1986) treated 1,108 Southeast Asian refugees under 35 years of age with prophylactic INH following the National Institutes of Health criteria and followed them up for 4 years. The annual incidence of active tuberculosis among them ranged from 2.04 to 2.86 cases per 1,000 persons, which amounts to 19 cases of active tuberculosis altogether in the 4-year period. Drug compliance was not optimal; only 6 took INH for longer than 6 months, and 10 took the drug for less than 3 months.

Short-Course Chemotherapy

By the mid-1960s, the question of how long a patient with tuberculosis should be treated had become a major issue. To achieve almost 100% effectiveness it had to continue 18 months to 2 years with regimens prevailing at the time; INH, streptomycin (SM), and p-aminosalicylic acid. However, maintenance of treatment for such a long period caused problems of compliance and even of finance, particularly in many developing countries. Therefore great interest was aroused by the reports from Singapore in 1971 that 6 months of daily INH and SM, followed by 6 months of daily INH alone, was very effective.

Singapore Study: Optimal Duration of Short-Term Therapy. A study was conducted in Singapore to determine the optimal duration of multidrug, short-term therapy (British Medical Research Council, 1979). All patients were treated with streptomycin-isoniazid-rifampin-pyrazinamide. Then patients were chosen at random to receive either isoniazid-rifampin-pyrazinamide or isoniazid and rifampin for 2 to 4 additional months. This study suggested that pyrazinamide contributed little to the therapeutic outcome and a short regimen (4 months) had an early relapse of 7.3%.

Hong Kong Studies: Use of Intermittent Therapy. The efficacy of intermittent medication, the use of pyrazinamide, and the optimal duration of short-term regimens were studied in Hong Kong (Fox, 1977; Fox & Mitchison, 1975). The value of daily administration of isoniazid-streptomycin-pyrazinamide was compared with biweekly or triweekly administration, both for 6-month and 9-month durations. The relapse rate was rather high for each 6-month schedule, ranging from 13% to 18%. However, the 9-month schedule brought down the relapse rate to 3% to 4%, suggesting that intermittent therapy had promise if continued for 9 months rather than 6 months.

American Thoracic Society and Centers for Disease Control Recommendations. As results became available for several studies, including East African, French, and British, the American Thoracic Society and the Centers for Disease Control issued the following recommendations for the short-course chemotherapy of tuberculosis:

1. A "core" of isoniazid and rifampin, taken for a minimum of 9 months, is an acceptable alternative to the longer-term treatment schedules used in the past. Daily doses should be 300 mg for isoniazid and 600 mg for rifampin. Ethambutol at 15 mg/kg/day should be added if the physician is concerned about drug resistance.
2. Following an initial phase of daily treatment (2 weeks to 2 months), treatment should be continued with isoniazid and rifampin, either daily (if self-administered) or twice weekly (if supervised).
3. Treatment should continue for 9 months or longer, until the sputum culture has been negative for 6 months. Because more than 90% of patients taking isoniazid-rifampin become culture negative by 3 months of treatment, in most instances total duration will not exceed 9 months. Longer treatment is encouraged for patients suspected of not taking their treatment regularly, for those with disseminated disease, and for those with complicating medical conditions (e.g., patients being treated with corticosteroids).
4. Patients should remain under surveillance for 12 months after completing therapy. This duration is recommended until sufficient information has been obtained about the efficacy of short-course treatment under field conditions in the United States.

Summary

Tuberculosis is one of the most common serious personal health problems facing Indochinese refugees and poses a significant public health problem for the host community. Among Indochinese refugees entering the United States in 1978 and 1979, approximately 2% had Class A tuberculosis, and another 2% had Class B tuberculosis. As of 1981 the estimated prevalence of tuberculosis at arrival in the United States was 1,138 in every 100,000 refugees, and an additional 407 out of 100,000 refugees developed tuberculosis after their settlement in the United States.

Tuberculin skin testing with 5 TU PPD is the screening test of choice in the United States; it should be administered to refugees and immigrants as part of their routine health assessment. As many as 50% to 60% of screened refugees are found to be tuberculin positive. Conversion rates of 20% to 43% after an initially negative skin test have been noted. The tuberculin skin test is interpreted without regard to a history of prior BCG inoculation. Intermediate skin reactions (5 mm to 9 mm) should suggest atypical mycobacterial infection.

Management of refugees and immigrants with tuberculosis should be closely coordinated with local tuberculosis authorities. The collection of appropriate specimens, proper processing of specimens for culture and sensitivity, selection of the most effective therapeutic agents, and decisions regarding duration and modification require expertise and resources beyond the means of the individual practitioner.

There are some differences between "imported" and "domestic" tuberculosis management. Drug resistance represents a major problem in the treatment of Southeast Asian refugees. Approximately one third of isolates of *M. tuberculosis* from those refugees have been found to be resistant to one or more antituberculous agents. Some 25% of strains tested have been found to be resistant to INH, which is widely used in the Far East. Thus the CDC recommends that initial therapy include three agents (INH, rifampin, and ethambutol) pending the results of culture and sensitivity testing. In children, as well as adults, streptomycin may substitute for ethambutol in case visual acuity cannot be evaluated. Chemoprophylaxis for the asymptomatic tuberculin converters may be accomplished with INH alone or INH plus rifampin, or with no treatment at all until the patient becomes symptomatic.

References

American National Tuberculosis and Respiratory Disease Association & the Center for Disease Control (1971). A joint statement on the preventive treatment of tuberculosis. *American Review of Respiratory Diseases, 104,* 460-465.

American Public Welfare Association. (1981). A statistical report. *Refugee Reports,* 2(21), 8.

American Thoracic Society. (1974). Preventive therapy of tuberculous infection: A statement by an ad hoc committee. *American Review of Respiratory Diseases, 110,* 371-374.

Atkinson, M. L., & Farer, L. S. (1979). TB testing for hospital employees: New recommendations. *Hospital Medical Staff, 8,* 16-20.

Banks, D. E. (1982). Asbestos-related diseases of the lung. *West Virginia Medical Journal, 76,* 263-268.

Barrett-Connor, E. (1978). Latent and chronic infections imported from Southeast Asia. *Journal of the American Medical Association, 239,* 1901-1906.

British Medical Research Council. (1979). Singapore tuberculosis: Clinical trial of 6 month and 4 month regimens of chemotherapy in the treatment of pulmonary tuberculosis. *American Review of Respiratory Diseases, 119,* 579-585.

Catanzaro, A. (1985). Multiple puncture skin test and Mantoux test in Southeast Asian refugees. *Chest, 87,* 346-350.

Centers for Disease Control. (1975). Update on refugee health status. *Morbidity and Mortality Weekly Report, 24,* 267-268.

Centers for Disease Control. (1979). Health status of Indochinese refugees. *Morbidity and Mortality Weekly Report, 28,* 385-398.

Coleman, D. L., & Root, R. K. (1981). Pulmonary infections in Southeast Asian refugees. *Clinical Chest Medicine, 2,* 133-143.

Costello, H. D., Caras, G. J., & Snider, D. E., Jr. (1980). Drug resistance among previously treated tuberculosis patients: A brief report. *American Review of Respiratory Diseases, 121,* 313-316.

Dean, A. G. (1979). Suggestions for medical screening of Southeast Asian refugees. *Minnesota Medicine, 60,* 753-754.

Drug-resistance among Indochinese refugees with tuberculosis. (1981). *Morbidity and Mortality Weekly Report, 30,* 273.

Dubos, R., & Dubos, J. (1952). *The white plague: Tuberculosis, man, and society.* Boston: Little, Brown.

Fairshter, R. D., Randazzo, G. P., & Garlin, J. (1975). Failure of INH chemoprophylaxis after exposure to INH resistant tuberculosis. *American Review of Respiratory Diseases, 112,* 37-42.

Fox, W. (1977). The modern management and therapy of pulmonary tuberculosis. *Proceedings of the Royal Society for Experimental Biology and Medicine, 70,* 4-15.

Fox, W., & Mitchison, D. A. (1975). Short course chemotherapy for pulmonary tuberculosis. *American Review of Respiratory Diseases, 11,* 325-352.

Glassroth, J., Robins, A. G., & Snider, D. E., Jr. (1980). Tuberculosis in the 1980's. *New England Journal of Medicine, 301,* 1441-1450.

Houk, V. N. (1972). Tuberculin: Past, present, and future. *Journal of the American Medical Association, 222,* 1421-1422.

Koplan, J. P., & Farer, L. S. (1980). Choice of preventive treatment for isoniazid-resistant tuberculosis infection. *Journal of the American Medical Association, 224,* 2736-2740.

Landis, S., & Held, H. R. (1975). Effect of light on tuberculin purified protein derivative solutions. *American Review of Respiratory Diseases, 111,* 52-61.

Mayer, G. J. (1979). Pulmonary paragonimiasis. *Journal of Pediatrics, 95,* 75-76.

Minh, V. D., Engle, P., Greenwood, J. R., Prendergast, T. J., Salness, K., & St. Clair, R. (1981). Pleural paragonimiasis in a Southeast Asian refugee. *American Review of Respiratory Diseases, 124,* 186-188.

Minh, V. D., Prendergast, T. J., & Engle, P. (1982). Tuberculosis in refugees from Southeast Asia. *Chest, 82,* 133-135.

Nolan, C. M., Aitken, M. L., Elarth, A. M., Anderson, K. M., & Miller, W. T. (1986). Active tuberculosis after isoniazid chemoprophylaxis of Southeast Asian refugees. *American Review of Respiratory Diseases, 133,* 431-436.

Primary resistance to antituberculosis drugs: United States. (1981). *Morbidity and Mortality Weekly Report, 29,* 345.

Robinson, C. (1980). *A special report: Physical and emotional health care needs of Indochinese refugees.* Washington, DC: Indochina Refugee Action Center.

Tuberculosis among Indochinese refugees: An update. (1981). *Morbidity and Mortality Weekly Report, 30,* 603.

Turkey, J. W., Dufour, E. H., & Seibert, F. (1950). Lack of sensitization follow skin tests with standard tuberculin (PPD-S). *American Review of Tuberculosis, 62,* 77-86.

Waldman, E. B., Lege, B., Oseid, B., & Carter, J. P. (1979). Health and nutritional status of Vietnamese refugees. *Southern Medical Journal, 72,* 1300-1303.

Wong, E. K., & Leopold, I. H. (1979). Zinc deficiency and visual dysfunction. *Metabolic and Pediatric Ophthalmology, 1,* 1-4.

11

Parasitic Infestations

RICHARD S. HANN

Parasitic infestations are common in Indochinese refugees as well as among Asians and Pacific Islanders who are entering the United States. The prevalence rates for intestinal parasitic infestations have been shown to be as high as 80% of screened refugees with at least one parasite per stool sample, and 55% with more than one parasite recovered (Barrett-Conner, 1989; Borchard, 1981; Center for Disease Control, 1979b, 1979c; Jones, Thomas, & Brewer, 1980; Skeels, 1982; Wisenthal, Nickels, Hashimoto, Endo, & Ehrhard, 1980).

Although the distribution and frequency of parasites identified vary among ethnic groups and countries of origin, the most commonly recovered parasites are as follows:

- nematodes
    Ancylostoma duodenale (hookworm)
    Necator americanus (hookworm)
    Ascaris lumbricoides (roundworm)
    Trichuris trichuria (whipworm)
    Enterobius vermicularis (pinworm)
    Strongyloides stercoralis
- trematodes
    Clonorchis sinensis (oriental liver fluke)
    Paragonimus westermani (lung fluke)

- cestodes
  Taenia species (tapeworm)
- protozoa
  Giardia lambria
  Entamoeba histolytica

In one of the studies done among refugees from Vietnam, Laos, and Cambodia, hookworm was by far the most common (38%) parasite found, with *Giardia* (9%), *Ascaris* (7%), and *Strongyloides* (6%) also frequent (Catanzaro & Moser, 1982). Three fourths of the *Ascaris* and one half of *Trichuris* infestations were in Vietnamese, 61% of *Clonorchis* infestation was found in Laotians, and the majority of hookworms (73%), *Giardia* (47%), and *Strongyloides* (80%) was found in Cambodians.

Certain parasites, such as *Clonorchis sinensis* and *Paragonimus westermani*, show rather distinct regional distribution even in the same country. Laotians who lived along the Mekong River frequently ate raw fish and crabs, the intermediate hosts for *C. sinensis* and *P. westermani*, respectively. Clonorchiasis is also endemic along the Nakdong River, and paragonimiasis is more or less widespread along small brooks in Korea (Sadun & Buck, 1960).

Age has been associated with both parasitic prevalence and parasitic type. Catanzaro and Moser (1982) found that two thirds of their subjects younger than 4 years had no parasites, those between 5 and 18 years had the highest prevalence of *Strongyloides* (48%), and the oldest group had the majority of the hookworm (51%) and *Clonorchis* (68%) infestations.

Although most individuals with intestinal parasites are asymptomatic, each of these parasites is capable of causing clinically significant diseases. Of equal concern is the potential public health risk. Most intestinal nematode ova require 1 to 2 weeks of incubation in appropriate soil conditions before infective larvae develop; this incubation period is precluded by sewage and sanitation standards in the United States. Similarly, most tissue trematodes require specific intermediate hosts (snails) that are nonexistent in the United States. In contrast, protozoan cysts, which are shed in stool, are directly infectious; both *Giardia* and *Entamoeba histolytica* are capable of person-to-person and food- and waterborne transmission, providing at least a theoretical basis for concern for public health. Likewise, cestode ova and cysts are directly infectious if ingested and could be hazardous to the public.

Paragonimiasis

Paragonimiasis is a chronic infection caused mainly by *Paragonimus westermani*. There are several other species of genus *Paragonimus* that may cause the disease, but they are not a problem in Asian Pacific Americans. Infection with *P. westermani* is endemic in Southeast Asia and the Far East. Approximately 1% of Laotian Hmong immigrants to the United States harbor *P. westermani*. The adult worms have life spans of four to five years, which they normally spend encysted in the lung parenchyma of the host. Thus the disease is characterized by cough and hemoptysis. Their eggs (50 by 90 nm) reach the bronchial trees, from which they are coughed up and excreted in sputum or swallowed and passed in the feces. The eggs must embryonate several weeks in fresh water before hatching to the miracidia.

The infection is acquired through ingestion of cysts in the second intermediate host, a freshwater crab or crayfish. The metacercariae excyst in the duodenum, penetrate the wall into the peritoneal cavity, and then migrate.

In mammals, paragonimiasis goes mainly to the lungs, where it elicits a granulomatous reaction resulting in pulmonary infarction or necrosis. Sclerosis and calcification eventually result (Yokogawa, 1965). The pulmonary damage is caused in part by hypersensitivity to worm products (Yokogawa, Cort, & Yokogawa, 1960). Besides the lung, *P. westermani* has been found in such diverse sites as the liver, diaphragm, scrotum, heart, brain, and many other tissues. Involvement of the brain, although rare, poses serious medical problems.

Pulmonary manifestations of paragonimiasis include a cough (in 95% of patients), occasionally productive of rusty sputum; chest pain (20%); and wheezing (13%). Radiographic findings of the chest include infiltrates, nodules, pleural thickening, pneumothorax, and pleural effusions. Eosinophilia is a prominent feature.

The ova may be found in the stool, sputum, or, rarely, in the urine. A sensitive technique for recovering eggs from sputum is to collect a 24-hour specimen and dilute it in a three-volume sodium hydroxide (2%), centrifuged and examined microscopically.

A complement fixation test using a buffered saline extract of adult worms as the antigen is useful for therapeutic follow-up but is cross-reactive with other trematode infection. A titer of greater than 1:8 is diagnostic. It becomes negative 3 to 9 months after clinical recovery. An intradermal test is also available that is very sensitive but lacks specificity. It remains positive 10 to 20 years after clinical resolution (Yokogawa, 1965).

For treatment, one may use bithionol (Lorothiodol, Winthrop Lab), a derivative of dichlorophenol developed in 1961 (Yokogawa et al., 1963). The recommended dose of bithionol is 40 mg/kg every other day by mouth for 10 to 15 doses (Center for Disease Control, 1979a). Diarrhea occurs in one-third of the patients and is the main side effect (Kim, 1970).

The drug of choice is praziquantel. A total of 75 mg/kg is given in three divided doses over a single 24-hour period. Concomitant bacterial infection must be treated.

Prevention of superinfection by the same parasite is important because the disease is self-limiting. The most effective and practical control measure is to cook all shellfish adequately before it is eaten.

Clonorchiasis

Clonorchiasis is an infection of the biliary passage caused by *Clonorchis sinensis,* the most important liver fluke. Clonorchiasis is widely distributed in Southeast Asia and also in the Far East. It is commonly found in Vietnam, Laos, Japan, Cambodia, China, and Korea. Most infections are acquired from the ingestion of uncooked freshwater fish that contains encysted metacercariae. The parasites excyst in the duodenum and migrate up the biliary tract or pancreatic duct. Eggs released in the stool (one adult fluke produces more than 2,000 eggs per day) infect appropriate snails, which release cercariae to infect fish.

Some 25% of the population of Hong Kong and a small proportion of Chinese immigrants and Southeast Asian refugees to the United States have been shown to be infected. The disease may also be acquired in the United States through the ingestion of infected dried, frozen, or pickled fish imported from the Far East. Most cases are asymptomatic. The disease becomes symptomatic only in a minority of adults in whom the accumulated worm load eventually produces pathological effects. The mature worms can live as long as 50 years in the biliary tree of the host, causing proliferation of the biliary epithelium, increased mucin production, adenoma formation, chronic pericholangitis, and periductal fibrosis. Cholangiocarcinoma may occur in patients with severe, long-standing infections. They may also infect the pancreatic ducts and may cause squamous metaplasia, periductal fibrosis, and acute pancreatitis (Komiya, 1966).

For a definitive diagnosis, the eggs should be demonstrated in the feces or the duodenal contents. A complement fixation test can be used to detect antibody response of the host. Occasionally, abdominal radiographs will demonstrate intrahepatic calcification. A liver scan may show multiple areas of diminished uptake in acute heavy infestation.

The drug of choice is praziquantel (Rim, Lyu, Lee, & Joo, 1981). A total of 75 mg/kg is given in three divided doses over a single 24-hour period. Thorough cooking of freshwater fish will prevent infection.

Strongyloidiasis

Infestation with *Strongyloides stercoralis* is widely distributed in tropical zones, with a prevalence of 0.4% to 4% in the southeastern United States. One third of cases are asymptomatic. However, an overwhelming autoinfection with the parasite is potentially lethal, particularly in the immunosuppressed host.

Transmission of *S. stercoralis* depends on soil, climate, and sanitation. Larvae ordinarily hatch in the mucosa, bore through the epithelium to the intestinal lumen, and are passed in feces, or they may metamorphose into the infectious filariform, which may cause autoinfection. Thus the patient's worm burden is dependent not only on the size of larval inoculation but also on the degree of autoinfection.

Approximately two thirds of infested people will have symptoms ranging from pruritus and vomiting to abdominal pain and mucous diarrhea, which may lead to protein-losing enteropathy. Some patients (5% to 22%) will develop a urticarial rash beginning perianally and extending to the buttock, abdomen, and thigh (Smith, Goette, & Odam, 1976).

Autoinfection may result in massive invasion of larvae into the lung and other tissue, particularly in immunocompromised hosts (Purtilo & Meyers, 1974; Scowden, Schaffiner, & Stone, 1978), leading to disseminated strongyloidiasis with resultant meningitis, sepsis, and shock.

Diagnosis is made by the demonstration of the larvae of *S. stercoralis* in the stool or duodenal fluid. A concentration technique using zinc sulfate should be used for stool examination (Melvin & Brooke, 1974, p. 183), and Enterotest can be employed for duodenal sampling.

The drug of choice is thiabendazole (Mintezol). A dose of 25 mg/kg twice a day for 2 days can eradicate the parasites in most infections except the hyperinfection syndrome, for which 2 to 3 weeks of medication is necessary. Still, the mortality rate is very high in the latter situation.

Giardiasis

Infection with *Giardia lambria* is found in up to 18% of Southeast Asian immigrants; it runs somewhere between 3.9% and 16% in the rest of U.S. citizens. It is the most prevalent enteric parasite in the United States and the leading infectious agent identified in waterborne outbreaks of diarrhea (Moore et al., 1969; Veazie, 1969). Giardiasis is widespread throughout the world, including Southeast Asia and the Far East.

Transmission occurs by oral ingestion of *Giardia* cysts from fecally contaminated water that is treated by a faulty purification system or by inadequate chlorination and not also subjected to flocculation, sedimentation, and filtration (Craun, 1979, p. 127). Children in day-care centers may transmit the cysts to each other and to their homes. Food has been shown to transmit the cysts (Osterholm et al., 1981). Reservoir of *Giardia* is not limited to humans; a wide range of animals, including beavers and apes, have been implicated in some waterborne outbreaks.

The ingested cysts have an incubation period of 1 to 2 weeks. Only 25% to 50% of ingestants will develop acute diarrhea syndrome; the majority will clear their infection within several weeks. Only a minority will continue to a chronic diarrhea syndrome resulting in severe malaise, steatorrhea, malabsorption, and weight loss.

Several effective drugs are available for the treatment of giardiasis. Quinacrine in a dose of 100 mg tid (or 6 mg/kg/day in children) for 7 days is considered by some to be the best treatment. Metronidazole, in a dose of 250 mg tid (or 15 mg/kg/day in children) for 7 to 10 days is also very effective. Furazolidone has been advocated as an alternative drug for the pediatric age group in a dose of 8 mg/kg/day for 10 days.

The prevention of giardiasis can be achieved by the proper handling and treatment of water and good personal hygiene practice in day-care centers and other custodial facilities. Because asymptomatic cyst passers (13%), particularly food handlers and children, are a risk to others and may themselves become symptomatic, they should also be treated.

Enterobiasis

Enterobiasis, an infection with *Enterobius vermicularis*, is highly prevalent throughout the world, particularly in countries of the temperate zone. It is the most common of all helminthic infection in the United States, with an estimated 42 million cases (Warren, 1974). It is particularly common among children and also most prevalent in congested areas, in institutionalized groups, and among family members.

Diagnosis is easily made by discovery of pinworms in the perianal region or by microscopic examination of transparent tape pressed against the perianal skin in the early morning.

The drug of choice is mebendazole (Vermox) in a single oral dose of 100 mg, resulting in a cure rate of 90% to 100% (Brugmans et al., 1971). All individuals living with infected persons should receive the same treatment.

Ascariasis

Ascariasis, infestation of *Ascaris lumbricoides*, is cosmopolitan in distribution, affecting roughly 1 billion people; it is most prevalent in tropical countries. Transmission of *A. lumbricoides* is usually hand to mouth. Ascariasis is most common in preschool children and young schoolchildren and affects approximately 4 million people in the United States.

Diagnosis is relatively easy, and is done by a direct smear examination of stools. The drug of choice for intestinal ascariasis is mebendazole (Vermox) in a dose of 100 mg bid for 3 days. In case of intestinal or biliary obstruction with the worms, piperazine citrate (Antepar) syrup is instilled through a nasogastric tube in several divided doses.

Hookworm Infestation

Human infestation with the two species of hookworm, *Ancylostoma duodenale* and *Necator americanus*, is widespread, affecting a quarter of the world's population, mostly in the tropical and subtropical zones. The infective larvae are positioned on the top of soil, so transmission is aided by the human habit of walking barefoot, with resultant pruritis called "ground itch" and papular erythema at the site of larvae penetration.

Diagnosis is made by direct fecal smear. The current drug of choice is mebendazole (Vermox) in a dose of 100 mg bid for 3 days and supplementary iron therapy for the anemia ("Drugs for Parasitic Infections," 1982).

Taenia Solium Infestation and Cysticercosis

Taeniasis solium, an infestation with *Taenia solium*, is worldwide but most common in Southeast Asia, Eastern Europe, South America, Africa, Mexico, and the Far East. The hog is the usual intermediate host, and humans are the only definitive hosts of *T. solium*. When autoinfected with the embryo, humans serve as the intermediate host, which leads to the development of cysticercosis. In cysticercosis, the embryo is carried by vascular channels to any part of the body, including the striated muscles, the eyes, and the brain (Loo & Braude, 1982), where it forms the cysticercus, an ovoid, grayish-white opalescent structure of about 1 cm in diameter.

Diagnosis of taeniasis solium is made by the recovery of eggs in perianal scrapings or in the feces. To differentiate from *T. saginata*, the beef tapeworm, proglottides or the scolex should be examined. On the other hand, cysticercosis should be suspected in those who have lived in an endemic area and who develop neurological findings. Radiographs of soft tissue will reveal calcified cysticerci. Computerized tomogram will reveal the cysts in the brain. Indirect hemagglutination is the best serological test available.

There are a few effective drugs for taeniasis solium. Nicolosamide (Yomesan) in a dose of 2 gm is very effective. Stool should be examined at 3 and 6 months for test of cure. An alternative drug is paromomycin (Humatin), 1 gm orally every 15 minutes for four doses. Mebendazole may be tried in doses of 300 mg bid for 3 days. To avoid development of cysticercosis, a saline purge should be administered 1 hour after the medication. Treatment of cerebral and ocular cysticercosis is usually surgery.

To prevent taeniasis solium and cysticercosis, pork should be thoroughly cooked before consumption; the habit of the eating uncooked pork should be abandoned.

Amebiasis

Amebiasis is very common in the tropics, especially in Southeast Asia, where more than 40% of the population may be infected (Martinez-Palomo & Martines-Baez, 1983). It is caused by *Entamoeba histolytica*, of which humans are the principal host and reservoir. Most carriers are asymptomatic, and intestinal ulceration, dysentery, and hepatic abscess are most prevalent in adult males. Although it is worldwide in distribution, the prevalence of amebiasis in the United States is only 1% to 5%, and over the past three decades the incidence of invasive disease has decreased sharply; an increasing proportion of such cases are now acquired outside this country.

The cysts of amoeba are the source of transmission and are usually spread directly from person to person under poor hygienic conditions. Also, food- and waterborne transmission may occur, occasionally in epidemic form.

The parasites may reach the liver, causing hepatic abscess, and they may extend to the lungs and pleural cavity, resulting in consolidating pneumonia or lung abscess.

The diagnosis is made by identifying the parasite in the stool or tissues. Sigmoidoscopy is of value in symptomatic cases. The diagnosis of extraintestinal amebiasis is difficult. A therapeutic trial of antiamebic drugs is very rewarding in suspected liver abscess (Thompson, Forlenza, & Verma, 1985). The drug of choice is metronidazole (Flagyl) in dosage of 75 mg tid for 5 to 10 days for intestinal amebiasis and smaller doses for hepatic amebiasis.

Malaria

Malaria is transmitted to humans by *Anopheles* mosquitoes. Malaria survives only in areas of the world where both the anopheline and infected human population remain above certain critical densities required for the sustained transmission. Thus malaria is no longer a numerically significant problem in the United States. However, when malaria does occur in this country today, it is primarily among the refugee population and, secondarily, in travelers from or military personnel stationed in endemic regions.

In 1980, there were 1,864 cases of malaria reported in the United States, a 113% increase over the previous year and nearly a 500% increase over 1975. More than 99% of those cases were imported: 82% occurred in foreign-born individuals and 55% (1,034) in Southeast Asian refugees. The malaria case rate in 1980 was 6.7 per 1,000 Southeast Asian refugees, with a slight preponderance in males (7.8/1,000) compared with females (4.6/1,000). The majority of cases occurred in the young, with the highest case rate in the 10 to 29 year age group (8.2/1,000).

Surveillance studies suggest that 2% to 5% of Southeast Asian refugees are infected at the time of entry to the United States. Clinical manifestations usually develop within 6 months of arrival, but in one third of the vivax cases are delayed beyond that point. In 1979, one fifth of morbidity and two mortalities were caused by the virulent *Plasmodium falciparum*, most of which could have been prevented with chemoprophylaxis.

Besides *P. falciparum*, three other species of parasites cause malaria: *P. vivax*, *P. ovale*, and *P. malariae*. Of these, *P. vivax* and *P. malariae* are the predominant forms found in Southeast Asia. *P. vivax* is responsible for three fourths of malaria cases found in the United States, of which 82% are found in Indochinese refugees.

P. vivax and *P. ovale* parasitize only young erythrocytes, and *P. malariae* only old erythrocytes, whereas *P. falciparum* is capable of invading erythrocytes of any age, thereby achieving high degrees of red cell destruction leading to fulminant and fatal courses.

Routine screening of all Southeast Asian refugees and travelers to these endemic areas who present with unexplained fever or other manifestations compatible with malaria is mandatory.

A definitive diagnosis of malaria is made by demonstrating the parasites in the peripheral blood. The intensity of parasitemia varies greatly from hour to hour, particularly with *P. falciparum*. Blood smears should be examined every 8 hours for 2 or 3 days before the disease is ruled out.

P. vivax and *P. ovale* persist in the liver in the exoerythrocytic stage, and thus complete cure is rather difficult. Primaquine base, 15 mg by mouth daily for 14 days, will effect a radical cure in most cases. If relapse occurs after the initial course, the dosage is doubled for a second course. Because primaquine may cause hemolysis in patients with glucose-6-phosphate dehydrogenase deficiency, which is rather prevalent in Indochinese (10% to 12%), the enzyme should be screened before primaquine is administered.

Because of the emergence of drug-resistant (choloroquine-resistant) *P. falciparum* in Southeast Asia, including Indonesia, Burma, Malaysia, China, and the Philippines (Mandell, Douglas, & Bennet, 1979), patients from these and other endemic areas with documented or suspected falciparum malaria should receive a combination of quinine, pyrimethamine, and one of the sulfonamides or sulfones. Recurrence may take place within 30 to 90 days, then retreatment with the same or an alternate regimen may be instituted. A variety of other combinations have been used. Fansidar, a fixed-drug combination containing 25 mg pyrimethamine and 500 mg sulfadoxine, has been particularly effective in both prophylaxis and curative therapy. However, strains of *P. falciparum* that are resistant to this combination have been reported in Thai-Kampuchean border camps, Indonesia, New Guinea, and Brazil (Hurwitz, 1981; "Imported Plasmodium Falciparum Malaria," 1980; "Prevention of Malaria," 1978).

Chemoprophylaxis with choloroquine will suppress symptoms, but it does not prevent the infection of malaria. Medication should be started 1 week prior to entry to the endemic area in a dose of 300 mg, continued weekly during the stay and for up to 6 weeks after leaving the area. This will eradicate *P. malariae* and sensitive strains of *P. falciparum*. The addition of primaquine during the final 2 weeks of the regimen will eradicate *P. ovale* and *P. vivax* as well. Cases with the retinopathy have been reported in individuals who have taken chloroquine in this dose over periods of 12 to 20 years.

For chloroquine-resistant *P. falciparum*, Fansidar should be given with chloroquine in the same fashion. Fansidar is contraindicated in pregnant women, persons allergic to sulfonamides, and children under 2 months of age.

Eradication of malaria from endemic areas is far from complete. Research is currently being conducted on the biological control of *Anopheles* mosquitoes and on the development of malaria vaccine.

Summary

Parasitic infestations are common among Asians and Pacific Islanders. Incidence of intestinal parasitic infestations among those entering the United States has been shown to be as high as 80%, and multiple parasitic infestations have been found in as many as 55% of the Indochinese refugees screened. Among parasites, hookworm is by far the most common (38%), followed by *Giardia* (9%), *Ascaris* (7%), and *Strongyloides* (6%). The predilection of the parasitic infestations varies significantly among different ethnic groups; Hmong (75%) are highest, followed by Cambodians (76%) and Vietnamese (47%). The distribution of parasite type is also significantly varied among different ethnicities; *Ascaris* and *Trichuris* are more common in Vietnamese, *Clonorchis* species are more prevalent in Laotians, and Cambodians show more multiple infestations by *Strongyloides*, hookworm, and *Giardia*.

Youngsters less than 4 years old are least infested, and school-aged children are most heavily infested, by *Trichuris*, *Giardia*, and *Strongyloides*. Adults have a majority of the hookworm and *Clonorchis* infestations.

Most intestinal nematode ova require 1 to 2 weeks of incubation in appropriate soil conditions before infective larvae develop, which is precluded by sewage and sanitation standards in the United States, and the absence of intermediate hosts of most tissue trematodes eliminates the potential risk of the dissemination of paragonimiasis (lung fluke) and clonorchiasis (liver fluke). Only some protozoa (i.e., *Giardia*, *E. histolytica*) and cestode (tapeworm) ova and cysts pose a potential risk to the public health. The drug of choice for paragonimiasis and clonorchiasis is praziquantel, with a total dose of 75 mg/kg in three divided doses over a single 24-hour period. Thiabendazole (Mintezol) in a dose of 25 mg/kg twice a day for 2 days can eradicate *Strongyloides stercoralis* in most infections, except the hyperinfection syndrome, for which 2 to 3 weeks of medication is necessary. Mebendazole (Vermox) is the drug of choice for enterobiasis, intestinal ascariasis, and hookworm infestation. Metronidazole (Flagyl) is very effective against *Giardia lambria* and is the drug of choice for amebiasis. Nicolosamide (Yomesan) is very effective against *Taenia solium*.

Although malaria is not a significant problem in the United States, it may occur among refugees and in travelers from or military personnel stationed in endemic regions. Thus more than 99% of cases are imported, 55% occur in Southeast Asian refugees, more occur in males than in females, and the highest incidence is in the 10 to 29 age group. Vivax malaria is the predominant form (82%) among refugees in the United States.

Plasmodium vivax requires radical curative therapy with primaquine in order to prevent relapse, whereas chloroquine-resistant *P. falciparum* should be treated with Fansidar, a combination of 25 mg pyrimethamine and 500 mg sulfadoxine, for both prophylaxis and curative therapy.

References

Barrett-Connor, E. (1989). Latent and chronic infections imported from Southeast Asia. *Journal of the American Medical Association, 239,* 1901-1906.

Borchard, K. A. (1981). Intestinal parasites in Southeast Asian refugees. *Western Journal of Medicine, 135,* 93.

Brugmans, J. P., Thienport, D. C., Van Wijngaarden, I., Vanparijs, O. F., Schuermans, V. L., & Lauwers, H. L. (1971). Mebendazola in enterobiasis: Radiochemical and pilot clinical study in 1278 subjects. *Journal of the American Medical Association, 217,* 313-324.

Catanzaro, A., & Moser, R. J. (1982). Health status of refugees from Vietnam, Laos, and Cambodia. *Journal of the American Medical Association, 247,* 1303-1308.

Center for Disease Control. (1979a). Drugs for parasitic infections. *Morbidity and Mortality Weekly Report, 21,* 105-112.

Center for Disease Control. (1979b). Health status of Indochinese refugees. *Morbidity and Mortality Weekly Report, 28,* 385-398.

Center for Disease Control. (1979c). Survey of intestinal parasites: Illinois. *Morbidity and Mortality Weekly Report, 28,* 346.

Craun, G. F. (1979). Waterborne outbreaks of giardiasis. In *Waterborne transmission of giardiasis.* Cincinnati, OH: Environmental Protection Agency.

Drugs for parasitic infections. (1982). *Medical Letter on Drugs and Therapeutics, 24,* 5.

Hurwitz, E. S. (1981). Resistance of Plasmodium falciparum malaria to sulfadoxine pyrimethamine (Fansidar) in a refugee camp in Thailand. *Lancet, 1,* 1068.

Imported Plasmodium falciparum malaria in U.S. physicians: California. (1980). *Morbidity and Mortality Weekly Report, 29,* 146.

Jones, M. J., Thomas, J. H., Jr., & Brewer, N. S. (1980). Infectious disease of Indochinese refugees. *Mayo Clinic Proceedings, 55,* 482-488.

Kim, J.S. (1970). Treatment of Paragonimus westermani infections with bithionol. *American Journal of Tropical Medicine and Hygiene, 19,* 940-942.

Komiya, Y. (1966). Clonochis and clonochiasis. *Advanced Parasitology, 4,* 53-106.

Loo, L., & Braude, A. (1982). Cerebral cysticercosis in San Diego: A report of 23 cases and a review of the literature. *Medicine, 61,* 341.

Mandell, G. L., Douglas, R. G., & Bennet, J. E. (1979). *Principles and practice of infectious diseases* (Vol. 2). New York: John Wiley.

Martinez-Palomo, A., & Martines-Baez, M. (1983). Selective primary health care: Strategies for control of disease in the developing world: X. Amebiasis. *Review of Infectious Diseases, 5,* 1093.

Melvin, D. M., & Brooke, M. M. (1974). *Laboratory procedures for the diagnosis of intestinal parasites* (Publication No. CDC 75-8282). Atlanta, GA: U.S. Department of Health, Education and Welfare.

Moore, G. T., Cross, W. M., McGuire, D., Mollohan, C. S., Gleason, N. N., Healy, G. R., & Newton, L. H. (1969). Epidemic giardiasis at a ski resort. *New England Journal of Medicine, 281*, 402-407.

Osterholm, M. T., Forfang, J. C., Ristinen, T. L., Dean, A. G., Washburn, J. W., Godes, J. R., Rude, R. A., & McCullough, J. G. (1981). An outbreak of foodborne giardiasis. *New England Journal of Medicine, 304*, 24.

Prevention of malaria in travelers. (1978). *Morbidity and Mortality Weekly Report,* 27(Suppl. 10), 81.

Purtilo, D. M., & Meyers, W. M. (1974). Fatal strongyloidiasis in immunosuppressed patients. *American Journal of Medicine, 56,* 488.

Rim, H. J., Lyu, K.-S., Lee, J. S., & Joo, K. H. (1981). Clinical evaluation of the therapeutic efficacy of praziquantel (Embay 8440) against Clonorchis sinensis infection in man. *Annual of Tropical Medicine and Parasitology, 75,* 27-33.

Sadun, E. H., & Buck, A. A. (1960). Paragonimiasis in South Korea; Immunodiagnostic, epidemiologic, clinical, roentgenologic and therapeutic studies. *American Journal of Tropical Medicine and Hygiene, 9,* 562-599.

Scowden, E. B., Schaffiner, W., & Stone, W. J. (1978). Overwhelming strongyloidiasis: An unappreciated opportunistic infection. *Medicine, 57,* 527.

Skeels, M. R. (1982). Intestinal parasitosis among Southeast Asian immigrants in New Mexico. *American Journal of Public Health, 72,* 57.

Smith, J. D., Goette, D. K., & Odam, R. B. (1976). Larva currens: Cutaneous strongyloidiasis. *Archives of Dermatology, 112,* 1161.

Thompson, J. E., Forlenza, S., & Verma, R. (1985). Amebic liver abscess: A therapeutic approach. *Review of Infectious Diseases, 7,* 171.

Veazie, L. (1969). Epidemic giardiasis. *New England Journal of Medicine, 281,* 853.

Warren, K. S. (1974). Helminthic disease endemic in the United States. *American Journal of Tropical Medicine and Hygiene, 23,* 723.

Wisenthal, A. M., Nickels, M. K., Hashimoto, K. G., Endo, T., & Ehrhard, H.-B. (1980). Intestinal parasites in Southeast Asian refugees. *Journal of the American Medical Association, 244,* 2543.

Yokogawa, M. (1965). Paragonimus and paragonimiasis. *Advanced Parasitology, 3,* 99-159.

Yokogawa, S., Cort, W., & Yokogawa, M. (1960). Paragonimus and paragonimiasis. *Experimental Parasitology, 10,* 139-205.

Yokogawa, S., Iwasaki, M., Shigeyasu, M., Hirose, H., Okura, T., & Tsuji, M. (1963). Chemotherapy of paragonimiasis with Bithionol. *American Journal of Tropical Medicine and Hygiene, 12,* 859-859.

12

Substance Use and Abuse

NOLAN ZANE

JEANNIE HUH KIM

The use and abuse of alcohol and other drugs has become a major health problem in the United States. It is estimated that during any given month, 14 million people in the nation have consumed some type of illicit drug and that 2.7% of the population 12 years or older are in need of treatment for substance abuse problems (Glantz & Pickens, 1992). As might be expected, the consumption of legal drugs is even more prevalent. In a recent national survey of high school seniors, 81% of the sample reported having used alcohol (National Institute on Drug Abuse, 1991). Everyday use of alcohol was reported by 4% of the seniors, and 32% of the students reported having five or more drinks during a single occasion within the previous 2 weeks. These trends are cause for great concern, because in addition to their obvious effects on individuals' health and social, psychological, and vocational functioning (Ball, Shaffer, & Nurco, 1983; Kandel, Davies, Karus, & Yamaguchi, 1986; Ross, Glaser, & Germanson, 1988; Roy et al., 1991), alcohol and other drug abuse problems incur substantial health care costs for society. Rice, Kelman, and Miller (1991) estimate that total losses to the economy

AUTHORS' NOTE: The research reported in this chapter was supported in part by the National Research Center on Asian American Mental Health (NIMH R01 MH44331). Correspondence concerning this chapter should be sent to Nolan Zane, Graduate School of Education, University of California, Santa Barbara, CA 93106-9490.

316

that are related to alcohol and drug abuse are $85.5 billion and $58.3 billion, respectively.

In contrast to the increased salience of alcohol and other drug issues for the nation at large, there exists a common perception that these problems have relatively little impact on Asian Pacific American communities, given the apparently low prevalence of alcohol and other drug use in these communities. The prevalence of drug abuse in these communities is a very controversial topic because of its important implications for research funding and health services to these communities. Because there is a pressing need to understand the extent of drug use and abuse among Asian Pacific Americans, the purpose of this chapter is to provide a detailed review of the research on substance use and abuse within this population, with attention to (a) the prevalence of substance use and abuse, (b) the effectiveness of prevention and treatment programs in serving these communities, and (c) the major methodological limitations of such studies. We also discuss certain strategies that may improve substance abuse research with Asian Pacific American populations.

Extent of Substance Abuse
Among Asian Pacific Americans

The relatively small amount of research that has been conducted on Asian Pacific Americans suggests that this population uses and abuses substances less frequently than do members of other racial/ethnic groups (e.g., Iiyama, Nishi, & Johnson, 1976; Johnson, Nagoshi, Ahern, Wilson, & Yuen, 1987; McLaughlin, Raymond, Murakami, & Gilbert, 1987; Sue & Morishima, 1982; Sue, Zane, & Ito, 1979; Trimble, Padilla, & Bell, 1987; Tucker, 1985). These data trends have been found using both treated case and untreated case methods for examining rates of alcohol and drug abuse. In the former, prevalence rates are estimated from utilization data of those seeking treatment for substance abuse problems; in the latter, rate estimates are based on surveys of samples drawn from noninstitutionalized populations.

Estimates From Untreated Cases

Research using untreated cases has involved primarily small-area surveys of either student or community populations. The majority of the studies have considered Asian Pacific Americans as one homogeneous population and have not examined inter-Asian group variations that may exist in substance use and abuse. Consequently, it is difficult to determine the extent to which these findings can be generalized to specific Asian Pacific populations. Recent surveys of students have shown that Asian Pacific Americans report the lowest use of cigarettes, alcohol, marijuana, and cocaine and other hard drugs when compared with other ethnic groups, particularly whites (Kandel, Single, & Kessler, 1976; Maddahian, Newcomb, & Bentler, 1985, 1986; McCarthy, Newcomb, Maddahian, & Skager, 1986; Newcomb, Maddahian, Skager, & Bentler, 1987).

Kandel et al. (1976) studied student drug use in New York and collected data in two waves, in autumn 1971 and spring 1972. The samples included 8,206 and 7,250 students, respectively, and identified African American, American Indian, Asian Pacific American, white, and Hispanic ethnic groups. Asian Pacifics ($n = 63$) reported the lowest levels of drug use for alcohol (liquor, beer, or wine), cigarettes, marijuana and hashish, barbiturates, cocaine, and heroin. In the case of hard liquor, 18% of the Asian Pacific adolescents reported having at least one drink in their lifetimes, compared with 74% of American Indians, 59% of African Americans, 50% of Hispanics, and 68% of whites. For the sample of Asian Pacific Americans, beer or wine (53%), cigarettes (39%), and hard liquor (18%) were the most frequently used substances.

Newcomb et al. (1987) surveyed middle school students in California and assessed substance abuse frequency, perceived harmfulness of marijuana, perceived parental attitudes toward drug use, and various emotional states. A number of risk dimensions, such as emotional distress, low educational aspirations, and poor psychological adjustment, were used to predict the likelihood of later substance abuse. In this study, the group designated *Asians* ($n = 77$) was found to have the lowest risk for future substance abuse.

Only a few studies have included sizable samples of Asian Pacific Americans. In New York, Welte and Barnes (1987) sampled 27,000 junior and senior high school students, of which 2% were Asian Pacifics. They found that the average use in one's lifetime of any nonalcohol drug for Asian Pacifics was comparable to that for whites and Hispanics, higher than that for African Americans and West Indians, and lower than that for American Indians. A substantial proportion of Asian Pacific students reported having used the following drugs: marijuana, 23%; over-the-counter drugs (including solvents, glue, air fresheners, and nonprescription cough medicine), 31%; pills (barbiturates, amphetamines, and tranquilizers), 20%; and hard drugs (heroin, cocaine, and hallucinogens), 12% (Welte & Barnes, 1985). However, Asians had the lowest percentage of drinkers (Barnes & Welte, 1986). Only 45% of Asian Pacific students reported drinking at least once in the past year. This rate was considerably lower than the next-lowest group, the West Indians (61%). Asian Pacifics ranked among the lowest groups in terms of the proportion of heavy drinkers (i.e., those who drink once a week and consume five or more drinks per occasion). Asian Pacifics (6%) were comparable to Hispanics (8%), blacks (5%), and West Indians (4%), but lower than whites (16%) and American Indians (18%). However, the Asian Pacific heavy drinkers did consume more alcohol per day when they did drink (1.46 ounces per day compared with 0.76 ounces for whites). All of the heavy drinkers among Asian Pacifics were males, whereas the other ethnic groups had small proportions of females who were heavy drinkers. Overall, the rate of heavy drinking among males was 18%, compared with 8% for females. The proportions of heavy drinkers among females in these ethnic groups were as follows: white, 11%; American Indian, 9%; Hispanic, 4%; black, 2%; and West Indian, 2%.

Two studies were conducted in Los Angeles among seventh and eighth graders, and these also included sizable samples of Asian Americans. In one study Asian Pacific students ($n = 275$) reported low lifetime marijuana use (2.6%), but their lifetime cigarette use (11.7%) and alcohol use (10.5%) were quite comparable to or greater than levels found for other ethnic groups studied (Hansen, Johnson, Flay, Graham, & Sobel, 1988). For example, white cigarette use and alcohol use were 12.7% and 9.7%, respectively. However, Sasao (1987) reported on another study that found that Asian Pacifics ($n = 596$) had lower rates of lifetime drug use for cigarettes (10.6%), alcohol (13.9%), and marijuana (2.6%) when compared with blacks, Hispanics, or whites. For example, the white use rates for these drugs were 34.2%, 36.2%, and 10.6%, respectively. Although both of these studies had considerable numbers of Asian Pacifics within their samples, they did not differentiate between specific Asian Pacific ethnic groups. Similar patterns were found in a statewide biennial survey of drug and alcohol use among students in grades 7, 9, and 11 (Skager, Fisher, & Maddahian, 1986; Skager, Frith, & Maddahian, 1989). At all grade levels, Asian Pacific students had significantly lower rates of alcohol use than the other ethnic groups included within the study.

Other research has focused on college-age samples, and the data trends have been similar to those found for younger Asian students. Adlaf, Smart, and Tan (1989) studied the rates of drug use among eight ethnic student groups in Ontario, Canada. After controlling for certain demographic variables such as acculturation level, religion, age, provincial region, and gender, the Asian Pacific group, consisting of Chinese and Japanese respondents, reported the lowest levels of tobacco, alcohol, and cannabis use. The researchers' definition of *ethnicity* differed somewhat from that used in most other studies. Ethnic group identification was operationalized as the ethnicity of the participant's "ancestors on the male side on coming to this continent." Accordingly, participants of mixed parentage/ancestry were included in the various ethnic samples. Most studies have not included mixed-ethnic individuals.

Sue et al. (1979) examined the drinking patterns of Asian Pacific and Caucasian college students in Washington. Asian Pacific students reported lower rates of drinking, had more negative attitudes toward drinking, and used fewer cues in the regulation of their own drinking than did the Caucasian students. More Asian Pacific students (15%) than Caucasians (9%) reported abstinence or light drinking, but Caucasians were two times more likely to be heavy or very heavy drinkers than Asians (66% and 34%, respectively). These results suggest that cultural factors play an important role in consumption patterns. More acculturated Asian Pacific individuals (based on generation in the United States and ability to speak the ethnic language) reported higher levels of drinking. Asian Pacific students reported that they and their parents held more negative attitudes toward drinking than did their Caucasian counterparts. However, Asians held less negative attitudes than Caucasians toward the harmfulness of alcohol on the body. Akutsu, Sue, Zane, and Nakamura (1989) also found that Asian Pacific American students reported lower levels of alcohol consumption than Caucasian students. Self-reported physiological reactions to alcohol as well as drinking attitudes accounted more for ethnic differences in drinking than did general cultural values.

Klatsky, Siegelaub, Landy, and Friedman (1983) studied interethnic differences in alcohol consumption of 59,766 individuals who participated in the multiphasic health examinations at Kaiser Permanente medical programs from 1978 through 1980. They found that Asian Pacific Americans, both men and women, reported significantly less drinking than individuals from other ethnic groups. Among the Asian groups, the Japanese reported the most alcohol use and the Chinese reported the least drinking. Among Asian women, Filipino women reported the least alcohol use and Japanese women reported drinking more alcoholic beverages than those in other Asian subgroups. The lower drinking rates among the Asian Pacific Americans were partly attributable to the sizable proportion of abstainers among the foreign-born Asians (Chinese 38.8%, Japanese 29.4%, and Filipinos 12.6%). Klatsky, Friedman, Siegelaub, and Gerard (1977) obtained information collected from a large ambulatory population using the Kaiser Permanente Medical Care Program in Oakland and San Francisco. They found that, when compared with whites and blacks, Asian Pacific males and females ($n = 4,319$) had the highest level of abstinence from alcohol.

The studies constituting small-area community samples suggest that Asian Pacific Americans from different geographic regions use and abuse substances less frequently than do non-Asian Pacific Americans. Such ethnic group comparisons are difficult to interpret because Asian Pacific sample sizes are usually small—with some exceptions, such as the studies by Klatsky and his colleagues. Small sample size becomes especially problematic because Asian Pacific samples are not homogeneous (i.e., sampled from only one specific Asian Pacific ethnic group). Consequently, it is unclear if these findings of lower comparative use are generalizable to any particular Asian Pacific American group. Based on the time periods and geographic regions of most of the aforementioned studies, it appears that the most frequently sampled groups may have been the most acculturated ones, primarily Japanese and Chinese Americans. The tendency for Asian Pacific Americans to have lower comparative alcohol and other drug use may apply only to these groups, but again, this tendency should be considered with caution in view of the lack of inter-Asian differentiation in the research.

More informative studies are those that have made some attempt to distinguish various Asian Pacific American groups. No national survey of alcohol or drug use has been conducted for these different populations. Research focused on specific Asian Pacific ethnic groups has tended to sample West Coast populations, primarily from Hawaii and California. McLaughlin et al. (1987) examined inter-Asian Pacific differences in substance use as part of a statewide alcohol, drug, and mental health survey in Hawaii that sampled 2,503 households. Using in-person interviews, the researchers assessed lifetime prevalence of alcohol and other drug use among Chinese Americans

(3.7%), Japanese Americans (21.6%), Filipino Americans (11.4%), Native Hawaiians (18.9%), and white Americans (28.5%). Caucasians reported higher lifetime prevalence than most Asian Pacific groups for most drugs, including alcohol, cocaine, heroin, amphetamines, tranquilizers, barbiturates, and major analgesics (e.g., morphine). However, drug use among Asian and Pacific Islander Americans was not uniform across groups. Hawaiians tended to have higher lifetime prevalence than the other Asian Pacific groups for alcohol, cocaine, amphetamines, and marijuana. Also, their alcohol lifetime prevalence was comparable to the Caucasian rate. Compared with the other Asian Pacific groups, Japanese and Chinese had a higher prevalence of tranquilizer use. The results underscore the importance of examining inter-Asian Pacific differences in substance use, but it is unclear if the differences observed can be generalized to Asian communities outside of Hawaii. Hawaiian Asian Pacific groups may be quite different from their mainland counterparts in terms of their nonminority status, acculturation, English-language proficiency, community cohesiveness, social-political identification, and so on (Kitano & Daniels, 1988; Sue & Morishima, 1982).

As part of a statewide Asian drug service needs assessment in California, a bilingual community telephone survey was conducted in order to assess the prevalence of perceived levels of alcohol and other drug use (Sasao, 1991). The sample included 409 Chinese, 416 Japanese, 399 Korean, 149 Filipino, 322 Vietnamese, and 78 Chinese-Vietnamese community residents from both Southern and Northern California. The Japanese group had the highest percentage of individuals who reported lifetime use of cigarettes and tobacco products (45.4%), followed by Filipinos (38.0%), Vietnamese (36.3%), Koreans (36.1%), Chinese (24.9%), and Chinese-Vietnamese (24.4%). Compared with the national statistics reported in the 1988 National Household Survey on Drug Abuse (National Institute on Drug Abuse, 1990), the lifetime use of cigarettes appears to be lower for Asian Pacific Americans than for the general population (approximately 80%). With respect to the proportion of respondents who had 10 or more alcoholic drinks in their lifetime, the Japanese had the highest level of lifetime use (68.8%), followed by Koreans (48.6%), Chinese (41.8%), Vietnamese (43.2%), Filipinos (39.3%), and Chinese-Vietnamese (38.5%). These rates were lower than the national prevalence (85%). Of those who reported drinking alcohol in the past month, the Chinese, Japanese, Korean, and Filipino groups tended to drink less than both the Vietnamese and Chinese-

Vietnamese. Most Asian Pacific drinking appeared to be socially based, as a large majority of drinkers in each Asian Pacific group (Chinese, 85%; Japanese, 92%; Koreans, 77%; Filipinos, 90%; Vietnamese, 86%; Chinese-Vietnamese, 81%) reported that they tended to drink on social occasions.

Using purposive random sampling from a local Japanese phone directory, Sasao (1989) conducted a bilingual telephone survey ($n = 127$) of a predominantly Japanese community in Southern California to assess the perception of substance abuse as a community problem and the lifetime and 30-day prevalence of cigarette, alcohol, and marijuana use. Substance abuse was perceived as a significant social and health issue in this community. Results indicated that lifetime alcohol use (73%) and cigarette use (55%) of both U.S.-born and Japanese-born respondents are slightly lower than that found for the general U.S. population. Telephone surveys have been criticized for sampling biases owing to low respondent participation, reliability and validity problems, and anonymity and confidentiality issues. However, in this study the interview completion rate was high (82%). In addition, there were important differences found between U.S.-born and foreign-born Japanese. The latter had a higher rate of refusing to participate and exhibited less knowledge and social concern about substance abuse. Many of the foreign-born respondents were spouses of Japanese businessmen, who tended to have lived in the United States for only a few years. The two subgroups also defined *substance abuse* differently. Specifically, Japanese-born respondents tended to use this term for hard drugs such as marijuana, LSD, and heroin and did not include alcohol use and cigarette use as potential substance abuse problems. However, U.S.-born Japanese defined substance abuse as involving the use of both alcohol and cigarettes. These differences underscore the heterogeneity related to acculturation and other variables that often exists within one particular Asian Pacific American group.

Studies by Kitano and his colleagues have focused on the alcohol drinking patterns among several Asian Pacific populations (Chi, Lubben, & Kitano, 1988, 1989; Kitano & Chi, 1985; Kitano, Lubben, & Chi, 1988; Lubben, Chi, & Kitano, 1989). Using Los Angeles phone directories, these researchers selected surnames of Chinese, Japanese, and Korean respondents in proportion to the Los Angeles population of each group. Snowball sampling was used to obtain Filipino respondents. In the final sample there were 298 Chinese,

295 Japanese, 280 Korean, and 230 Filipino Americans. The demographic characteristics of the participants indicated that most of them were married men who ranged in age from 30 to 60 years. The majority were foreign-born, with the exception of the Japanese. The investigators found that the alcohol drinking practices of young Asian Pacific males were comparable to national norms (Cahalan & Cisin, 1976), and they question the myth of Asian Pacific Americans as nondrinkers. Also, it appears that certain Asian Pacific groups have high proportions of heavy drinkers. The Japanese group studied had the highest percentage of individuals who were heavy drinkers (25.4%), followed by the Filipinos (19.6%), the Koreans (14.6%), and the Chinese (10.4%). Analyses of attitude items converged with Sue et al.'s (1979) findings, in which more permissive attitudes associated with greater acculturation were related to heavier alcohol consumption. These findings suggest that, at least in the case of alcohol consumption, Asian Pacific American substance use has been underestimated (see D. Sue, 1987).

In spite of some evidence of heavy drinking in these samples, very little problem behavior was reported. There were a number of instances of respondents' being arrested for drinking, but otherwise there was little to implicate alcohol drinking in problems such as job loss, personal impairment, and drastic changes in lifestyles. Much of the drinking tended to occur with friends and on special occasions. There appeared to be social controls on drinking behavior. Kitano and his colleagues attribute the diversity and variability in alcohol drinking practices among Asian Pacific American groups to cultural patterns brought with them from their countries of origin. In a related finding, Maddahian et al. (1985) found that Asians were the largest group that tried *only* alcohol and no other substances. The Kitano et al. study was one of the first large-sample surveys conducted to determine the alcohol drinking practices of different Asian Pacific American groups. However, the telephone survey methodology may have excluded certain individuals in the population who may be at highest risk for alcohol problems. For example, single, recent-immigrant males living alone or in crowded communal arrangements with no private phones may not have been sampled adequately.

In another large epidemiological survey (*n* = 2,418) conducted in Hawaii, Wilson, McClearn, and Johnson (1978) examined the prevalence of alcohol use among four different ethnic groups: Chinese, Japanese, whites, and Asian-whites (mixed parentage with one white and one Asian parent). There were more than 600 respondents in each group, with the exception of Asian-whites (443 respondents). The effects of certain sociodemographic variables (e.g., social class, gender) were controlled for in the design of this study. Asian Pacific subgroups were found to be more likely than whites to be abstainers (Chinese, 18%; Japanese, 17%; Asian-whites, 7%; whites, 4%). Whites had the highest consumption of alcohol and flushed less than either the Chinese or Japanese, whereas the two Asian Pacific groups were similar to each other in their patterns of drinking and flushing. Individuals of mixed Asian-white ancestry had mean alcohol consumption levels that were comparable to those of the white group. However, Asian-whites resembled Asian Pacifics more than whites in their tendency to flush. This set of findings is interesting because some researchers have noted that the tendency for Asian Pacifics to flush reflects an alcohol-related physiological sensitivity. They hypothesize that this ethnic difference in physiological response accounts for the tendency for Asian Pacific individuals to have lower drinking rates than whites (Agarwal, Eckey, Harada, & Goedde, 1984; Ewing, Rouse, & Aderhold, 1979; Goodwin, 1979). However, after reviewing the research on ethnic-based physiological determinants of drinking, both Chan (1986) and Johnson and Nagoshi (1990) conclude that the physiological model cannot adequately account for much of the ethnic variation in drinking rates. Moreover, Wilson et al. (1978) indicate that whereas Asian-whites more closely resemble Asians in their physiological sensitivity to alcohol, their drinking patterns are more similar to those of whites. It appears that cultural variables (in this case, marital assimilation) may have a more significant influence on the extent of alcohol use than physiological factors. Using almost the same ethnic classifications, Johnson et al. (1987) found similar results in another sample from Hawaii.

In a binational study of alcohol consumption patterns, an extensive epidemiological survey was conducted using Japanese in Japan, Japanese Americans in Hawaii, and Japanese and Caucasians in Santa Clara County, California (National Institute on Alcohol Abuse and Alcoholism & National Institute on Alcoholism in Japan, 1991). The samples from Japan were selected by stratified random sampling from four areas in Japan and included 1,224 individuals (579 males, 646 females). The 514 Japanese Americans interviewed in Hawaii (271 males, 243 females) were drawn using a randomly generated telephone list. The Japanese Americans in Santa Clara

County were selected based on Japanese surnames found in the Santa Clara County telephone directory. The study used a revised World Health Organization survey questionnaire to assess alcohol drinking and relevant predictors or correlates of drinking (e.g., frequency, reasons for drinking, alcohol-related problems). The proportions of current drinkers (those who drank alcohol within the past year) in all of the study sites were somewhat high when compared with rates for the adult population of the United States as a whole. Japanese men (91%) had the highest percentage of current drinkers, followed by Caucasian men (85%), Japanese American men in Santa Clara (84%), and Japanese American men in Hawaii (80%).

In general, women drank less and their pattern of ethnic variation differed from that found for men. Caucasian women had the highest proportion of current drinkers (81%), followed by Japanese women in Santa Clara (75%), Japanese women in Hawaii (68%), and Japanese women (61%). With regard to frequency of drinking alcoholic beverages, the data show that patterns of alcohol use vary across the different locations. A large proportion of Japanese men in Japan (62%) reported drinking at least three times a week; only 7% of this group said they drank less than once a month. Almost half of Caucasian male drinkers (44%) reported drinking three or more times a week, whereas 13% indicated that they drank less often than once a month. These figures indicate that the alcohol drinking patterns of Caucasian men in Santa Clara County are very similar to the national rates (National Institute on Drug Abuse, 1990). However, the data reveal that Japanese Americans use alcohol less frequently. Less than one third of the male Hawaii (32%) and Santa Clara County (29%) Japanese samples reported drinking as often as three times a week, whereas close to one fourth (20% and 26%, respectively) reported drinking less often than once a month.

Different drinking patterns were found for women. Caucasian women in Santa Clara (32%) had the highest proportion of individuals drinking three or more times a week. These women drank more than either Japan Japanese or Japanese Americans, and their consumption was higher than that of Caucasian women in the U.S. national sample (21%). Japanese women in Japan had the next-highest proportion of frequent drinkers (21%), and Japanese American women had the lowest proportion of frequent drinkers in either of the Japanese American groups (9% for both Hawaii and Santa Clara County). Also, Parrish et al. (1990) found that drinking norms of the ethnic groups in this cross-national study were major determinants of alcohol consumption.

The Asian Pacific population is diverse, and certain Asian Pacific American groups are considered at high risk for developing health and/or mental health problems. For example, many Southeast Asian refugees have experienced extensive trauma as a result of their forced evacuation from their home countries, prolonged stays in refugee camps, and hazardous migration to the United States (Beiser, Turner, & Ganesan, 1989; Charron & Ness, 1983; Cohon, 1981). Unfortunately, not many studies have been conducted on these high-risk groups. In one of the few studies undertaken, Yee and Thu (1987) examined the prevalence and nature of substance use problems among Southeast Asians in Texas. They sampled 840 adult refugees, mainly Vietnamese (90%), and employed household interviews to elicit information on individual drug use and mental health status. A majority of the sample (52%) reported occasional problems involving alcohol and/or tobacco use. It appears that drugs were used by those in this sample for coping purposes. Close to half of the respondents reported that they used alcohol and/or smoked to cope with stressful situations or with personal problems resulting from stress.

A community survey of San Diego Job Corps members found that Indochinese youth had the lowest level of drinking (use in the past six months), compared with whites, blacks, and Hispanics (Morgan, Wingard, & Felice, 1984). Two thirds (66%) of Indochinese males and 43% of Indochinese females drank, compared with an average of 87% for males and 88% for females for the other groups. Indochinese youth began drinking later than other groups. The average initiation age was 18 for both Indochinese males and females, compared with 11 years for Caucasian males and 14 years for Caucasian females. The Indochinese who did drink had very low levels of other drug use. None had used cocaine, and only 3% used marijuana, whereas 53% of the whites who drank had used marijuana and 7% had used cocaine.

In contrast to most of the previous studies, Wong (1985) found relatively high rates of substance use among Chinese youth in a community associated with high-risk indicators, San Francisco's Chinatown. Using a chain referral method to sample 123 Chinese youths who ranged in age from 13 to 19, Wong estimated that the prevalence of substance abuse among these youth was higher than that found among other non-Asian youth in the previous study conducted in San Francisco with the same methodology. The lifetime use of cigarettes, marijuana, cocaine, and Valium by the Chinese sample was similar to that reported by the non-Asian Pacific samples (i.e., whites, blacks, Hispanics). The proportions who indicated they had ever used various drugs were as follows: beer, 77%; cigarettes, 75%; marijuana, 59%; wine, 54%; hard liquor, 49%; quaaludes, 42%; cocaine, 40%; hashish, 22%; Valium, 16%; and LSD, 15%. Limited use was reported for amphetamines (5%), amyl nitrate (2%), opium (2%), PCP (1%), and glue (1%). Males and females had roughly comparable levels of use for most drugs, but females more often reported use of Valium, codeine, and quaaludes. No one reported use of heroin. The Chinese sample tended to use quaaludes more frequently than did the other groups. By comparison with previous community surveys of drug use among other ethnic groups in San Francisco, quaalude use was twice as high among Chinese American youth as among white and Latino youth and five times greater than among black youth. On the other hand, Chinese Americans had lower use of heroin, PCP, amphetamines, and Valium than other groups. The nonrandom sampling method used in this study raises serious questions about the representativeness of the sample obtained and how comparable this study is to previous surveys that have employed more systematic sampling strategies.

In one of the few studies on actual alcohol abuse, Yamamoto, Lee, Lin, and Cho (1987) used DSM-III diagnostic criteria to examine alcohol abuse among elderly Asian Pacific Americans (age 65 and older) in Los Angeles. This research is one of the few studies conducted on elderly Asian American substance use problems. Filipino males were found to have the highest rate of alcohol abuse/dependence (10.5%). Rates for Chinese and Japanese men were considerably lower, 4.3% and 5.7%, respectively. In accord with previous research, males in each of the ethnic groups had much higher prevalence rates of alcohol abuse/dependence than did females. The sample sizes were small (48 Chinese, 129 Japanese, and 65 Filipino), and the sample may not have been representative of the elderly Asian population in Los Angeles because convenience sampling was used, in which the Asian respondents were drawn from lunch programs, retirement homes, and community parks.

The various studies that have been reviewed here suggest that, in general, Asian Pacific Americans have higher rates of abstinence and lower rates of heavy alcohol and/or drug use than do individuals from other racial/ethnic groups. However, important variations occur among the specific ethnic groups of Asian Pacific Americans.

Estimates From Treated Cases

The use of treated cases, or utilization data, to estimate prevalence can be problematic, considering the host of socioeconomic, administrative, and other nosocomial factors that may influence utilization patterns (Kramer & Zane, 1984). Nevertheless, this method provides an alternative source for investigating Asian Pacific substance use and abuse. For the past few years in both San Francisco and Los Angeles, Asian Pacific Americans have consistently underutilized drug abuse treatment services compared with their respective proportions in the local populations. Low rates of alcohol-related hospital admissions for these populations have been reported. It has been noted that low utilization rates may reflect the tendency of Asian Pacific individuals not to seek services for help rather than a lower need of such services (e.g., Murase, 1977). Asian Pacific individuals with problems such as substance abuse or mental illness may not seek formal treatment because of the shame and stigma associated with these problems, lack of knowledge about available help, and shortages of bilingual, bicultural staff to provide appropriate care (Sue & Morishima, 1982). Indeed, in the case of mental health services, when such services are provided by bilingual, bicultural personnel, utilization rates for Asian Pacific Americans have been shown to increase dramatically (True, 1975; Wong, 1977; Zane, 1989).

Using a key informant approach, Asian, Inc. (1978) estimated that the substance use of Chinese and Filipino Americans is lower than that of the general population, whereas the level of use for Japanese Americans is similar to that found in the general San Francisco population. Phin and Phillips (1978) conducted a national study of drug abuse programs and found that Asian Pacific Americans (55%) and whites (63% to 67%) were admitted primarily for heroin abuse. Asian Pacific clients reported higher levels of barbiturate use than did whites (45% and 11%, respectively). Namkung (1976) found that in the California prison population, 95% of the Asian Pacific inmates incarcerated were there for drug-related crimes. The utilization research has suffered from limitations similar to those found in the untreated cases studied. The research has not distinguished among different Asian Pacific groups in the context of relatively small samples, has failed to identify and/or control for important demographic variables (e.g., socioeconomic status, living arrangement, family size) that may be confounded with ethnicity, and has relied predominantly on self-report instruments. The self-report measures have often been used without adequate testing for conceptual equivalence among items, regional dialect differences in language translations, and literacy levels of respondents in *both* Asian and Pacific Islander countries of origin languages and English.

In summary, on the basis of research on either untreated or treated cases it is difficult to obtain good estimates of the level of substance use and abuse for various Asian Pacific American populations. Zane and Sasao (1992) recently identified a number of trends in the research, and these appear to remain unchanged, even with the inclusion of more recent studies. First, use of various drugs, including alcohol, nicotine, cocaine, and marijuana, appears to be lower for many Asian Pacific groups when compared with rates for whites and other ethnic minority groups. However, it may be more important to note the considerable variation in substance use among the different Asian Pacific populations. For example, Hawaiians tend to use alcohol and other drugs more frequently than do other Asian Pacific groups, and their alcohol use is comparable to that of whites. Second, although the general drinking rates of Asian Pacific Americans are lower than national norms, it appears that alcohol use has been underestimated, particularly for certain groups, such as Japanese American males and Filipino American males. Third, some evidence suggests that for Chinese and Japanese Americans barbiturate and tranquilizer use may be an increasing problem. Fourth, cultural factors appear to play an important role in limiting and, at other times, enhancing substance use among certain Asian Pacific groups.

Treatment of Substance Abuse

To date, few studies have directly examined the outcomes (in terms of decreased drug use) of Asian Pacific American clients in substance abuse treatment. Phin and Phillips (1978) compared the treatment of outcomes of Asian Pacific and white Americans using retention in treatment, drug use patterns, change in employment, and legal status as indices of treatment outcome. Asian Pacific clients reported that treatment had positive effects on living conditions and/or health and led to decreased drug use. Compared with whites, Asian Pacific clients stayed in therapy longer but had higher rates of continuing drug abuse. These outcome data are difficult to interpret because the Asian Pacific and white samples were not comparable in age or drug abuse patterns at admission to treatment.

Culturally Responsive Services and Programs

Given that Asian Pacific Americans tend to underutilize substance abuse treatment programs, it is not surprising that emphasis has been placed on developing programs that are responsive to the specific needs of these communities and their youth. Various strategies and solutions have been proposed to develop effective services for Asian Pacific Americans. Murase (1977) has identified certain features that may enhance cultural responsiveness of services to these communities. These include delivering services from community-based sites, incorporating community input into service delivery decisions, using bilingual and bicultural staff, linking with indigenous formal and informal community care/support systems, and developing intervention methods that address culturally salient aspects of Asian Pacific American functioning (e.g., value of family, face concerns, survival-related issues, flexibility in the use of time).

In terms of program development, a number of parallel services in substance abuse prevention and treatment have developed in areas highly impacted by Asian Pacific populations. Parallel services are programs that focus on providing services to particular ethnic groups; they operate independent of the mainstream services used by the general public (S. Sue, 1977). They are parallel to mainstream services in that they are similar in function and organizational structure to those services, but they are separate in operation and usually in location.

A number of parallel programs in substance abuse prevention or treatment have been developed. For example, in San Francisco, the Asian Youth Substance Abuse Project (AYSAP) involves a coordinated effort among several Asian Pacific communities to implement a community-based intervention for the prevention of alcohol and drug abuse among high-risk youth (Asian Youth Substance Abuse Project, 1991). Operating from a consortium of seven community-based agencies, AYSAP has designed a set of coordinated program activities that draw from a number of empirically validated prevention approaches, including social competence, empowerment, parenting skills, and community resource development. The great variation among the specific prevention approaches used in each community agency clearly reflects the diversity that exists among Asian Pacific populations.

The results of a program evaluation of AYSAP suggest that certain types of prevention programs are effective in different Asian Pacific communities (Asian Youth Substance Abuse Project, 1993). A significant increase in knowledge about the effects of drugs and a significant decrease in engagement in high-risk behaviors (e.g., truancy, cheating on exams) were reported by Japanese youth who participated in a year-long, after-school drug-free alternatives program focused on providing recreational and youth group support activities. A life skills program focused on leadership development for Vietnamese youth from a high-risk community (i.e., economically depressed, large number of latchkey children, high crime rate) appears to have significantly increased social skills, assertiveness, and goal-directed behaviors. Process evaluation findings suggest that this success is largely attributable to the high dosage and structure of the program. Youth participated in the program for 4 hours each weekday for more than 2 months. Detailed curricula were applied in which structured exercises (e.g., frequent role-playing) were used to develop skills. It appears that the program served a primary prevention function in that most of the youth participating tended to be the "clean" members of families in which one parent and/or sibling were using substances.

Similarly, a life skills summer program for Japanese youth used peer role models and support groups to develop social skills and discourage engagement in high-risk behaviors. Significant decreases in drug use and risk behaviors were reported by youth participants. There were also significant increases in social skills, drug knowledge, and perceived environmental risk (e.g., people offering drugs, asking youth to help cheat on tests). Paradoxically, a significant decrease in self-esteem was found. This program relied heavily on prevention staff to serve as youth mentors in the support groups. Often staff acted as sounding boards for youth who were coping with interpersonal problems and drug issues. In the support groups, the actions of positive role models among the peers were recognized and peer pressure was applied to reinforce members for not engaging in risk behaviors.

Filipino youth participating in a brief counseling program reported significant improvements in psychosocial functioning, self-esteem, and family support. Increases in interpersonal adjustment also approached significance. Staff rated youth participants as significantly improved with respect to psychological adjustment. A program targeted for Filipino youth appears to have been particularly effective in improving various aspects of interpersonal functioning for these youth. Filipino family members participating in a counseling program reported significant increases in psychosocial functioning and significant decreases in social acculturation (e.g., having more contact with Asian friends) and hierarchical role relationships with children. A major objective of the Filipino family counseling program was to encourage parents to adopt a less restrictive approach to child rearing and child management. The self-reported decrease in hierarchical role relationships with children suggests that the parents developed less restrictive attitudes.

A community education program directed toward Vietnamese and other Southeast Asians in a high-risk community involved an aggressive door-to-door education campaign with an extensive bilingual mass-media campaign. Independent community surveys conducted prior to and after the program found significant increases in community perception of drug use and drug problems of both youth and adults. Also, a significant increase was found in knowledge about the effects of different drugs. There was no reported increase in drug use with respect to alcohol drinking, smoking, and marijuana or cocaine use. Thus the increase in the perception of more drug problems and drug use in the community appears to reflect an increase in awareness as opposed to actual changes in use. The effects attributed to this program were particularly marked considering that changes were detected with independent community surveys.

AYSAP appears to have succeeded in developing a number of culturally responsive prevention strategies. First, it was critically important to link peer- and family-oriented prevention approaches into the natural support systems of particular Asian Pacific communities and to structure prevention interventions so that they complemented this support system. For example, the Filipino community program provided substance abuse education and family empowerment interventions within a religious context. This program used the church as the major community medium or forum for prevention work. For many Filipinos the church is the most natural place to discuss personal problems. Self-disclosure in this spiritual setting often counters the shame and stigma associated with revealing family problems and substance abuse. The value of fatalism is dominant in Filipino culture, but spiritual practices are seen as a culturally appropriate way of changing one's behavior. This prevention program capitalized on these beliefs to introduce

alternative ways of dealing with family problems that often place
youth at risk for abusing drugs. Previous prevention programs
were often minimally successful because they failed to recognize
the prominent role that spiritualism plays in the Filipino community.

Second, the key to empowering many Asian families involved
providing Asian immigrant parents with the skills and mastery
experiences they needed to help their children adjust to American
cultural norms and expectations. For example, the prevention program for the Vietnamese community implemented an empowerment strategy for Vietnamese parents. The prevention approach
assumed that Vietnamese parents often felt ineffective because they
could not help their children with schoolwork or school-related
problems. The great emphasis placed on education in Asian families tended to exacerbate these feelings of powerlessness. Many
parents were also very determined to improve the family economically, but in this process they lost focus on their relationships with
their children and with each other. All these factors combined to
disempower parents. The prevention approach attempted to reverse this maladaptive trend by teaching parents their role in the
American educational system and by validating parental roles. In
role validation, parents were encouraged to see themselves as cultural experts who can only enrich their children's bicultural heri-
tage and functioning. Mass-media campaigns reinforced anti-drug
use messages and challenged the belief that refugees and immigrants are better off when they become totally acculturated.

Third, an important issue that often complicates prevention efforts in Asian Pacific communities is extreme shame over substance
abuse as well as over problems that place youth at risk (e.g., intergenerational conflict, mental health problems). A number of prevention
programs have developed innovative strategies to minimize shame
and loss of face in Asian Pacific families. For example, a program
focused on the Japanese American community adopted a graduated approach to handle intergenerational conflicts in Japanese and
other Asian Pacific families. In many Asian Pacific communities
intermediaries are often used to manage interpersonal conflicts.
Intermediaries present or advocate for a person's position without
personalizing the issue with the other party. In this way, loss of face
is minimized and opposing views are presented so as not to violate
the hierarchical relationships in a family. In this prevention effort,
workers often served as intermediaries to help maintain communi-

cation among family members. Essentially, the program presented the youth view to parents and the parental view to youth in a number of workshops and community forums. In this program a culturally syntonic problem-solving approach was utilized to support Japanese American families at risk.

Finally, community education programs that involved more personalized contacts rather than primarily relying on mass-media mechanisms appeared to be more effective with certain Asian Pacific communities. For example, the Vietnamese prevention program conducted a door-to-door education campaign in a high-risk community. A personalized approach was considered more effective and efficient because Vietnamese and other Asian Pacifics tend to minimize or deny that substance abuse and other related problems exist in their communities. This program combined the personalized education approach with mass-media anti-drug use messages and community events centered on disseminating information on the effects of drugs and on the treatment and support services available to the community.

The successful development of substance abuse programs by parallel service agencies implies that drug abuse treatment may require modification in some way to make it effective and culturally responsive to the needs of Asian Pacific clients. Evaluations of other parallel programs like AYSAP are needed to determine if similar culturally responsive features result in effective prevention programs for other Asian Pacific American youth.

Methodological Limitations of Past Research

Past research has not been very informative because it has often been unclear which Asian Pacific groups have been studied. This is a serious methodological shortcoming, because Asian and Pacific Islander groups that appear at highest risk for developing substance abuse problems have seldom been studied or have not been identified separately in previous research. There have been dramatic changes in the Asian Pacific American population. Whereas the Japanese and Chinese constituted the largest groups in 1970, it is estimated that by the year 2000 Filipinos will be the largest group, followed by Chinese, Vietnamese, Koreans, and Japanese. Moreover, many of the fastest-growing groups (i.e., Southeast Asian refugees, Koreans, and Filipinos) are also the ones with the highest risk factors for drug use and abuse. Given these substantial changes in population and sociodemographics, it is likely that the estimates provided by past and current data will soon be gross underestimates of substance use and abuse among Asian Pacific Americans.

In general, the lack of empirical information seriously limits our understanding of Asian Pacific Americans and their particular patterns of substance abuse (Austin, Prendergast, & Lee, 1989; Johnson & Nishi, 1976; Trimble, Padilla, & Bell, 1987). The data that are available on Asian Pacific use patterns also has major limitations. As noted earlier, most of the research has sampled the relatively more acculturated Asian Pacific groups, such as Chinese and Japanese, who tend to be at lower risk for use and abuse. The research also has used primarily student samples, which tend to be at lower risk than older populations. The groups who may be at greatest risk for substance abuse problems (e.g., refugees, recent immigrants, adolescents) have been inadequately sampled, which prevents any meaningful disaggregated analyses. Further, studies have seldom controlled for socioeconomic and other demographic differences that may be confounded with ethnic or cultural variation.

Finally, the reliance on self-report measures for assessing substance use may be questionable. Researchers have noted how cultural differences may influence assessment procedures, particularly those involving self-reports (e.g., Sue & Sue, 1987). A number of cultural differences between Asian Pacific and white Americans may affect self-report responses. First, symptom tolerance—how much impact a symptom or problem has on an individual's life—is a phenomenon that has not received much attention. Studies have shown that cross-cultural differences exist in how much physical pain or distress can be tolerated. For example, in the case of Japanese Americans, Kitano (1976) has noted the importance of the cultural attitude of *ski-ka-ta-ga-nai*, which refers to a fatalistic feeling that things are the way they are. If this is the case, there may be cultural differences in the ways substance use or abuse problems are perceived and, consequently, reported. Second, shame and stigma are often associated with substance abuse problems, and these factors may inhibit self-reporting of such problems. Shame is a salient interpersonal dynamic for most Asian Pacific cultures. Kim (1978) notes that *haji* for Japanese, *hiya* for Filipinos, *mentz* for Chinese, and *chaemyun* for Koreans are the terms used to convey the concept of shame. This concept has been used to explain the underutilization of mental health services, and the underreporting of mental health problems, as well as the reluctance to self-disclose among Asian Pacific Americans (Sue & Morishima, 1982). Third, cultures differ in their tolerance for the public display of excessive behaviors, including those associated with intoxication. In most Asian cultures behavioral signs of drug intoxication are considered socially inappropriate and are greatly discouraged. Given this context of intense social disapproval of excessive behaviors, signs of intoxication may be more suppressed or hidden by Asian Pacific users. As a result, there may be social norms for the underreporting of substance use and/or abuse.

A Model for Examining Cultural Differences in Substance Abuse Research

A research model developed by Zane and Sue (1986) can be used to facilitate research in Asian Pacific communities. Through point research, one can investigate if Asian Pacific Islanders and white Americans differ on a particular measure of substance use or risk for substance use and abuse. By using linear research, we can determine if the differences are consistent across different measures. Finally, the parallel research strategy allows us to test explanations for any observed ethnic or cultural differences on the measures.

Point research is the most frequently used approach and involves the employment of an instrument derived in one culture with members of another culture. In many cases the scores on the instruments are compared between the different cultures and interpreted from the norms developed from one culture. The problem in point research is that the cross-cultural validity of instruments is often unknown and application of the norms from one group to another may be inappropriate.

Linear research was developed because of the problems associated with point research. It involves the use of a series of studies that systematically test hypotheses generated by the construct of interest. As with point research, the assessment instruments are developed in one cultural group and used on another. However, instead of depending on one study, the researcher performs two or more studies to gain more points of reference on which to compare the cultural groups. If the hypotheses are supported by the separate studies, the construct may be considered to be cross-culturally valid and can be used meaningfully for cultural comparisons.

Parallel research is a strategy that develops means of conceptualizing the behavioral phenomena from both cultures in question. A parallel design is essentially two linear approaches, each based on its own cultural viewpoint. The advantage of this design is that the framework or perspective of one cultural group is not imposed on another. In this way, similarities and differences of the construct or concept under investigation can be determined. For example, applied to substance abuse research, the parallel strategy has the advantage of directly examining specific cultural factors that would, for example, affect self-reporting of substance use. If the results of the two parallel approaches converge, the researcher can be relatively confident that the prevalence rates found reflect good estimates of rates in that particular ethnic community.

Conclusions

In this review we have noted that the majority of studies have found that certain Asian Pacific groups, particularly Chinese and Japanese, may use and abuse substances less frequently than American whites and other ethnic minority groups. However, there has been little research to determine if all Asian Pacific groups have similar use patterns. Moreover, few studies have been conducted on groups that may be expected to show higher use rates, namely, those at greater risk for health and mental health (e.g., Southeast Asian refugees). There clearly is a need for more research on the recent immigrant and refugee groups, because, in addition to their high-risk status, many of these groups are also the fastest-growing populations among Asian Pacific Americans.

Despite the methodological difficulties described earlier and the limited scope of past research (in terms of the various Asian Pacific groups sampled), there has been a tendency to focus on the lower drinking rates of certain Asian Pacific groups as evidence of lower need for substance abuse services. This interpretation appears to be unwarranted. Relative need depends on two variables: prevalence and the availability of appropriate services. Even when prevalence is relatively low, relative need may be high if appropriate care is not made available to individuals in need of service. It is highly possible that the relative need for substance abuse services is similar to that for other ethnic groups, including whites, when one considers the other major empirical trend in Asian Pacific substance abuse. Many studies have documented that Asian Pacific Americans tend to underutilize substance abuse and mental health services; this underutilization reflects problems in service delivery rather than a low need for such services. The lack of appropriate culturally responsive services may create a situation in which many individuals who need services are not receiving them. Under these conditions, the relative need of Asian Pacific Americans for substance abuse services remains high. There appears to be a critical shortage of culturally responsive substance abuse treatment and prevention programs for these groups. More programs such as the Asian Youth Substance Abuse Project are clearly needed to respond to the substance abuse issues that have developed in many Asian Pacific communities.

On the other hand, the relatively low rates of alcohol and other drug use found among certain Asian Pacific groups should be more closely examined for their possible important implications for the prevention of substance abuse problems. There has been no systematic program of research to (a) determine if the lower rates of drinking and other drug use are reliable trends for certain Asian Pacific groups and, if this is the case, (b) investigate the cultural, community, and other social factors that account for these tendencies. The examination of sociocultural factors that influence drinking and other drug use in Asian Pacific communities that have relatively low rates of use may provide some keys for making substance abuse prevention programs more effective. Intergroup comparisons within Asian Pacific American communities on community norms, cultural values, attitudes toward drinking and drunkenness, and culture-based self-regulatory practices (e.g., how family members monitor drinking of each other) may identify specific sociocultural variables that could be manipulated or affected by these programs to discourage and control substance use. In this manner, substance abuse research on Asian Pacific populations can guide the systematic development of culturally responsive prevention approaches as well as provide guidelines for better community-based prevention strategies in general.

References

Adlaf, E. M., Smart, R. G., & Tan, S. H. (1989). Ethnicity and drug use: A critical look. *International Journal of the Addictions, 24*, 1-18.

Agarwal, D. P., Eckey, R., Harada, S., & Goedde, H. W. (1984). Basis of aldehyde dehydrogenase deficiency in Orientals: Immunochemical studies. *Alcohol, 1,* 111-118.

Akutsu, P. D., Sue, S., Zane, N. W. S., & Nakamura, C. Y. (1989). Ethnic differences in alcohol consumption among Asians and Caucasians in the United States. *Journal of Studies on Alcohol, 50,* 261-267.

Asian, Inc. (1978). *Assessment of alcohol use service needs among Asian Americans in San Francisco.* Unpublished manuscript.

Asian Youth Substance Abuse Project. (1991). *End of year report.* Washington, DC: Office of Substance Abuse Prevention.

Asian Youth Substance Abuse Project. (1993). *Final report.* Washington, DC: Office of Substance Abuse Prevention.

Austin, G. A., Prendergast, M. L., & Lee, H. (1989). Substance abuse among Asian American youth. *Prevention Research Update, 5,* 1-28.

Ball, J. C., Shaffer, J. W., & Nurco, D. N. (1983). Day to day criminality of heroin addicts in Baltimore: A study in the continuity of offense rates. *Drug and Alcohol Dependence, 12,* 119-142.

Barnes, G. M., & Welte, J. W. (1986). Patterns and predictors of alcohol use among 7-12th grade students in New York State. *Journal of Studies on Alcohol, 47,* 53-62.

Beiser, M., Turner, J., & Ganesan, S. (1989). Catastrophic stress and factors affecting its consequences among Southeast refugees. *Social Science and Medicine, 28,* 183-195.

Cahalan, D., & Cisin, I. H. (1976). Drinking behavior and drinking problems in the United States. In G. Kissin & H. Begleiter (Eds.), *Social aspects of alcoholism* (pp. 77-115). New York: Plenum.

Chan, A. W. K. (1986). Racial differences in alcohol sensitivity. *Alcohol and Alcoholism, 21,* 93-104.

Charron, D., & Ness, R. (1983). Emotional distress among Vietnamese adolescents: A statewide study. *Journal of Refugee Resettlement, 1,* 7-15.

Chi, I., Lubben, J. E., & Kitano, H. H. L. (1988). Heavy drinking among young adult Asian males. *International Social Work, 31,* 219-229.

Chi, I., Lubben, J. E., & Kitano, H. H. L. (1989). Differences in drinking behavior among three Asian-American groups. *Journal of Studies on Alcohol, 50,* 15-23.

Cohon, D. (1981). Psychological adaptation and dysfunction among refugees. *International Migration Review, 15,* 255-275.

Ewing, J. A., Rouse, B. A., & Aderhold, R. M. (1979). Studies of the mechanism of Oriental hypersensitivity to alcohol. In *Currents in alcoholism* (Vol. 5, pp. 45-52). New York: Grune & Stratton.

Glantz, M., & Pickens, R. (1992). Introduction. In M. Glantz & R. Pickens (Eds.), *Vulnerability to drug abuse.* Washington, DC: American Psychological Association.

Goodwin, D. W. (1979). Protective factors in alcoholism. *Journal of Drug and Alcohol Dependency, 4*(1/2), 99-100.

Hansen, W. B., Johnson, C. A., Flay, B. R., Graham, J. W., & Sobel, J. L. (1988). Affective and social influence approaches to the prevention of multiple substance abuse among seventh grade students: Results from Project SMART. *Preventive Medicine, 17,* 135-154.

Iiyama, P., Nishi, S. M., & Johnson, B. (Eds.). (1976). *Drug use and abuse among U.S. minorities.* New York: Praeger.

Johnson, R. C., & Nagoshi, C. T. (1990). Asians, Asian-Americans, and alcohol. *Journal of Psychoactive Drugs, 22,* 45-52.

Johnson, R. C., Nagoshi, C. T., Ahern, F. M., Wilson, J. R., & Yuen, S. H. L. (1987). Cultural factors as explanations for ethnic group differences in alcohol use in Hawaii. *Journal of Psychoactive Drugs, 19*, 67-75.

Johnson, B., & Nishi, S. (1976). Myths and realities of drug use by minorities. In P. Iiyama, S. M. Nishi, & B. Johnson (Eds.), *Drug use and abuse among U.S. minorities*. New York: Praeger.

Kandel, D. B., Davies, M., Karus, D., & Yamaguchi, K. (1986). The consequences in young adulthood of adolescent drug involvement. *Archives of General Psychiatry, 43*, 746-754.

Kandel, D. B., Single, E., & Kessler, R. C. (1976). The epidemiology of drug use among New York State high school students: Distribution, trends, and change in rates of use. *American Journal of Public Health, 66*, 43-53.

Kim, B. L. C. (1978). *The Asian-Americans: Changing patterns, changing needs*. Montclair, NJ: Association of Korean Christian Scholars in North America.

Kitano, H. H. (1976). Japanese-American mental illness. In S. C. Plog & R. B. Edgerton (Eds.), *Changing perspectives in mental illness* (pp. 256-284). New York: Holt, Rinehart & Winston.

Kitano, H. H. L., & Chi, I. (1985). Asian Americans and alcohol: The Chinese, Japanese, Koreans, and Filipinos in Los Angeles. In D. Spiegler, D. Tate, S. Aitken, & C. Christian (Eds.), *Alcohol use among U.S. ethnic minorities* (pp. 373-382). Rockville, MD: National Institute on Alcohol Abuse and Alcoholism.

Kitano, H. H. L., & Daniels, R. (1988). *Asian Americans: Emerging minorities*. Englewood Cliffs, NJ: Prentice Hall.

Kitano, H. H. L., Lubben, J. E., & Chi, I. (1988). Predicting Japanese American drinking behavior. *International Journal of the Addictions, 23*, 417-428.

Klatsky, A. L., Friedman, G., Siegelaub, A. B., & Gerard, M. J. (1977). Alcohol consumption among white, black, or Oriental men and women. *American Journal of Epidemiology, 105*, 311-323.

Klatsky, A. L., Siegelaub, A. B., Landy, C., & Friedman, G. D. (1983). Racial patterns of alcoholic beverage use. *Alcoholism: Clinical and Experimental Research, 7*, 372-377.

Kramer, M., & Zane, N. (1984). Projected needs for mental health services. In S. Sue & T. Moore (Eds.), *The pluralistic society: A community mental health perspective* (pp. 47-76). New York: Human Sciences.

Lubben, J. E., Chi, I., & Kitano, H. H. L. (1989). The relative influence of selected social factors on Korean drinking behavior in Los Angeles. *Advances in Alcohol and Substance Abuse, 8*(1), 1-17.

Maddahian, E., Newcomb, M. D., & Bentler, P. M. (1985). Single and multiple patterns of adolescent substance use: Longitudinal comparisons of four ethnic groups. *Journal of Drug Education, 15*, 311-326.

Maddahian, E., Newcomb, M. D., & Bentler, P. M. (1986). Adolescents' substance use: Impact of ethnicity, income, and availability. *Advances in Alcohol and Substance Abuse, 5*(3), 63-78.

McCarthy, W. J., Newcomb, M. D., Maddahian, E., & Skager, R. (1986). Smokeless tobacco use among adolescents: Demographic differences, other substance use, and psychological correlates. *Journal of Drug Education, 16*, 383-402.

McLaughlin, P. G., Raymond, J. S., Murakami, S. R., & Gilbert, D. (1987). Drug use among Asian Americans in Hawaii. *Journal of Psychoactive Drugs, 19*, 85-94.

Morgan, M. C., Wingard, D. L., & Felice, M. E. (1984). Subcultural differences in alcohol use among youth. *Journal of Adolescent Health Care, 5*, 191-195.

Murase, K. (1977). Delivery of social services to Asian Americans. In National Association of Social Workers (Ed.), *The encyclopedia of social work*. New York: National Association of Social Workers.

Namkung, P. S. (1976). Asian American drug addiction: The quiet problem. In P. Iiyama, S. M. Nishi, & B. Johnson (Eds.), *Drug use and abuse among U.S. minorities*. New York: Praeger.

National Institute on Alcohol Abuse and Alcoholism & National Institute on Alcoholism in Japan. (1991). *Alcohol consumption patterns and related problems in the United States and Japan: Summary report of a joint United States-Japan alcohol epidemiological project*. Washington, DC: Government Printing Office.

National Institute on Drug Abuse. (1990). *National Household Survey on Drug Abuse: Population estimates 1988*. Washington, DC: Government Printing Office.

National Institute on Drug Abuse, Division of Epidemiology and Prevention Research. (1991). *Monitoring the future, 1990: National high school senior drug abuse survey, 1990*. Rockville, MD: Author.

Newcomb, M. D., Maddahian, E., Skager, R., & Bentler, P. M. (1987). Substance abuse and psychosocial risk factors among teenagers: Associations with sex, age, ethnicity, and type of school. *American Journal of Drug and Alcohol Abuse, 13*, 413-433.

Parrish, K. M., Higuchi, S., Stinson, F. S., Dufour, M. C., Towle, L. H., & Harford, T. C. (1990). Genetic or cultural determinants of drinking: A study of embarrassment at facial flushing among Japanese and Japanese-Americans. *Journal of Substance Abuse, 2*, 439-447.

Phin, J. G., & Phillips, P. (1978). Drug treatment entry patterns and socioeconomic characteristics of Asian American, Native American, and Puerto Rican clients. In A. J. Schecter (Ed.), *Drug dependence and alcoholism: Vol. 2. Social and behavioral issues*. New York: Plenum.

Rice, D. P., Kelman, S., & Miller, L. S. (1991). Estimates of economic costs of alcohol and drug abuse and mental illness, 1985 and 1988. *Public Health Reports, 106*, 280-291.

Ross, H. E., Glaser, F. B., & Germanson, T. (1988). The prevalence of psychiatric disorders in patients with alcohol and other drug problems. *Archives of General Psychiatry, 45*, 1023-1031.

Roy, A., DeJong, J., Lamparski, D., Adinoff, B., George, T., Moore, M., Garnett, D., Kerich, M., & Linnoila, M. (1991). Mental disorders among alcoholics: Relationship to age of onset and cerebrospinal fluid neuropeptides. *Archives of General Psychiatry, 48*, 423-427.

Sasao, T. (1987). *Patterns of drug use and health-related practices among Japanese Americans: A Southern California study*. Unpublished manuscript.

Sasao, T. (1989, August). *Patterns of substance use and health practices among Japanese Americans in Southern California*. Paper presented at the Third Annual Meeting of the Asian American Psychological Association, New Orleans.

Sasao, T. (1991). *Statewide Asian drug service needs assessment: A multimethod approach*. Sacramento: California Department of Alcohol and Drug Abuse.

Skager, R., Fisher, D. G., & Maddahian, E. (1986). *A statewide survey of drug and alcohol use among California students in grades 7, 9, and 11*. Sacramento: Office of the Attorney General, Crime Prevention Center.

Skager, R., Frith, S. L., & Maddahian, E. (1989). *Biennial survey of drug and alcohol use among California students in grades 7, 9, and 11: Winter 1987-1988*. Sacramento: Office of the Attorney General, Crime Prevention Center.

Sue, D. (1987). Use and abuse of alcohol by Asian Americans. *Journal of Psychoactive Drugs, 19,* 57-66.

Sue, D., & Sue, S. (1987). Cultural factors in the clinical assessment of Asian Americans. *Journal of Consulting and Clinical Psychology, 55,* 479-495.

Sue, S. (1977). Community mental health services to minority groups: Some optimism, some pessimism. *American Psychologist, 32,* 616-624.

Sue, S., & Morishima, J. K. (1982). *The mental health of Asian Americans.* San Francisco: Jossey-Bass.

Sue, S., Zane, N., & Ito, J. (1979). Alcohol drinking patterns among Asian and Caucasian Americans. *Journal of Cross-Cultural Psychology, 10,* 41-56.

Trimble, J. E., Padilla, A., & Bell, C. S. (1987). *Drug abuse among ethnic minorities.* Rockville, MD: National Institute on Drug Abuse.

True, R. (1975). Mental health services in a Chinese American community. In W. Ishikawa & N. Hayashi (Eds.), *Service delivery in Pan Asian communities.* San Diego: Pacific Asian Coalition.

Tucker, M. B. (1985). U.S. ethnic minorities and drug use: An assessment of the science and practices. *International Journal of the Addictions, 20,* 1021-1047.

Welte, J. W., & Barnes, G. M. (1985). Alcohol: Gateway to other drug use among secondary-school students. *Journal of Youth and Adolescence, 14,* 487-498.

Welte, J. W., & Barnes, G. M. (1987). Alcohol use among adolescent minority groups. *Journal of Studies on Alcohol, 48,* 329-336.

Wilson, J. R., McClearn, G. E., & Johnson, R. C. (1978). Ethnic variation in use and effects of alcohol. *Drug and Alcohol Dependence, 3,* 147-151.

Wong, H. Z. (1977, June). *Community mental health services and manpower and training concerns of Asian Americans.* Paper presented to the President's Commission on Mental Health, San Francisco.

Wong, H. Z. (1985). *Substance use and Chinese American youths: Preliminary findings on an interview survey of 123 youths and implications for services and programs.* Unpublished manuscript, the Richmond Area Multi-Services, Inc., San Francisco.

Yamamoto, J., Lee, C. K., Lin, K., & Cho, K. H. (1987). Alcohol abuse in Koreans. *American Journal of Social Psychiatry, 4,* 210-214.

Yee, B. E. K., & Thu, N. D. (1987). Correlates of drug use and abuse among Indochinese refugees: Mental health implications. *Journal of Psychoactive Drugs, 19,* 77-83.

Zane, N. (1989, August). *Parallel services for ethnic minority clients: A review of the evidence.* Paper presented at the annual meeting of the American Psychological Association, New Orleans.

Zane, N., & Sasao, T. (1992). Research on drug abuse among Asian Pacific Americans. *Drugs and Society, 6,* 181-209.

Zane, N., & Sue, S. (1986). Reappraisal of ethnic minority issues: Research alternatives. In E. Seidman & J. Rappaport (Eds.), *Redefining social problems* (pp. 289-304). New York: Plenum.

PART III

Health Service and Policy

13

Access to Health Care

LAURIN MAYENO
SHERRY M. HIROTA

Equal access to health care in the United States is a relatively recent societal aspiration. Prior to the 1950s, access to medical care was conceived of as an individual issue between the patient and his or her physician (Anderson & Aday, 1978). However, in 1946 the Hill-Burton Program, which provided funding for health care facilities in return for the equity in the provision of services to all people, marked a nationwide conceptual and sociopolitical shift from individual to societal responsibility for health care access, and from health care as an individual privilege based on economic means to an individual's right, regardless of the person's ability to pay. Given the societal goal of providing equal access to health care to all who live in the United States, it is not surprising that, in a pluralistic and multicultural society such as the United States, particular problems have arisen in implementing this goal.

Barriers to health care facing Asian Pacific Americans were identified as far back as 15 years ago, yet many persist today, exacerbated by lack of funding and an absence of cultural sensitivity in health care policy and planning. The neglect becomes even more

AUTHORS' NOTE: We would like to acknowledge the many organizations and individuals who provided information and insights toward the preparation of this chapter. Special acknowledgment goes to Rene Ciria Cruz for his editorial assistance and to Abdi Jibril, Michael Lu, and Eddie Yuen for their assistance in research and information gathering.

alarming when viewed in light of the fact that the Asian Pacific population is the fastest-growing minority group in the United States. The U.S. Bureau of the Census reported that in 1990, the Asian Pacific population reached 7.3 million, nearly double the 3.7 million in 1980 (Asian Week, 1991). In one decade, the Asian Pacific American population had increased by 141%. Although this growth trend is expected to continue, so that by the year 2000 Asian Pacific Americans will exceed 10 million (Gardner, Robey, & Smith, 1985), efforts to mitigate health access difficulties for these populations continue to lag behind the demographics.

Access to health care can be examined in a variety of ways. For the purposes of this chapter, the aspects of access to health care we will discuss are the availability of health care facilities and culturally responsive services and personnel, the health care utilization patterns, and the use and availability of health care services relative to Asian Pacific communities' needs for such services. By illustrating the seriousness of the access problem, we outline the challenge of addressing the particular needs of Asian Pacific Americans vis-à-vis health care delivery. We begin with an identification of some of the factors that influence access to health care. We then present some of the limited data available to describe barriers to health care access. Finally, we examine current policies that affect access to health care for these populations and put forth some recommendations for policy formulation.

Factors That Influence Access to Health Care

Because of the diversity of the Asian Pacific American population, the examination of health access issues is an extremely complex undertaking. For all Asian Pacific groups, socioeconomic and cultural factors play crucial roles in influencing access to health care. The roles of such factors as language and culture vary among the different ethnic groups. In light of this, the limitations of this chapter are obvious. Far from being an in-depth exploration of access issues that affect each subgroup, this report is a thumbnail sketch of some of the major factors that affect health care access.

Asians Pacific Americans are affected by the same barriers to health care that exist for other segments of our society, such as skyrocketing costs, fragmentation of the health care system, and inadequate health care facilities in urban and rural areas. These problems are further exacerbated by factors that are unique to, or have particular impact on, different Asian Pacific groups. In this section we discuss socioeconomic factors that are shared by other groups, but whose particular impact on Asian Pacific populations must be understood; and ethnicity-specific factors such as language, culture, and immigration status.

Socioeconomic Factors

It is widely known that socioeconomic factors affect access to health care. There is limited recognition, however, that these factors have a significant impact on Asian Pacific communities. Thus it is necessary to discuss socioeconomic factors here, if only to dispel the common impression that Asians, as a model minority, "have it made" and are on the higher rungs of the proverbial socioeconomic ladder.

Poverty

A bipolar pattern of socioeconomic status among Asian Pacific Americans masks the reality of poverty in which many of them live. Although 7.5% of the population had annual family incomes above $50,000 in 1980, there were also significant concentrations in lower income brackets. Lin-Fu (1988) points out that "Asian Pacific Americans had the highest mean income deficit of any racial-ethnic group" (p. 21). In other words, Asian Pacific Americans whose family incomes were below the federal poverty level were poorer than any other group. Asian Pacifics also had the highest proportion (24.2%) of unrelated persons (persons who are not in the same family) aged 15 and older with incomes below $2,000. This compares with 12.7% for Whites, 21.7% for African Americans and Hispanics, and 23.9% for Native Americans.

Poverty levels vary considerably among Asian Pacific ethnic groups. For example, the 1980 U.S. Census showed that 67.2% of Laotians, 65.5% of Hmong, 46.9% of Cambodians (Khmer), 35.1% of Vietnamese, 27.5% of Samoans, 13.1% of Koreans, and 13.1% of Thais were below the federal poverty level, compared with 9.6% of the total U.S. population (U.S. Bureau of the Census, 1988).

Local surveys have revealed poverty rates even higher than those shown by the Census Bureau for some groups. In a San Diego, California, survey of 739 Hmong, Khmer, Laotians, Chinese/Vietnamese, and Vietnamese, 75.8% lived below the poverty level. The lowest proportions were found among the Vietnamese (57.1%) and the highest among the Hmong (93.7%). In contrast, the 1980 poverty rate in the area for whites was 9.3%; for African Americans, 20.3%; and for Latinos, 20.8% (Rumbaut, Chavez, Moser, Pickwell, & Wishnik, 1988). A San Francisco Bay Area survey of 215 Vietnamese revealed similar rates: 53% of survey respondents were found to be below the federal poverty level (Jenkins, McPhee, Bird, & Bonilla, 1990).

Unemployment

Unemployment rates are also high for some Asian Pacific American groups. Data from the 1980 census showed the following rates of unemployment, compared with 7% for the total U.S. population: Hmong, 20%; Laotian, 15.3%; Cambodian (Khmer), 10.6%; Samoan, 9.7%; Vietnamese, 8.2%; Tongan, 7.6% (U.S. Bureau of the Census, 1988). Data from a 1989 survey of Southeast Asian refugees showed a labor force participation (working or seeking work) of 37% for individuals aged 16 and older, compared with 66% for the U.S. population. Notably, 94.2% of those not seeking employment cited health as a reason and 53.4% cited limited English capabilities as a reason. Refugees who said they spoke no English had a labor force participation rate of only 7% (U.S. Department of Health and Human Services, Office of Refugee Resettlement, 1990). These figures clearly demonstrate that the "model minority" image has little to do with the reality of large segments of the Asian Pacific American population. In fact, many Asian Pacific Americans share the socioeconomic characteristics of other populations who are at high risk for health problems and medical underservice.

Lack of Health Insurance

In Oakland, the owner of the factory will not provide any health insurance. If you have worked for him for a long time maybe he will buy half of the insurance for you or if you have really good relations with him he might buy insurance for you. But many women cannot buy insurance for even the rest of the family because the factory cannot afford it and it makes it really difficult. (Asian Pacific Islander Health Coalition, 1990)

Most statistics on the millions of Americans without health insurance do not include breakdowns for Asians Pacific Americans and therefore fail to reveal this population's true condition. A major study on the uninsured in the United States (Robert Wood Johnson Foundation, 1987) and a study commissioned by the California Legislature (Brown, Valdez, Morgenstern, Bradley, & Hafner, 1987) collapsed Asian Pacifics together with whites. The first author of that study later explained that information for uninsured Asian Pacifics was not available (E. R. Brown, personal communication, April 29, 1988).

In the absence of specific data, these reports leave the impression that these populations are relatively well insured. However, a report on health insurance coverage among Californians in 1989 concluded that Asian Pacifics were among the groups least likely to have access to employer-provided health benefits. According to this study, 20% of nonelderly Asian Pacifics and "others" in California, and 21% nationally, were uninsured (Brown, Valdez, Morgenstern, Wang, & Mann, 1991).

A 1985 survey conducted by the Boston Redevelopment Authority found that Asian Pacifics and Hispanics were much more likely than whites to be without health insurance. Whereas 12% of whites and 19% of blacks were uninsured, 27% of Hispanics and 27% of Asian Pacifics lacked insurance (Gold & Socolar, 1987; Gold, Socolar, Goldfied, & Newschaffer, 1987). Several local surveys also identified a startling lack of health insurance among Asian Pacific Americans, as shown in Table 13.1. The Boston study showed that among this group a large percentage of the uninsured are, in fact, employed but have low incomes. Of the residents in Boston's Chinatown, 61% of the uninsured were employed, yet two thirds of the uninsured had annual incomes of less than $10,000.

Southeast Asian refugees tend to have greater access to health insurance coverage, though time limited, through the Medicaid provisions under the Refugee Assistance Program. Refugee health experts estimate that Medicaid covers roughly one third of the Southeast Asian refugee population (Phan, 1984). In the San Diego study mentioned above, 68% of the adults interviewed reported being covered by MediCal (California's version of Medicaid), and 18% had private insurance. Nevertheless, 67% reported that they were worried that their MediCal would be cut, and utilization of health care services was still low because of language and cultural barriers (Rumbaut et al., 1988).

Table 13.1 Asian Pacific Americans Without Health Insurance, as
              Shown by Local Surveys

Ethnicity/Location (Source)	Number Surveyed	% No Insurance
Asian Americans		
Boston (Gold & Socolar, 1987)	450	27
Chinese		
Oakland (Lew & Chen, 1990)	296	35.1
Chicago (Yu et al., 1990)	200	30.5
Koreans		
Los Angeles (Korean Health Survey		
Task Force, 1989)	350	50
Chicago (Rhee, 1989)	500	40.9
Southeast Asians		
San Diego (Rumbaut et al., 1988)	739	37
Vietnamese		
San Francisco Bay Area (Jenkins et al., 1990)	215	15
Asian women		
Southern California (National Council of		
Negro Women, 1991)	304	21

Education/Literacy

In addition to the language barriers, limited reading skills (in
English or native languages) also have a negative impact on access.
The ability to read and comprehend signs in health facilities, health-
related information, and applications or registration forms is crucial for navigating the health care access path. Limited education
and literacy serve to obstruct the path to health care access.

Among the Southeast Asian respondents in Rumbaut et al.'s
(1988) San Diego study, 54.2% of Hmong, 55.3% of Khmer, 48.9% of
Laotians, 58.8% of Chinese, and 25.4% of Vietnamese could not read
English. In the Oakland Chinese Community Survey, although the
majority of the 296 respondents were Chinese speaking, 38% could
not read Chinese (Lew & Chen, 1990). In a survey of 200 Chinese
Americans in Chicago's Chinatown, 23% of respondents could read
"a little" or "none" (Yu, Huber, Wong, Tseng, & Liu, 1990). These
findings underscore the fact that even bilingual written materials
have limited value for helping Asian Pacific Americans overcome
language barriers.

The stereotype of a highly educated population is untrue for many Asian Pacific Americans. Lin-Fu (1988) examined 1980 U.S. Census data and noted that for Asian Pacific women aged 25 and over, 7.47% had less than 5 years of elementary school education. This is three times the rate for their white counterparts. In the Chicago Chinatown survey, only 41% of respondents had any high school education, 31% had elementary school education or less, and only 18.5% had some college education. A total of 9.5% had no education or only an informal education (Yu et al., 1990). It is evident, based on the information presented here, that the problems of health care access can be addressed only through the utilization of forms of communication that are accessible to individuals with limited or no reading skills.

Ethnicity-Specific Barriers

The Language Gap

The inability to speak English is a major obstacle for immigrants as most practitioners are not bilingual. As a result, even the simple exchange of information is very difficult without an interpreter. Often, interpreters are not available at crucial times in the delivery of health care. These events further isolate the immigrant, and lead to the fragmentation of care. (U.S. Department of Health, Education and Welfare, 1980, p. 17)

Language is one of the most formidable ethnicity-specific obstacles to health care access. Available statistics indicate the severity of the language problem. Local surveys among Korean and Chinese Americans have shown English skills to be more limited than U.S. Census figures indicate. Table 13.2 compares U.S. Census data with data from local surveys. The discrepancies between census and community data can most likely be attributed to two factors. First, the community surveys were conducted in areas with concentrations of Asian Pacifics, where there was greater likelihood that individuals would speak a primary language other than English. Second, because of language barriers, individuals with primary languages other than English were less likely to complete the census questionnaire and therefore were more likely to be undercounted.

A total of 60% of the Southeast Asians in the San Diego survey mentioned above cited language as a major problem in obtaining health care. The language problem was much more acute among

Table 13.2 Asian Pacific Americans With Limited or No English
            Speaking Skills: Comparison of Local Survey and U.S.
            Census Data

Ethnicity	U.S. Census %	Local Survey Number Surveyed (Location)	%
Chinese	23	300 (Oakland)	88
Korean	24	500 (Chicago)	93
		345 (Los Angeles)	76
Vietnamese	38	215 (San Francisco Bay Area)	46
Cambodian (Khmer)	59	Not available	
Hmong	63	Not available	
Laotian	69	Not available	

SOURCES: Lew and Chen (1990), Rhee (1989), Korean Health Survey Task Force (1989), Jenkins et al. (1990), U.S. Bureau of the Census (1988).

Khmers (85%), Hmong (83%), and Chinese/Vietnamese (54%) than for Vietnamese, of whom 28% cited language as a major problem (Rumbaut et al., 1988).

Agencies often make limited and insufficient attempts to overcome the language barrier. Many facilities use bilingual staff who are not trained in medical terminology or rely on family members to interpret. Literal interpretations that are not understandable in the patient's cultural context are also commonplace. Often, a sole bilingual staff person is burdened with providing bilingual access for patients at every point in the health care delivery system. Health facilities with some bilingual staffing during the daytime often lack emergency access on a 24-hour basis. Unless a comprehensive, systemwide approach is taken, language barriers will persist as major obstacles to health care access.

Lack of Cultural Competence

For many Asian Pacific Americans, Western biomedical health care practices conflict sharply with traditional health and healing practices. Among Southeast Asian refugees, factors such as traditional concepts of illness, folk remedies, and unfamiliarity with the U.S. health care system combine with linguistic barriers to create a pattern of "unexpressed health needs" (Phan, 1984). For example, it may be difficult to get Southeast Asians to accept an appointment system, as the concept of waiting two or three weeks to see a physician seems inappropriate (Hoang & Erickson, 1985).

The Native Hawaiian Health Needs Study concluded that "the lack of acceptability of services to Native Hawaiians due to cultural differences" was a major reason for underutilization of health services (Native Hawaiian Health Research Consortium, 1985, p. M-7). The study recommended the development of programs that integrate traditional Hawaiian health care practices with Western ones. It was found that in rural areas, Native Hawaiians had maintained a strong commitment to traditional practices and reliance on traditional Hawaiian healers.

Many times, the cultural beliefs of Asian Pacific Americans are blamed for their underutilization of services. This perspective ignores the responsibility of health systems to respond to the increasingly multicultural character of society. Cultural barriers are built into the very structure of the Western biomedical model, which emphasizes isolating and treating different ailments, rather than a holistic approach. This tendency toward specialization in the U.S. health care delivery system is an obstacle to anyone seeking care. To seek care effectively, one must possess sufficient knowledge about the health care system and perseverance to seek and obtain care. Furthermore, one must have the ability and flexibility to make appointments with and to visit various health care providers regarding different problems. Without these abilities, one may become lost in confusion or bandied back and forth between specialists, assuming one has the resources and communication skills to get care at all. This fragmented health care system is even more formidable for those who possess different conceptions of health care and healing, use different health care-seeking practices, and lack prior experience in dealing with such systems. Lacking the tools and the language capability to navigate the system, many recent immigrants and refugees simply fall through the cracks.

In addition to this structural problem is a lack of culturally appropriate practices at the provider level. There is a lack of bicultural and culturally competent staff to provide appropriate care. This is perpetuated by an educational system for preparing health professionals in which cultural awareness is almost entirely absent. Health professions training institutions are not compelled by accrediting bodies, such as the Council on Post-Secondary Accreditation, to provide education on cultural awareness. Accreditation is meant to inform the public that the level of quality and integrity of an educational institution is acceptable. In addition, examinations for licensing of health professionals do not include questions related to cultural awareness. Therefore training institutions tend to focus their curricula on required topics and neglect the issue of cultural competence.

Comprehensive community-based primary care has been shown to be an effective model for overcoming cultural barriers to care. Strong links to the community and an emphasis on hiring bilingual/bicultural staff help to remove cultural and language barriers. In addition, the emphasis on comprehensive, case-managed care provides continuity in place of the fragmentation and isolation that exists throughout the general system. When referring patients out for tertiary care, some health centers utilize community health workers to advocate for their patients and to ensure continuity of care.

Immigration Status

Confusion regarding eligibility for services, fear of deportation, and concerns about jeopardizing immigration status are powerful deterrents to the utilization of health care services among immigrant populations. Undocumented immigrants are often afraid to leave their homes for fear of being apprehended by immigration authorities. Furthermore there is fear that presenting oneself to a health care facility may result in deportation. Those who are seeking permanent residency or citizenship for themselves or their families may be unclear as to whether they qualify for publicly funded services such as Medicaid and may fear that the use of health services will jeopardize their immigration status.

In fact, immigrants may be denied permanent residency if they are considered by the Immigration and Naturalization Service (INS) to be potential "public charges." This leads to the reluctance of many immigrants to utilize programs such as Medicaid. Although the use of public services alone is not grounds for exclusion (the INS uses an overall evaluation of the applicant's status to assess whether he or she is a potential public charge), there is sufficient ambiguity in this area to prevent many immigrants from seeking public benefits for health care.

Generally, legal permanent residents, refugees, and individuals granted asylum are eligible for federal public benefits programs, but eligibility requirements for public services as applied to undocumented aliens and nonimmigrant documented aliens are inconsistent at all levels of government and differ among public programs.

Documenting the Problem

Anecdotal data regarding language and cultural barriers to health care have been accumulating rapidly. These problems are obvious and well known to many providers and consumers, yet formal documentation that goes beyond anecdotes is scarce. The lack of data on Asian Pacific American health status and health access problems has been acknowledged in such national documents as *Healthy People 2000* (U.S. Department of Health and Human Service, Public Health Services, 1990) and *Civil Rights Issues Facing Asian Americans in the 1990s* (U.S. Commission on Civil Rights, 1992). Most national, state, and local data systems do not disaggregate information by Asian Pacific ethnic subgroups, foreign- or U.S.-born, or limited English speaking. This makes it difficult to assess leading causes of death and disease among Asian Pacific Americans, as well as utilization patterns that are critical to addressing access issues.

In the past several years, some progress has been made in efforts to reflect more adequately the health problems in Asian Pacific American communities through the completion of several local surveys and studies. The themes of this research are consistent: high levels of poverty, lack of English-speaking capability, inability to acquire health insurance (with few exceptions), lack of routine or preventive medical care, and low levels of preventive health education. Most of these surveys focus on one Asian Pacific ethnic group or another in a defined geographic area. Although they cannot make up for the paucity in national data, the documentation they provide is significant.

Low Utilization Rates

An immediate indication of access problems is the low rate of utilization of health services by Asian Pacific Americans. A superficial look at these low utilization rates could give the impression that there are few health problems among these populations. However, as True (1985) points out, whereas low utilization is often equated with or related to low morbidity or absence of need, studies have established that other factors, including barriers to care, affect utilization rates.

In an analysis of 1979 data from the National Ambulatory Medical Care Survey (NAMCS), Yu and Cypress (1982) found that Asian Pacific Americans had the lowest rate of visits to office-based physicians (1.55) compared with all races (2.58). This finding was based on a limited sampling, 442 records representing 5,559,524 visits, with no breakdown by Asian Pacific ethnic groups. In various local surveys, the findings show an even greater disparity than that reflected in the NAMCS data.

A study of Korean Americans in Chicago found that 49% of the 500 respondents surveyed did not have regular sources of medical care (Rhee, 1989). In Los Angeles, the Korean Health Survey found that physician utilization by Koreans was one third the rate of whites. Some 22% of 345 Koreans surveyed reported failing to seek appropriate medical care (Korean Health Survey Task Force, 1989). In the Oakland Chinese Community Survey, 27% of the 296 respondents had never had a routine checkup (Lew & Chen, 1990). A 1991 survey of 304 Chinese, Filipino, Korean, and Vietnamese women in Southern California found that 59% had not had annual gynecological exams (National Council of Negro Women, 1991).

Even where lack of health insurance does not appear to be a problem, access barriers continue to affect utilization patterns. The San Diego study of Southeast Asian refugees showed that despite the fact that 9 out of 10 had health coverage (mainly MediCal), 44.5% had never had a general checkup. Hmong had the lowest utilization rate, with 62% never having had a general checkup. Vietnamese had relatively better utilization, with 30.4% never having had a general checkup.

The pattern was similar for dental care. Some 21% of the Southeast Asian refugees in the San Diego survey had not been to the dentist since their arrival in the United States (mean 3.6 years). Reasons for low utilization cited by the respondents included language barriers, transportation problems, long waits, and lack of insurance. Folk healing practices, fear, and a history of negative experiences in the health care system are also factors contributing to the poor utilization of health care services (Rumbaut et al., 1988).

High Rates of Emergency Room Use

When Asian Pacific Americans do seek medical attention, they may tend to use the most expensive end of the health care system, namely, the emergency room. NAMCS data show that visits to emergency rooms represented 18.8% of the total visits by Asian Pacifics, compared with 11.7% for whites (Yu & Cypress, 1982). A study of 98 Vietnamese and Laotian refugee families in the Amarillo, Texas, area demonstrated a tendency to use emergency rooms over other sources of health care. Only 20% of the families interviewed had private physicians; 41% of the Laotian families and 69% of the Vietnamese families used emergency rooms as the first place for treatment (Fasano, Hayes, & Wilson, 1986).

Lack of Prenatal Care

Low utilization of health services is also reflected in the inadequate prenatal care that some Asian Pacific Americans receive. When data are broken down by ethnic groups, it is evident that some Southeast Asian groups lack adequate prenatal care. This is demonstrated by data from California and Hawaii, the only states that provide data broken down by specific Asian Pacific ethnic groups.

Hawaiian data from 1989 show that 30.1% of all mothers with live births had no prenatal care in the first trimester. The proportions were higher for Hawaiians and part-Hawaiians (40.7%), Filipinas (32.7%), and Samoans (62.6%) (Hawaii Department of Health, 1991). For 1984 to 1985, 25.4% of California women giving birth received no prenatal care in the first trimester. By comparison, lack of prenatal care was high for some of the Asian Pacific groups: 30.3% of Vietnamese, 43.1% of Laotians, 47.6% of Cambodians, and 57.2% of Samoan women received no first-trimester prenatal care. For "other specified," a category that included Hawaiians, Guamanians, Pacific Islanders, Eskimos, and Aleuts, 35.9% received no first-trimester prenatal care. Data from the "other" category are the only indication of prenatal care utilization among Pacific Islanders, although they have the limitation of including the non-Pacific Islander ethnic groups of Eskimo and Aleut.

The data for the same cohort also show that 1% of California women were not attended by a physician, midwife, or nurse/assistant during delivery. For Laotians this figure was 3.7%, and for Cambodians, 2% (California Department of Health Services, 1988). In spite of shortcomings in national data, the above-cited evidence makes it clear that there is a lack of access to preventive health care among Asian Pacific American populations. This is demonstrated by low physician utilization rates, a tendency to rely on emergency rooms for services, and lack of adequate prenatal care.

Low Utilization Not Linked to Low Morbidity

Existing data indicate that higher rates of disease among Asian Pacific Americans are not linked to low morbidity. For example, Buehler, Stroup, Kaucke, and Berkelman (1989) analyzed 1987 data from the Epidemiological Surveillance Project of the Centers for Disease Control and found that "for malaria and tuberculosis, the rates among Asians and Pacific Islanders were markedly higher than the rates among other ethnic groups" (p. 458). Buehler et al. also note that, had an index on morbidity been employed in the Secretary's Task Force on Black and Minority Health, infectious diseases would have been included in the listing of priority diseases and conditions. This would have resulted in a much clearer recognition of health status disparities between Asian Pacific and white Americans. Further, Buehler et al. indicate that poor access to medical care affects the quality and completeness of disease reporting. This may contribute to underreporting of disease among Asian Pacific Americans who lack access to health care.

Disease Prevention, Identification, and Treatment

Whereas low utilization rates may be indicative of access barriers, inadequate measures for the prevention, identification, and treatment of diseases endemic to Asian Pacific populations highlight the breadth of the problem. Several local studies have shown that Asian Pacific Americans do not receive adequate preventive education, nor are there sufficient provisions for the identification or treatment of diseases known to affect their communities. For example, more than 50% of the Southeast Asian families in the Amarillo, Texas, study mentioned above were unaware or unsure of where their children's routine immunizations had been administered or where they were available (Fasano et al., 1986).

Hepatitis B

The handling of hepatitis B exemplifies the lack of adequate approaches to diseases that are common to Asian Pacific Americans. Phan (1984) recounts: "In La Crosse, Wisconsin a few months ago a Hmong delivered a twin in the elevator, another one delivered in a car. Both were found surface antigen positive for hepatitis

B. Only at that time was it found that other children in the household also carried hepatitis B" (p. 9). Although the prevention of the transmission of hepatitis B is not a problem unique to these communities, hepatitis B is more common in Asian Pacifics than in other ethnic populations, and so prevention is an important health concern; access to systematic hepatitis B screening and immunization is thus clearly crucial. Many carriers of hepatitis B are asymptomatic and unaware of the threat to their own health or the health of others. In the case Phan describes, it is probable that transmission to all of the children could have been avoided if the mother had had access to proper care. These children now live with the possibility of developing active hepatitis, which could lead to severe liver damage and premature death. With proper screening and immunization, the risk of transmission to the newborn and other household members can be almost completely eliminated.

Perinatal transmission, which usually occurs during birth, is still one of the most common means of hepatitis B transmission among Asian Pacifics in the United States. Women who receive late or no prenatal care are less likely to be screened and are therefore more likely to transmit the virus to their babies at birth. Inadequate prenatal care among some Asian Pacific ethnic groups and high rates of unattended deliveries add to the risk of transmission.

Approximately half of the hepatitis B surface antigen-positive women (hepatitis carriers) who gave birth in the United States in 1988 were Asian Pacific Americans. An estimated 54% of all hepatitis B carrier infants born in the United States were born to Asian Pacific women, the majority of whom were foreign-born (Margolis, Alter, & Hadler, 1991). These statistics are staggering considering that only 3.2% of the total births for that year were to Asian Pacifics (Margolis et al., 1991). A quick calculation (54/3.2 = 16) shows that the risk of perinatal hepatitis B transmission is 16 times as high for Asian Pacific infants as it is for the total U.S. population. Given the high risk of contracting hepatitis B among these populations, community awareness is crucial. However, in a survey of Vietnamese in the San Francisco Bay Area, a surprising 94% of respondents (n = 215) had never heard of hepatitis B (Jenkins et al., 1990).

Tuberculosis

The high incidence of tuberculosis among Asian Pacific Americans underscores the need for a more sophisticated screening process. In 1989, 17.6% of total reported U.S. tuberculosis cases were among Asian Pacifics (Centers for Disease Control, 1990). Considering that these populations constitute only 2.9% of the total U.S. population (Asian Week, 1991), the incidence of this disease is more than six times as high among Asian Pacifics as it is in the U.S. population as a whole ($17.6/2.9 = 6.09$).

As the prevalence of tuberculosis can also be linked to high endemicity in countries of origin or refugee camps, any immigrant or refugee seeking legal entry into the United States is routinely screened for active tuberculosis. Active tuberculosis is grounds for exclusion. However, this one-time screening misses individuals who are infected with tuberculosis but are asymptomatic, who may later develop active tuberculosis and infect other people. Of the Cambodian adults who were screened in 1986 in Rhode Island, 61% had positive tuberculin skin test, indicating exposure to tuberculosis (Chow & Krumholtz, 1989). This finding is significant, because the patients screened had resided in the United States for at least 3 years.

A more sophisticated screening process, possibly with several stages, would be useful in preventing the spread of tuberculosis, because an individual found to have a positive tuberculin skin test can receive therapy to prevent active tuberculosis. A total of 39% of the cases among Asian Pacific Americans in 1989 were potentially preventable (cases among persons under 35 years of age are considered potentially preventable, because preventive treatment is considered to pose minimal risk for this age group), compared with 16% for non-Hispanic whites (Centers for Disease Control, 1990).

Cancer

Current low levels of cancer screening among Asian Pacific Americans are bound to hinder diagnosis and treatment in that population group. The San Francisco Bay Area survey of Vietnamese mentioned above showed that levels of screening for cancer in various sites were consistently lower than for the U.S. population. The study sample was also consistently higher than the U.S. population as a whole in being overdue for cancer screening (Jenkins et al., 1990). Table 13.3 compares data from local surveys of Chinese and Vietnamese populations to data from the National Health Interview Survey (NHIS).

Table 13.3   Cancer Screening Data From Local Surveys Compared With NHIS (in percentages)

	United States	San Francisco Bay Area Vietnamese	Oakland Chinese
Never had a Pap smear	9	32	45
Never had a mammogram	62	83	74

SOURCES: Jenkins et al.(1990), Lew and Chen (1990).

Hypertension

Hypertension is an ailment common to Asian Pacific Americans, yet studies have shown this population group to be consistently less knowledgeable about hypertension than the overall U.S. population (Stavig, Igra, & Leonard, 1988). This lack of understanding, of course, lessens the likelihood that these individuals will seek medical attention for problems related to hypertension.

A study of Asian Pacifics in California, based on 1979 data, showed that only 24.4% of Japanese and 20.6% of other Asian Pacifics with hypertension had seen physicians about their elevated blood pressure in the previous 6 months, compared with 40.5% of the entire California hypertensive population. The Oakland Chinese Community Survey showed that 15% of respondents had never had their blood pressure taken by a physician (Lew & Chen, 1990).

In summary, various local studies on questions ranging from utilization rates to approaches to endemic diseases readily reveal the alarming extent of health access problems for Asian Pacific Americans. Although the national data and research are insufficient to provide a clear picture of problems in access to health care among Asian Pacific populations, local investigations provide ample evidence that critical problems exist in access to health care for these populations. Beyond research, to define the extent of the problem fully, major changes are required in the area of policy in order to promote action in addressing these problems.

Policy Issues and Recommendations

The current debate on national health care reform has focused on universal health care. Although Asian Pacific Americans have a great stake in this debate, such reform will not automatically remove other significant barriers to care. As Strand and Jones (1985) point out, "While financial assistance may guarantee that health services are available to refugees, research on other immigrant populations indicates that effective health service access and utilization require additional forms of assistance that are informational, psychological and organizational" (p. 93).

Thus the parameters of the debate over health care reform must be broadened to include an examination of changes in the system that will increase availability, accessibility, and quality of care. The discussion must include developing strategies to make the health care delivery system more culturally competent and linguistically accessible. Within this context, special emphasis must be placed on reducing fragmentation of care and ensuring that comprehensive primary care services are both available and accessible. There must be a proactive approach to eliminating barriers to care, emphasizing community-based outreach and education.

While the Clinton administration addresses the bigger picture of national health care reform, several current policies that affect access to health care must also be examined. A starting point would be to work toward full compliance with existing laws. Current policies, if enforced, would lead to major improvements in access for Asian Pacific Americans. Legislation has existed for more than 25 years that is intended to guarantee protection from unequal treatment. Title VI of the Civil Rights Act of 1964 says that "no person in the United States shall, on the grounds of race, color, or national origin, be excluded from participation in, be denied the benefits of, or be otherwise subjected to discrimination under any program or activity receiving Federal financial assistance" (U.S. Department of Health and Human Services, Office for Civil Rights, 1990, p. 1).

Any program or activity that receives any form of federal financial assistance must adhere to this antidiscrimination policy. A wide array of services are included, such as extended care facilities, nursing homes, hospitals, state administrative agencies, Medicaid, Medicare Part A, community mental health centers, alcohol and drug treatment centers, family health centers and clinics, physicians and other health care professionals in private practice, state and local public assistance agencies, adoption agencies, foster care homes, day-care centers, senior citizens' centers, and nutrition programs (U.S. Department of Health and Human Services, Office for Civil Rights, 1990).

To assist several states in furnishing adequate health care to "all their people," the Hill-Burton Program was brought into existence in 1946 through the enactment of the Hospital Survey and Construction Act, Title VI of the Public Health Service Act. Nearly 7,000 facilities have received Hill-Burton funding in the form of grants, loans, and loan guarantees to construct and modernize health care facilities. More than 4,200 hospitals have received this assistance. In return for the assistance received, the facilities are required to give assurances that services will be provided to persons who are unable to pay, and that services will be made available to all persons residing in the geographic area of the facility ("A Hill-Burton Primer," 1985). The Office for Civil Rights (OCR) of the U.S. Department of Health and Human Services is responsible for monitoring compliance with the community service assurance of Hill-Burton. This is done through a survey that recipients of Hill-Burton funds must complete. If a facility does not meet antidiscrimination criteria, the OCR investigates and imposes various requirements on the facility.

On Language Access

Although Title VI does not explicitly mention discrimination based on language, this form of discrimination is included in the U.S. Department of Justice's interpretation and in enforcement activities of the OCR and has been affirmed by legal precedent (Nishikawa, 1989). This interpretation essentially places responsibility on federally funded programs to provide language access to populations in need.

The case that set precedent for others was *Lau v. Nichols* in 1974. In this case, the U.S. Supreme Court ruled that the San Francisco Unified School District discriminated against Chinese-speaking students by conducting classes only in English. There have also been numerous cases in the health care field. The Office for Civil Rights is responsible for enforcement of Title VI. The OCR investigates complaints related to language discrimination in health facilities and initiates discretionary investigations as well. Although some of these complaints have resulted in court action, most result in voluntary settlement agreements. In these agreements, health care facilities are obligated to take defined measures to improve language access. For example, as a result of a complaint filed against San Francisco General Hospital, the hospital was obliged to establish a bilingual services department and to hire on-call interpreters and bilingual health professionals (Asian and Pacific Islander American Health Forum, 1990).

Title VI of the Civil Rights Act of 1964 and numerous legal cases provide a very strong framework for language access, but there are important gaps to be noted. Despite established legal strictures, federally funded programs have repeatedly been found to discriminate on the basis of language. Because of resource constraints, the OCR is limited in its capacity to investigate complaints and to identify lack of compliance with Title VI and Hill-Burton. In fiscal year 1990, 11 complaints related to language discrimination were investigated nationally. According to Virginia Apodaca, regional manager of the OCR for Region IX (personal communication, November 22, 1991), this small number of complaints does not reflect a lack of discrimination. The OCR, on its own, also initiated 13 discretionary investigations related to language discrimination. Cases such as these are always initiated on the basis of some suspicion that potential problems may exist within the facility being investigated. The number of cases investigated is limited primarily by a lack of staff time within the OCR.

Coupled with the lack of enforcement is a lack of explicit legislative and administrative mandates to ensure compliance with Title VI. For example, legislation authorizing funds for different government-funded services and programs often lacks explicit language requiring adherence to Title VI. Further, adherence to Title VI is not explicit in administrative-level policies in all branches of federal government responsible for these programs.

Without a commitment of resources, agencies that rely heavily on public funds are hard-pressed to comply with legislative mandates to provide bilingual services. For example, facilities that provide services to Medicare and Medicaid recipients are required to comply with Title VI. However, most states do not provide reimbursement for interpretation services under these programs. Section 330 of the Public Health Services Act, which governs community health centers, states: "If a substantial number of individuals in the populations services by a center are of limited English-speaking ability, the services of appropriate personnel fluent in the languages" must be provided. However, hiring and training of bilingual or multilingual staff is an expensive undertaking. To date there has been only limited allocation of funds to cover the costs of providing these mandated services.

Further complicating the picture is ambiguity regarding what constitutes sufficient need to warrant bilingual services. As stated in the Justice Department definition, language services are required "where a significant number or proportion of the populations eligible to be served or likely to be directly affected by a federally assisted program" requires it (Nishikawa, 1989, p. 14). What constitutes a "significant" number or proportion is usually interpreted as a percentage of the population in a given catchment area, which would mean that there is no obligation to provide services for any group that does not constitute a "significant number."

However, one interpretation in the state of California goes as far as to require that services be provided whenever there is need. In a 1986 memo to MediCal field office administrators, the deputy director of medical care services for the state of California clarified that "hospitals which contract with the Department of Health Services for inpatient hospital services are required to ensure that bilingual translation and interpreter services are available to all non-English speaking beneficiaries regardless of the size of their group represented in the populations being served" (Rodriguez, 1986, p. 1). This example serves as a strong model by placing the responsibility for meeting language needs of all patients on the hospital.

Implementation of existing law is a cornerstone of any strategy to increase language access. At the government, top-down level, a concerted effort needs to be made on the part of the federal government to increase enforcement activities through the Office for Civil Rights. In addition, resources need to be made available to assist federally funded agencies in complying with these legal mandates. In addition, consistent policies and mandates that require the provision of bilingual services whenever needed should be developed and monitored on the legislative and administrative levels.

At a community, bottom-up level, an increase in the number of complaints generated from the Asian Pacific communities and organizations that advocate on their behalf would serve to document access problems for policy makers. When necessary, legal action should be taken to target patterns of language discrimination by health care facilities.

On Cultural Competence

Though not mentioned explicitly, discrimination based on culture is also prohibited by Title VI. If services are provided in a modality that is not accessible, given an individual's cultural belief system, thereby denying the benefits of these services, this is considered to have the *effect* of discrimination. Title VI states:

A recipient . . . may not, directly or through contractual or other arrangements, utilize criteria or methods of administration which have the effect
of subjecting individuals to discrimination because of their race, color, or
national origin, or have the effect of defeating or substantially impairing
accomplishment of the objectives of the program as respect individuals
of a particular race, color or national origin. (U.S. Department of Health
and Human Services, Office for Civil Rights, 1987, p. 2)

Although precedent has established that this law applies to cultural acceptability of services, it has not led to significant changes
in the cultural practices within the health care delivery system.
However, if only in isolated cases, the U.S. Congress has shown
some willingness to address the issue. Included in the Native Hawaiian Health Care Improvement Act of 1988 is the following
language: The Native Hawaiian Health Care Improvement Act is
"premised upon the findings and recommendations of the Native
Hawaiian Health Research Consortium report to the HHS Secretary
of December, 1985. That report clearly indicates that the underutilization of existing health care services by Native Hawaiians can be
traced to the absence of culturally relevant services, in which traditional Native Hawaiian concepts of healing are lacking" (Native
Hawaiian Health Care Improvement Act, 1988).

Although numerous articles and studies have explored the cultural characteristics of Asian Pacific American ethnic groups, no
major federal policy has comprehensively taken their particulari-
ties into account. The Native Hawaiian Health Care Improvement
Act may serve as a precedent for addressing the issue of cultural
competence for other ethnic groups.

Requiring cultural competence as a means of mitigating the
access problem poses a special challenge. Although *cultural appropriateness, cultural acceptability,* and *biculturalism* have become
commonly used terms, they have no widely held common definitions. The term *culturally competent*, which refers to service delivery systems, has begun to take hold in recent years. According to
one definition, a culturally competent system of care would do
the following:

1) value diversity; 2) have the capacity for cultural self-assessment; 3)
be conscious of the dynamics inherent when cultures interact; 4) have
institutionalized cultural knowledge; and 5) have developed adapta-
tions to diversity. Further, each of these five elements must function at

every level of the system. Attitudes, policies, and practices must be congruent within all levels of the system. Practice must be based on accurate perceptions of behavior, policies must be impartial, and attitudes should be unbiased. (Cross, Bazron, Dennis, & Isaacs, 1989, p. v)

This framework may be a useful starting point for identifying the required minimum standard in a service delivery system.

Ensuring compliance with Title VI ultimately requires a methodology for evaluating cultural competence. However, cultural competence is difficult to quantify. Evaluating whether or not a facility is providing culturally appropriate services requires the adaptation of qualitative evaluation methodology. The Multicultural Initiative Project at Portland State University has done considerable work to develop qualitative measures of cultural competence. With support from the National Institute of Mental Health, they have developed the Cultural Competence Self-Assessment Questionnaire, which is designed to help agencies conduct self-assessment and covers areas such as knowledge of communities, personal involvement, resources and linkages, staffing, service delivery and practice, organizational policies and procedures, and reaching out to communities (Mason, 1992). Efforts such as this can serve as a basis for formulating policy related to cultural competence.

On Financial Access

Constantly rising numbers of uninsured and underinsured have brought the issue of universal health care to the top of the national agenda. Many Asian Pacifics are among the tens of millions of underserved Americans who are unemployed or working in occupations that tend to be heavily uninsured. Those who are insured through Medicaid or Medicare obtain limited coverage that does not fully cover screening or immunization for diseases that are common among Asian Pacific Americans.

The provision of a comprehensive national health insurance will enable underserved Asian Pacific Americans, along with the unemployed and the uninsured, to hurdle the steep financial barriers to health care in this country. If we as a society conceive of access to health care as an individual right, regardless of ability to pay, such national health insurance needs to address the issue of providing coverage for all individuals residing in the United States, regardless of immigration status. Coverage must also be comprehensive and must include the costs of a full range of required services, including screening and treatment for diseases that are endemic among Asian Pacific Americans.

On Immigration Status and Eligibility for Benefits

In the absence of major health care reform, eligibility for government services remains a key issue. Here, there has been a dangerous intersection between immigration policy and health care, which has resulted in denial of services to many underserved individuals. Before 1970, immigration status was not a basis for denial of public benefits. However, this changed as states began to restrict access to these programs to certain classes of immigrants (Drake, 1986).

In discussing immigration status and eligibility, it is important to distinguish between refugees and immigrants (legally termed *aliens*). Only 57.6% of all Asian Pacifics in the United States are citizens (U.S. Bureau of the Census, 1988). Refugees are eligible for the same programs as U.S. citizens. However, they make up only about one sixth of the total Asian Pacific American population. For remaining noncitizen immigrants, there exists great confusion in eligibility for public services.

States are limited in their ability to restrict services to legal permanent residents. In *Graham v. Richardson* (1970), the U.S. Supreme Court held that state restrictions on welfare benefits for lawfully resident aliens as a class are inherently illegal and violate the equal protection clause as well as the supremacy clause (Drake, 1986). Nonetheless, some states maintain a 3-year residency requirement before a legal resident can obtain services, thus denying care to recent arrivals, a segment of the population most in need of health care.

The federal government can restrict services to certain classes of legalized immigrants. In *Matthews v. Diaz* (1975), a congressional restriction on Medicare Part B benefits to legal permanent residents who have lived in the United States for at least 5 years was upheld (Wheeler, 1988). The court observed that making distinctions among citizens, aliens, and classes of aliens was not a violation of constitutional protections (Drake, 1986).

Undocumented immigrants (officially referred to as *illegal aliens*) and nonimmigrants (aliens admitted temporarily, for specific reasons) are ineligible for most public services, with the exception of emergency medical care under Medicaid and services offered under the Hill-Burton Act (Wheeler, 1988). However, undocumented immigrants can utilize the services of federally funded community and migrant health centers.

The passage of the 1986 Immigration Reform and Control Act has sown additional confusion. Individuals granted temporary legalization under this act would be ineligible for most public benefits, including certain forms of Medicaid, for a 5-year period even though they are considered legal residents. This restriction is a result of concern in Congress that newly legalized immigrants may add additional strain to limited government resources (Wheeler, 1988).

The underpinnings of U.S. government policies that limit access to services on the basis of legal status and/or the length of time a person has held such status must be reexamined. These restrictions are based on the general assumption that immigrants pose a burden to the state or put a strain on public services. However, this assumption may be inaccurate. It has been rigorously challenged, for example, by Simon (1989) in a thorough examination of the economic impact of immigration. Simon concludes that the net impact of legal immigrants on public services is a beneficial one, because they pay more in taxes than the costs of the public services they utilize. An underlying reason for this is that most immigrants are young and are therefore less likely to draw on public benefits than would older persons. Furthermore legal immigrants use far fewer public services than do U.S. natives for the first 12 years of residence in the United States, after which point their utilization of public services equals that of U.S natives. Undocumented immigrants are ineligible for most public services and therefore use far fewer services than legal immigrants and U.S. natives. If adequate resources were directed to meeting the health care needs of these populations, perhaps their utilization of public services would more closely approximate their investment in tax dollars.

Conclusion

If the United States as a society aspires to the equal treatment of all people and enacts laws and policies to ensure that all have equal access to the goods of our society, then there should be consistency in the means to achieve those ends. As detailed in this chapter, there is a discrepancy between the societal consensus that all people should have access to health care, regardless of their ability to pay, and the implementation of policy statements intended to achieve that goal. The most fundamental assumption of this chapter is that all members of society should have access to quality health care. Quality health care should be accessible to everyone and should not vary depending on the language, culture, citizenship or residency, and legal or financial status of the care seeker. It is important to spell out this assumption because its practical implications are much more complex. Summarized below are the recommendations we have detailed above.

- Expand resources for compliance with and enforcement of Title VI of the Civil Rights Act of 1964.
- Increase complaints and litigation against facilities that discriminate on the basis of language and culture.
- Develop authorizing legislation and administrative policies to ensure compliance with Title VI.
- Develop policies to require the provision of culturally appropriate services.
- Increase the availability of community-based primary care that is culturally, linguistically, and financially accessible.
- Enact legislation to provide national health insurance for all who reside in the United States.
- Eliminate restrictions on eligibility to services based upon immigration status.
- Provide coverage for a full range of comprehensive services, including screening and treatment of diseases endemic among Asian Pacific Americans, case management, and interpretation services.
- Develop systems of care to serve populations and areas where systems are lacking.

Providing access to Asian Pacific Americans must be seen in the context of improving health care access for all Americans. However, the needs of all Americans cannot be addressed through a generic approach. The unique characteristics and needs of all special populations must be taken into account. The Asian Pacific experience calls for strategies that will increase cultural, linguistic, and geographic access to care even while attempts are made to eliminate the more fundamental financial obstacles that deprive tens of millions of Americans of their basic human need for health care.

As the national debate on health care reform continues, decision makers must recognize the great diversity that exists among Asian

Pacific ethnic groups and enlist expertise from each of the communities to help ensure a full understanding and decisive resolution of the health needs and problems that press upon this important segment of the American population.

References

Anderson, R., & Aday, L. A. (1978). Access to medical care in the U.S.: Realized and potential. *Medical Care, 16*, 533-546.

Asian and Pacific Islander American Health Forum. (1990). *Asian and Pacific Islander American Health Forum national agenda for Asian Pacific health.* San Francisco: Author.

Asian Pacific Islander Health Coalition. (1990). *California Asian health issues in the 1990s.* Oakland: California Commission for Economic Development.

Asian Week. (1991). *Asians in America: 1990 census classification by states.* San Francisco: Author.

Brown, E. R., Valdez, R. B., Morgenstern, H., Bradley, T., & Hafner, C. (1987). *Californians without health insurance: A report to the California Legislature.* Berkeley: University of California, California Policy Seminar.

Brown, E. R., Valdez, R. B., Morgenstern, H., Wang, C., & Mann, J. (1991). *Health insurance coverage of Californians in 1989.* Berkeley: University of California, California Policy Seminar.

Buehler, J. W., Stroup, D. F., Kaucke, D. N., & Berkelman, R. L. (1989). The reporting of race and ethnicity in the national notifiable diseases surveillance system. *Public Health Reports, 104*, 457-464.

California Department of Health Services, Health Data and Statistics Branch. (1988). *Selected maternal and infant health status indicators among American Indians, Asians and Pacific Islanders, California birth cohort, 1984-1985.* Sacramento: Author.

Centers for Disease Control. (1990). [Unpublished data].

Chow, R. T. P., & Krumholtz, S. (1989). Health screening of a Rhode Island Cambodian refugee population. *Rhode Island Medical Journal, 72*, 273-276.

Cross, T. L., Bazron, B. J., Dennis, K. W., & Isaacs, M. (1989). *Towards a culturally competent system of care: A monograph on effective services for minority children who are severely emotionally disturbed.* Washington, DC: CASSP Technical Assistance Center.

Drake, S. B. (1986, Summer). Immigrants' rights to health care. *Clearinghouse Review* (National Health Law Program, Los Angeles).

Fasano, M. B., Hayes, J., & Wilson, R. (1986). Traditional beliefs and use of health care services by Vietnamese and Laotian refugees. *Texas Medicine, 82*, 33-36.

Gardner, R. W., Robey, B., & Smith, P. C. (1985). *Asian Americans: Growth, change and diversity.* Washington, DC: Population Reference Bureau.

Gold, B., & Socolar, D. (1987). *Report of the Boston Committee on Access to Health Care.* Boston: Boston Committee on Access to Health Care.

Gold, B., Socolar, D., Goldfied, H., & Newschaffer, C. (1987). *Boston Committee on Access to Health Care: Second Report to Mayor Raymond L. Flynn.* Boston: Boston Committee on Access to Health Care.

Graham v. Richardson, 403 U.S. 365 (1970).

Hawaii State Department of Health. (1991). *State Title V annual report*. Honolulu: Author.

A Hill-Burton primer. (1985, May). *Clearinghouse Review* (National Health Law Program, Los Angeles), p. 13.

Hoang, G. N., & Erickson, R. V. (1985). Cultural barriers to effective medical care among Indochinese patients. *Annual Review of Medicine, 36*, 229-239.

Jenkins, C. N. H., McPhee, S. J., Bird, J. A., & Bonilla, N. (1990). Cancer risks and prevention practices among Vietnamese refugees. *Western Journal of Medicine, 153*, 34-39.

Korean Health Survey Task Force. (1989). *Korean health survey*. Unpublished manuscript, Korean Health Education, Information and Referral Center, Los Angeles.

Lew, R., & Chen, A. (1990, October). *A community survey of health risk behavior among Chinese Americans*. Paper presented at the annual meeting of the American Public Health Association.

Lin-Fu, J. (1988). Population characteristics and health care needs of Asian Pacific Americans. *Public Health Reports, 103*, 18-27.

Margolis, H. S., Alter, M. J., & Hadler, S. (1991). Hepatitis B: Evolving epidemiology and implications for control. *Seminars in Liver Disease, 2*, 84-86.

Mason, J. L. (1992). *Cultural Competence Self-Assessment Questionnaire*. Portland, OR: Portland State University, Research and Training Center on Family Support and Children's Mental Health.

Matthews v. Diaz, 426 U.S. 67 (1975).

National Council of Negro Women, Communications Consortium Media Center. (1991). *Women of color reproductive health poll*. Rochester, NY: Winters Group.

Native Hawaiian Health Care Improvement Act, 100 USC Report 100 500 (1988).

Native Hawaiian Health Research Consortium, Alu Like, Inc. (1985). *E Ola Mau: The Native Hawaiian Health Needs Study, medical task force report*. Honolulu: Author.

Nishikawa, A. (1989). *Barriers to health care: Improving services to non-English speaking patients in Sonoma County*. Unpublished document prepared for Community Hospital.

Phan, T. C. (1984). *Unexpressed health needs among refugees from Southeast Asian countries*. Unpublished manuscript, Wisconsin Department of Health and Social Services.

Rhee, S. O. (1989). *A study of the health needs and behavior of Korean-Americans in Chicago, Illinois* (Preliminary Report). Unpublished manuscript, Governors State University, University Park, Illinois.

Robert Wood Johnson Foundation. (1987). *Access to health care in the United States: Results of a 1986 survey* (Special Report No. 2). Princeton, NJ: Author.

Rodriguez, J. (1986, November 3). [Memorandum from deputy director, Medical Health Services, State of California].

Rumbaut, R. G., Chavez, L. R., Moser, R. J., Pickwell, S. M., & Wishnik, S. M. (1988). The politics of migrant health care: A comparative study of Mexican immigrants and Indochinese refugees. *Research in the Sociology of Health Care, 7*, 143-202.

Simon, J. L. (1989). *The economic consequences of immigration*. Cambridge, MA: Basil Blackwell.

Stavig, G. R., Igra, A., & Leonard, A. R. (1988). Hypertension and related health issues among Asians and Pacific Islanders in California. *Public Health Reports, 103*, 28-37.

Strand, P. J., & Jones, W. (1985). *Indochinese refugees in America: Problems of adaptation and assimilation*. Durham, NC: Duke University Press.

True, R. H. (1985). *Health care services delivery in Asian American communities* (Report of the Secretary's Task Force on Black and Minority Health, Vol. 2). Washington, DC: U.S. Department of Health and Human Services.

U.S. Bureau of the Census. (1988). *We, the Asian Pacific Americans*. Washington, DC: Government Printing Office.

U.S. Commission on Civil Rights. (1992). *Civil rights issues facing Asian Americans in the 1990s*. Washington, DC: Government Printing Office.

U.S. Department of Health and Human Services, Office for Civil Rights. (1987). *Regulations under Title VI of the Civil Rights Act of 1964, 45 Code of Federal Regulation, Public Welfare Part 80*. Washington, DC: Government Printing Office.

U.S. Department of Health and Human Services, Office for Civil Rights. (1990). *Your responsibilities as a health care or social service administrator under Title VI of the Civil Rights Act of 1964* (Fact Sheet). Washington, DC: Government Printing Office.

U.S. Department of Health and Human Services, Office of Refugee Resettlement. (1990). *Report to Congress: Refugee resettlement program*. Washington, DC: Government Printing Office.

U.S. Department of Health and Human Services, Public Health Service. (1990). *Healthy People 2000: National health promotion and disease prevention objectives* (Conference ed., summary). Washington, DC: Government Printing Office.

U.S. Department of Health, Education and Welfare. (1980). *Special report to Congress on the primary health care needs of immigrants*. Washington, DC: Government Printing Office.

Wheeler, C. (1988, November). Alien eligibility for public benefits: Part I. *Immigration Briefings*.

Yu, E., & Cypress, B. K. (1982). Visits to physicians by Asian Pacific Americans. *Medical Care, 20*, 809-820.

Yu, E., Huber, W., Wong, S., Tseng, G., & Liu, W. (1990). *Survey of health coverage needs in Chicago's Chinatown: A final report*. San Diego, CA: Pacific/Asian Mental Health Research Center.

14

Supply of
Health Care Professionals

LAURA UBA

This chapter addresses the availability of Asian Pacific American[1] health care professionals[2] available to meet the health care needs of Asian Pacific American populations. More specifically, this chapter focuses on the importance of such health care providers to the provision of health care to Asian Pacific Americans, the supply and distribution of such health care providers, and the policies that affect that supply.

Asian Pacific American
Health Care Providers

There is a need to examine the supply of Asian Pacific American health care providers because that supply has a bearing on the quantity and quality of health care services delivered to Asian Pacific Americans. The availability of such health care providers can affect the number of Asian Pacific Americans who use health care services. Asian Pacific Americans underutilize health services when there is a lack of ethnically-matched professionals (Thien, 1990) and increase their use of some types of health care services when those

AUTHOR'S NOTE: I would like to extend thanks to Maia Forman for her assistance in the data collection.

services are delivered by Asian Pacific Americans (Asian and Pacific Islander American Health Forum, 1986; Sue & McKinney, 1975) because many patients in this population, particularly the less acculturated, want an ethnic match with their physicians (Anderson, 1983; Ito & So, 1982a).

The supply of Asian Pacific American health care providers can also have a bearing on the quality (i.e., cultural sensitivity) of health care services delivered to Asian Pacific Americans. Insofar as these health care professionals may provide services that are culturally sensitive, their supply affects the availability of culturally sensitive services and therefore the quality of health care services available.

There is reason to believe that Asian Pacific Americans are more likely than their non-Asian Pacific American counterparts to provide services that are culturally sensitive to Asian Pacific Americans. For example, researchers have found that many Asian Pacific American patients prefer health care providers who are bilingual (Egawa & Tashima, 1982; Gould-Martin & Ning, 1981; UCLA Health Team, 1975). Further, Asian Pacific American health care professionals are more likely than their counterparts of other ethnicities to provide bilingual services in an Asian or Pacific Islander language. However, bilingualism is not the only way in which these professionals provide culturally sensitive health care services. Indeed, some Asian Pacific American patients prefer coethnics over white health care providers even if the Asian Pacific health care providers are not bilingual (Muecke, 1983a; True, 1985).

Asian Pacific American health care professionals also often share and understand culture-specific styles of interacting, traditions, and expectations commonly found among Asian Pacific Americans; such health care professionals would therefore be more likely to be culturally sensitive to those styles of interacting and traditions than would those who have not shared an Asian Pacific American cultural background. Such cultural familiarity may make these health care professionals sensitive to particular expectations and taboos; for example, a Southeast Asian health care provider would understand that some Southeast Asians would be insulted if the provider crossed his or her legs and let his or her foot point at the Southeast Asian patients (Olness, 1979). Gould-Martin and Ning (1981) found that some Asian Pacific Americans understate their physical complaints in an effort to be polite, unassuming, or stoic. Other researchers suggest that some Asian Pacific Americans think that speaking of a malady can cause the malady or make it worse

(Muecke, 1983a) or are reticent to ask physicians questions because they do not want to imply they are questioning the physicians' authority (Grizzel, Savale, Scott, & Detroit, 1980; U.S. General Accounting Office, 1990). The ability to understand these styles of interacting and to detect subtle social cues can affect how well health care professionals and patients communicate with each other, how quickly accurate diagnoses are reached, and the speed with which appropriate medical treatments are instigated.

In addition to awareness of culture-specific interaction patterns, Asian Pacific American health care professionals may be more likely than their counterparts of other ethnicities to be familiar with cultural beliefs held by some (especially immigrant) Asian Pacific Americans concerning illness, diagnosis, and treatment (Anderson, 1983; Muecke, 1983b; Silverman, 1979; U.S. General Accounting Office, 1990). Thus such health care providers may be more adept at educating patients about the limitations of folk medicine (True, 1985), translating Western medical concepts into concepts that can be understood from the patient's cultural perspective (Egawa & Tashima, 1982; Muecke, 1983a; Tung, 1980), and recognizing the residual effects of the traditional, non-Western treatments patients may have tried (Egawa & Tashima, 1982; Yeatman, Shaw, & Barlow, 1976).

Providing culturally sensitive health services increases the rapport between the patient and the health care provider. In turn, such cultural rapport can make a significant difference in the ability to provide effective services. Researchers have suggested that cultural rapport can increase the likelihood that patients will trust Western medicine (True, 1985); disclose concerns, symptoms, and questions (Gaw, 1975); and understand and comply with prescribed medical treatment plans (Gaw, 1975; Muecke, 1983a; Rosario, 1980). Moreover, inasmuch as cultural rapport facilitates patient-physician communication, it increases the physician's understanding of the patient's symptoms, concerns, and goals, which in turn can influence the physician's decisions about which medical avenues to pursue. Conversely, cultural insensitivity may drive patients away from needed services.

In summary, the availability of Asian Pacific American health care providers is important because such professionals can provide a cultural rapport with their patients that in turn may result in increased use of health services and improved quality of care. Such health care providers often have an understanding of Asian Pacific Americans that is not taught in medical schools and that other health care providers would have difficulty offering. However, cultural rapport should not be interpreted as extending too globally. Given the differences among Asian Pacific American cultures, Asian Pacific American health care providers of one ethnic group or acculturative history may not be able to establish the cultural rapport needed to meet the needs of patients of another ethnic group or acculturative history.

Supply of Asian Pacific American Health Care Providers

An overview of the supply of Asian Pacific American health care providers normally would include the number, medical specialties, languages spoken, sex, and geographic distribution of these health care providers in general and for each specific Asian Pacific ethnic group. However, such information is largely unknown. The raw data have never been collected by the Public Health Service (PHS), the National Institutes of Health (NIH), the Bureau of Health Professions, the Bureau of Labor Statistics, or the Association of American Medical Colleges (AAMC) in such a form that this information could be discerned.

However, based on some AAMC data and studies sampling the Asian Pacific American medical community, some characteristics of Asian Pacific Americans in health care professions can be tentatively derived. Consideration will be given here to the medical school education of Asian Pacific Americans, the number of such physicians, the health care fields that they gravitate toward, the types of institutions in which they work, their geographic distribution, and the specialties and work settings of Asian Pacific American professionals who tend to be oriented toward serving the health care needs of Asian Pacific American communities.

Medical Education

An analysis of data on applicants to medical schools from 1981 to 1990 reveals that Asian Pacific Americans are an increasing proportion (5.3% in 1981 to 14.9% in 1990) of those applying to medical schools and a corresponding proportion of those being accepted to medical schools (4.8% in 1981 to 14.9% in 1990) (AAMC, 1989a, 1989b, 1990). Asian Pacific Americans are the only ethnic group that had an increase in the number of applicants to medical school from 1983 to 1989. During that period there was an 86.9% increase in Asian Pacific American applicants to medical school (AAMC, 1989a). AAMC (1989b) data reveal that, on average, Asian Pacific Americans sent out more applications to medical schools (12.4 in 1987 and 13.2 in 1988) than did whites (9.2 and 9.3, respectively), Hispanics (11.2 and 11.7, respectively), or African Americans (10.0 and 10.1, respectively).

Further analysis of the AAMC data shows that from 1981 to 1989 the rate at which Asian Pacific Americans have been accepted to medical schools has been lower than that of white Americans and than that of all applicants. For example, in 1981, 47.1% of all applicants and 48.3% of white applicants were accepted, whereas 41.7% of Asian Pacific American applicants were accepted (AAMC, 1989b). More recently, however, the Asian Pacific American acceptance rate has been closer to the average. In 1990, the rate of acceptance of Asian Pacific Americans was slightly higher than that of all applicants, but it remained slightly lower than the rate of acceptance of whites (AAMC, 1990).

Although the AAMC does not keep track of GPA and MCAT scores of Asian Pacific Americans as it does for other minorities, there is evidence that the Asian Pacific American applicants to medical school are at least as qualified as others, if not more qualified. A comparison of the number of Asian Pacific Americans graduating from medical school in 1990 with the number of Asian Pacific Americans accepted into medical school 4 years earlier reveals that Asian Pacific Americans graduate at rates similar to other groups. The percentage of Asian Pacific Americans having to repeat an academic year is lower than that of all other students (AAMC, 1989b). Moreover, the rate at which Asian Pacifics graduate from prestigious medical schools also suggests high qualifications. For example, in 1988 Asian Pacific Americans constituted 8% of the graduating class at Johns Hopkins, 9% at Harvard, 10% at the University of Michigan, 14% at Stanford, 15% at George Washington, and 20% at UCLA.

Furthermore Asian Pacific Americans are an increasing proportion of medical school graduates. In 1983 they were 5.6% of medical school graduates; in 1990 the proportion was 9.3% (AAMC, 1989a, 1990). From 1983 to 1990, white Americans and Asian Pacific Americans have had similar proportions of females among medical school graduates. For example, in 1990, females constituted 32.4% of white medical school graduates, compared with 35.5% of Asian Pacific American medical school graduates (AAMC, 1990).

A comparison of the regions of the United States from which Asian Pacific Americans are graduating from medical schools indicates that the percentages of Asian Pacific Americans graduating from schools in the Northeast, South, and Central Plains are similar to the percentages of white Americans graduating from medical schools in those same regions. For example, 11% of Asian Pacific American male and 8% of Asian Pacific American female graduates of medical school in 1988 graduated from medical schools in New York; similarly, 10% of white American male and female graduates of medical school that year graduated from medical schools in New York. The one state in which there was a striking difference was California: 14% of Asian Pacific American males and 18% of Asian Pacific American females graduating from medical school in 1988 graduated from medical schools in California, whereas only 5% of white American males and females graduating from medical schools did so in California (AAMC, 1989b). There has been no significant difference in the percentages of Asian Pacific Americans attending private versus state-run medical schools (AAMC, 1989b).

Foreign Medical Education

An estimated 20.9% of all physicians in the United States are trained in other countries (Matsunaga-Nishi & Wang, 1985). In 1980 there were 37,717 foreign medical graduates from Asia in the United States, constituting 38.2% of all foreign medical graduates in the United States (Matsunaga-Nishi & Wang, 1985). Of all foreign medical graduates in the United States, 15.4% came from India, 12.9% came from the Philippines, and 4.4% came from Korea. At the same time, foreign medical graduates from India, the Philippines, and Korea accounted for 84.7% of the Asian Pacific foreign medical graduates working in the United States (Matsunaga-Nishi & Wang, 1985). What is most notable given these numbers is that, as the AAMC (1989b) counted only 43,450 Asian Pacific American physicians in the United States in 1980, the 37,717 foreign medical graduates from Asia constituted 86.8% of Asian Pacific American physicians.

Extrapolating from the fact that 60% (i.e., 4,121) of Asian Pacific American medical residents on duty in 1987 were foreign-educated (AAMC, 1989b), it appears that foreign medical graduates constitute a diminishing proportion of new Asian Pacific American physicians but still are more than half of the Asian Pacific American physicians in the United States. Furthermore, of all residents on duty in 1987, 8.5% were Asian Pacifics but only 3.3% were Asian Pacifics from U.S. or Canadian medical schools (AAMC, 1989b). This again suggests that the majority of new Asian Pacific American physicians in 1987 were foreign medical graduates. Together these facts suggest that many Asian Pacific American physicians do not have training that is comparable to that of U.S.-educated physicians (Robinson & Schriver, 1989).

Number of Health Care Providers

In 1980 Asian Pacific American physicians constituted 10% of all physicians (AAMC, 1989b). Of the Asian Pacific American physicians, 73% were males. The male Asian Pacific American physicians were 8.5% of all male physicians and the female Asian Pacific American physicians were 20.2% of all female physicians (AAMC, 1989b). Among specific Asian ethnic groups, Japanese Americans constituted .5% and Chinese Americans constituted 1.7% of all physicians (Bureau of Health Professions, 1984), whereas they make up, respectively, .031% and .035% of the U.S. population (Kitano & Daniels, 1988; U.S. General Accounting Office, 1990).

Health Care Fields

A 1985 study of Asian Pacific Americans in health care occupations in New York found that more than 50% were nurses (31.9%) and nurse's aides, orderlies, and attendants (26.1%), many of whom "were foreign-trained professionals who had not passed their licensure examinations" in the United States (Matsunaga-Nishi & Wang, 1985, p. 154). If clinical laboratory technicians and technologists (15.3%) and physicians (10.2%) were added to the aforementioned occupations, they would account for more than 80% of Asian Pacific Americans in health care occupations. The remainder of the Asian Pacific Americans in health care occupations in 1985 were dentists, pharmacists, dietitians, therapists, radiologic technicians, and dental hygienists.

Table 14.1 presents the proportion of Asian Pacific Americans in various health fields based on the 1980 U.S. Census. Ethnic Chinese and Japanese constituted 22% and 19%, respectively, of the Asian Pacific American population in 1980 (U.S. General Accounting Office, 1990). Yet, as Table 14.1 indicates, almost all of the Asian Pacific American dental hygienists, optometrists, physical therapists, and speech therapists were ethnic Chinese or Japanese.

To give another perspective on the distribution of Asian Pacific Americans in health care fields, Table 14.2 presents data on the types of professional doctoral degrees received by Asian Americans in 1984-1985. It is unclear whether Asian Pacific American physicians tend to choose different specialties than do other physicians. Matsunaga-Nishi and Wang (1985) have shown that Asian Pacific Americans are less represented in higher-income specialties than are physicians in general and instead are more often found in specialties such as psychiatry and anesthesiology than are physicians in general. Cuca (1980) found that fewer Asian Pacifics (8.1%) than whites (19.3%) wanted to specialize in family practice but that internal medicine was the preferred specialty of both Asian Pacifics (27.9%) and whites (34.6%). More recently, Babbott, Baldwin, Killian, and O'Leary-Weaver (1989) found no differences in chosen specialties between Asian Pacific and white physicians, both when the students started medical school and when they finished.

Since 1976 there have been severe restrictions on the employment of foreign medical graduates and aliens who have graduated from U.S. or Canadian medical schools (Robinson & Schriver, 1989). The amended Immigration and Nationality Act excludes alien physicians from receiving visas as temporary professional workers "if their duties [would] primarily entail direct patient care" (Robinson & Schriver, 1989, p. 359). However, such visas can be obtained if the physician's primary duty is teaching or doing research. Thus there are forces pushing Asian Pacific foreign medical graduates away from directly serving the health care needs of Asian Pacific Americans. The Immigration Act of 1990 will not affect this situation, because it simply recodifies extant laws on labor certification for foreign medical graduates.

There is conflicting information concerning whether foreign medical graduates go into the same specialties as U.S. medical graduates. Goodman and Wunderman (1981) found that those foreign medical graduates who do provide direct patient care generally choose the same specialties as U.S. medical graduates. By contrast, Matsunaga-Nishi and Wang (1985) found that foreign medical graduates are represented in surgery (13.8%) and general practice (9.4%) less often than the average medical graduate in the United States (18.1% and 12.8%, respectively) and that foreign medical graduates are

Table 14.1 Proportions of Asian Pacific Americans in Various Health Professions, According to 1980 U.S. Census (in percentages)

	White	African American	All Asian Pacific Americans	Chinese	Japanese
Dental hygienists	95.4	1.6	1.3	.4	.6
Dentists	93.6	2.3	2.5	.6	.8
Dietitians	84.6	6.7	6.3	1.4	1.0
Nurses					
registered[a]	88.3	5.7	3.9	.3	.3
practical	77.6	17.0	1.4	.1	.2
Optometrists	95.4	.9	2.2	.7	1.4
Pharmacists	91.2	2.3	4.4	1.9	.9
Physicians	82.8	2.6	10.6	1.7	.5
Technicians					
laboratory	79.5	11.1	5.7	1.4	.7
radiologic	86.2	7.7	1.8	.3	.4
Therapists					
physical	93.4	3.3	1.8	.7	.7
occupational	94.7	2.1	2.2	.5	1.1
speech	92.9	4.3	1.1	.3	.7

SOURCE: Bureau of Health Professions (1984).
NOTE: a. With 2 or more years of college.

represented in internal medicine (17.6%), anesthesiology (6%), and psychiatry (7.7%) more often than the average medical graduate (15.3%, 3.4%, and 5.9%, respectively). Kim (1981) found that 62% of Korean foreign medical graduates are in the less prestigious specialties of anesthesiology, general practice, obstetrics-gynecology,

Table 14.2 First Professional Degrees Received by Asian Americans in the United States, 1984 to 1985 (in percentages)

	Asian Americans	All Recipients
Medicine	32.1	21.1
Optometry	4.2	1.6
Chiropractic	1.7	3.7
Osteopathy	1.7	2.1

SOURCE: Peng (1988).

pathology, pediatrics, physical medicine and rehabilitation, psychiatry, and radiology.

Types of Institutions

A study in New York found that more than twice as many white American male physicians in New York (45.8%) were in private practice as were Asian Pacific American male physicians (20.9%), and almost twice as many white American female physicians (23.2%) as Asian Pacific American female physicians (12%) were in private practice (Matsunaga-Nishi & Wang, 1985). In 1988 there were 1,839 Asian Pacific Americans working as medical school faculty members. They constituted 6.0% of the male and 12.1% of the female medical school faculty who were medical doctors (AAMC, 1989b).

Because more prestige is associated with graduating from American medical schools than foreign medical schools, foreign medical graduates are not offered the choice residencies. Many Asian foreign medical graduates are hired by the public sector in the less prestigious and less lucrative inner-city hospitals, Medicaid-sponsored programs, and state psychiatric hospitals (Kim, 1981; Matsunaga-Nishi & Wang, 1985). Indeed, Matsunaga-Nishi and Wang (1985) found that more than 16% of foreign medical graduates in the United States are full-time, hospital staff physicians, compared with 9.1% of all physicians. Further, Asian foreign medical graduates and Asian Pacific Americans who are involved in diagnosis were found disproportionally in government employment such as city hospitals and state mental hospitals: 22.6% of Asian Pacific American men and 33.8% of Asian Pacific American women work for the government, whereas 10.5% of white American men and 21% of white American women do so.

Distribution

Asian Pacific Americans in health services, particularly nurses and technicians, tend to be concentrated in inner cities (Matsunaga-Nishi & Wang, 1985). For example, Matsunaga-Nishi and Wang (1985) found that 53.8% of Asian Pacific Americans (compared with 47.2% of all others) in health-diagnosing occupations in New York are in central cities. Although it appears that most Asian Pacific Americans live in urban areas, the degree to which various Asian

Pacific American groups actually live in inner cities has not been analyzed from census data.

There are indications that many communities do not have available to them health services provided by Asian Pacific American physicians. This is true even in California, which has a relatively large Asian Pacific American population. According to the 1980 census, there were 11 counties in California that had no Asian Pacific American physicians and there were 7 counties with only one Asian Pacific American physician (California Office of Statewide Health Planning and Development, 1981).

A physician-to-population balance index derived from the 1980 census reveals that about one third of California's counties had a below-balance physician-to-population index for Asian Pacific Americans (i.e., fewer Asian Pacific American physicians per Asian Pacific Americans in the county population than would be expected statistically). Of the California counties with more than 10,000 Asian Pacific Americans, there was a below-balance index in half of the counties. The average county in California had a population of 5.3% Asian Pacific Americans. Of the eight counties in which Asian Pacific Americans exceeded 5.3%, there was a below-balance physician-to-population index in seven. The exception was Los Angeles County, which had a higher concentration of Asian Pacific American physicians (California Office of Statewide Health Planning and Development, 1981).

Of the total number of Korean foreign medical graduates, the majority work on the Eastern seaboard (Kim, 1981). In particular, 35% work in New York, New Jersey, and Connecticut, whereas only 14% of the Koreans in the United States live in those states (Kim, 1981). Another 25% work in the Midwest, especially in Ohio, Michigan, and Illinois, three states that account for only 12% of the Korean population in the United States (Kim, 1981; Kitano & Daniels, 1988).

Health Professional Orientations

Ito and So's (1982b) study with a Los Angeles sample found that Chinese American and Japanese American physicians who are oriented toward the Asian American ethnic community tend to be in different specialties than Japanese and Chinese who are not oriented toward serving the ethnic community. That study found that those "who are oriented to their ethnic communities [i.e., have a patient load of more than 5% Asian Pacific American] tend to be in . . . family practice, internal medicine, obstetrics-gynecology, and pediatrics" (p. 9). Chinese American and Japanese American physicians who are not oriented toward their ethnic communities (i.e., have a patient load of less than 5% Asian Pacific American) tend to be found to be in specialties such as cardiology, neurology, and plastic surgery.

Further, Ito and So found that Chinese American and Japanese American physicians who are oriented toward serving the ethnic community tend to work in different settings than those who are not so oriented. In this Los Angeles sample, Chinese and Japanese American physicians whose proportions of Asian Pacific American patients were more than 5% tended to work in private practice, whereas those who served 5% or fewer Asian Pacific American patients were more likely to work in hospitals, clinics, and research institutions. None of these relationships held for Filipino American physicians.

In summary, Asian Pacific Americans as a group constitute a significant number of the nation's supply of physicians, yet it is not possible to determine whether all ethnicities included in the category of "Asian Pacific Americans" are well represented in the ranks of U.S. physicians because the number of physicians in each particular Asian Pacific American group is not known. It is quite possible, for example, that there are many Filipino American physicians but few Korean American physicians, or that there are many Southeast Asian physicians who are foreign medical graduates but few who are graduates of American medical schools.

Policies Affecting the Supply and Training of Asian Pacific American Physicians and Health Researchers

Two factors that affect the supply and training of Asian Pacific American physicians and health researchers are discussed in this section: the changes in foreign medical graduate policies and the adoption of the notion that Asian Pacific Americans are overrepresented among physicians and biomedical researchers.

Policies Affecting Foreign Medical Graduates

The 1976 Health Professions Educational Assistance Act (P.L. 94-484) brought about a decline in the number of foreign medical graduates in the United States. New requirements, such as the Visa Qualifying Examination, were instituted, and visa exemptions for physicians were no longer given (Kim, 1981; Matsunaga-Nishi & Wang, 1985), making it difficult for foreign-trained Asians to become licensed. In addition, P.L. 94-484 created difficulties in converting visitor visas to permanent visas (Goodman & Wunderman, 1981), making it difficult for foreigners to stay in the United States. Furthermore, as mentioned earlier, the amended Immigration and Nationality Act restricted the types of work alien physicians could do (Robinson & Schriver, 1989). Therefore there are proportionally fewer Asian foreign medical graduates now than there were before 1976.

Moreover, foreign medical graduates tend to work in nonuniversity-affiliated hospitals (Matsunaga-Nishi & Wang, 1985), so Asian Pacific American foreign medical graduates have fewer opportunities to learn research skills than do those working in university hospitals.

Adoption of a Population Parity/ Underrepresentation Criterion

To determine which minority groups need increased numbers of physicians to meet the health care needs of their ethnic communities, medical schools and government agencies have adopted the "population parity" model and "underrepresentation" model, respectively. The two models are essentially the same: Both broadly compare the number of physicians in an ethnic minority group to the total population of that ethnic group.

At NIH agencies, a "minority" (defined as black, Hispanic, Native American, or Asian Pacific American) is considered "underrepresented" when that minority is "disproportionately represented in biomedical and behavioral science careers, based on their minority group's representation in the total population" (National Heart, Lung and Blood Institute, 1989, pp. 72-73). According to the National Heart, Lung and Blood Institute (1989), "Asian Americans make up only 2% of the U.S. population but . . . comprise 6% of the science and engineering workforce, 10% of the physician population, and 7% of the Ph.D.s in science and engineering. Therefore, they are not considered underrepresented" (p. 73).

The notion that Asian Pacific Americans are not underrepresented in health care professions is at the root of many policies affecting the supply of Asian Pacific American health care providers. Consideration will be given below to the dubious bases for the assessment of Asian Pacific American overrepresentation and how this notion affects the supply of Asian Pacific American health care providers.

Flaws in Population Parity/Underrepresentation Models

The categorization of Asian Pacific Americans as overrepresented in health care professions is dubious on a number of counts. The method used to determine underrepresentation is questionable because, as will be discussed, it (a) aggregates all Asian Pacific Americans, (b) uses different criteria to define minorities, (c) bases calculations on census data of questionable validity, (d) makes spurious comparisons to determine that Asian Pacific Americans are overrepresented, and (e) bases the assessment on few data.

First, despite the facts that the Census Bureau's definition of Asian Pacific Americans includes people whose ethnicities or countries of origin are among 28 Asian countries or 25 Pacific Islander cultures, and that various Asian Pacific American groups differ in cultural background, assimilation, socioeconomic status, and immigration history, the criterion for underrepresentation and population parity used by the NIH and the AAMC aggregates all Asian Pacific Americans into one category, as though the differences among them are not sufficiently significant to warrant distinguishing among various ethnic groups that make up this large category. Such aggregation carries with it the assumption that, for example, a third-generation Filipina American nurse who knows some Tagalog will be able to provide needed culturally sensitive health services to a Chinese immigrant who can speak and understand only Mandarin. Each individual Asian Pacific American health care provider reflects a culturally specific background and thus cannot serve just any sector of the Asian Pacific American population with equal understanding and rapport. In fact, some Asians (e.g., Cambodians) are uncomfortable with health care providers of other particular Asian ethnic backgrounds (e.g., Vietnamese) because of political antagonisms between their Asian countries (Muecke, 1983a).

Moreover, the criterion's broad measure of representation does not examine whether there is overrepresentation of specific Asian

Pacific American ethnic groups. The AAMC (1989b) claims that a "group is considered underrepresented if the percentage of a *specific* racial/ethnic group in the physician population is less than that group's percentage in the total population" (p. 2; emphasis added). Yet at the same time, the AAMC does not distinguish among each of the specific Asian Pacific ethnic groups. The Public Health Service's affirmative-action goal is to ensure that various segments of the population have equal access to education in health professions (U.S. Department of Health and Human Services, 1987) and "to increase the number of underrepresented minority scientists participating in biomedical research" (National Institutes of Health, 1989, p. 1). However, because the different Asian Pacific groups have been aggregated into one Asian Pacific category and as a single group are declared overrepresented, individuals from specific Asian or Pacific Islander groups that may be underrepresented do not have access to education in health professions or research opportunities equal to that of other minorities.

Second, the criterion of underrepresentation is defined differently for different minorities. For example, the National Heart, Lung and Blood Institute specifies "Black citizens" when defining blacks but does not specify U.S. citizenship when defining *Asians*. Thus the large contingent of alien Asian foreign medical graduates in the United States skews and inflates the total count of Asian Pacific American physicians.

Third, the underrepresentation criterion is based on census estimates of the total number of Asian Pacific Americans. There have been suspicions that the census has undercounted them (U.S. General Accounting Office, 1990). Moreover, because it usually takes years for census data on Asian Pacific Americans to be analyzed, by the time census analyses are distributed they are often already outdated and may not reflect the number and composition of the Asian Pacific American population. Basing the underrepresentation calculation on old census data without projecting a count of the current population can be misleading.

Fourth, part of the argument for not considering Asian Pacific Americans underrepresented in health care professions has been a comparison between the number of Asian Pacific American Ph.D.s in engineering and science with the total Asian Pacific American population. The validity of this comparison is questionable, given that engineers and scientists often have little to do with delivering health care or health care research. This is especially the case among

Asian Pacific Americans, where only 4.4% of Ph.D.s are in health sciences (Peng, 1988).

Fifth, the notion that Asian Pacific Americans are not underrepresented in health care professions is based on questionable data. Data on Asian Pacific Americans have often been lost in the category of "other" when information has been collected and presented on African Americans, Hispanic Americans, and European Americans. Furthermore, there is no evidence that there is a sufficient variety of Asian Pacific American health care providers in terms of ethnicity, ethnicity by sex, medical specialty, languages spoken, and geographic distribution to serve the health care needs of Asian Pacific Americans. In addition, PHS funding agencies do not keep track of the ethnicities of recipients of biomedical research grants. Despite this lack of information, policies have been instituted that assume Asian Pacific Americans are overrepresented in biomedical and behavioral research.

The Notion of Underrepresentation and the
Supply of Asian Pacific Health Care Providers

Regarding all Asian Pacific Americans as overrepresented means that Asian Pacific Americans are not eligible for special AAMC or government minority programs or research grants. For example, because they are not considered to be underrepresented minorities, Asian Pacific Americans are excluded from NIH's Minority High School Summer Student Research Apprenticeship, which encourages "high school students to consider careers in . . . biomedical and behavioral sciences" (National Institutes of Health, 1989, p. 1). They are also excluded from the Health Careers Opportunity Program's Division of Disadvantaged grants "to improve access to health careers [and] to help institutions identify, motivate, recruit, place, and retain [minority and disadvantaged] students" (Carr, 1989, p. 81). Asian Pacific Americans are not eligible for NIH Research Supplements for Minority Undergraduate Students that support "undergraduate students to continue on to graduate level training in biomedical and behavioral sciences" (National Institutes of Health, 1989, p. 1) or National Heart, Lung and Blood Institute (1989) biomedical career development programs.

Because Asian Pacific Americans are not considered underrepresented minority medical students, the AAMC (1989b) does not try to help medical schools recruit, admit, retain, and graduate Asian

Pacific Americans as it does for other minorities. A comparison of the numbers of Asian Pacific Americans graduating in 1986, 1987, and 1988 to the numbers of them accepted to medical school 4 years earlier (AAMC, 1989b) shows that attrition rates for Asian Pacific Americans (6.6%, 7.2%, and 7.0%) were higher than for whites (3.8%, 4.9%, and 5.3%, respectively). Whether the higher Asian Pacific American dropout rates are a result of lack of financial support is not clear. However, Asian Pacific American medical school applicants tend to come from poorer families than do white applicants. For example, in 1988, 6% of Asian Pacific American medical school applicants came from families making less than $15,000 per year, compared with 3% of white applicants. Further, whereas 43.3% of Asian Pacific American applicants came from families making $30,000 or more per year, 49.7% of the white applicants came from such families (AAMC, 1989b). It is possible that Asian Pacific Americans have dropped out at higher rates because they could not receive the federal grants they needed to continue their education.

Asian Pacific Americans are not eligible for biomedical research grants designed to increase the number of minorities in biomedical and behavioral research. For example, they are excluded from the U.S. Department of Health and Human Services Research Supplements for Minority Investigators, which provide opportunities "to participate in on-going research projects and to develop their own independent research potential" (U.S. Department of Health and Human Services, 1990, p. 2). Asian Pacific Americans are excluded from receiving National Heart, Lung and Blood Institute grants for "programs focusing primarily on health problems unique to one or more minority populations [and] programs focusing on a minority health issue through comparative studies of a minority population with another population" (National Heart, Lung and Blood Institute, 1989, p. 78). Because Asian Pacific Americans, who might be interested in studying issues in Asian Pacific American health, are excluded from receiving these grants, there is even less knowledge of health issues facing these ethnic populations.

In summary, despite the dearth of information on Asian Pacific American health care providers and the demographic misrepresentation caused by the aggregation of all Asian Pacific American groups under one category, many have assumed that there is a sufficient supply of Asian Pacific American health care providers and have adopted policies that seem to undermine the continuing supply of such professionals. Declaring Asian Pacific Americans an overrepresented minority has resulted in policies that exacerbate the problems in meeting the health needs of Asian Pacific American communities because less research is done on Asian Pacific American health and fewer Asian Pacific Americans are available to provide primary care. These policies also limit opportunities to improve the health status of Asian Pacific Americans by restricting funds for research, training, education, and services.

Policy Change Recommendations

Among the policy changes that might help make the supply of Asian Pacific Americans in medical practice and in biomedical research more equitable would be the establishment of data collection practices that disaggregate the various Asian Pacific American ethnic groups and distinguish between Asian Pacific Americans who are foreign medical graduates and those who are not. Including Asian Pacific foreign medical graduates in the total count of Asian Pacific American physicians gives a misleading impression of the number of Asian Pacific American physicians available to meet the needs of Asian Pacific American communities, because a disproportionate number of foreign medical graduates work on the staffs of public hospitals. In addition, rather than basing the number of minority researchers and physicians strictly on affirmative action standards, the number of minority researchers and physicians should also be based on the health care needs of various ethnic communities. That there are many Asian Pacific American physicians and biomedical researchers does not necessarily indicate that the health concerns of all Asian Pacific American populations are adequately addressed.

In addition, there is a need for much more information on Asian Pacific Americans on which to base policies. More specifically, data are needed on the number of Asian Pacific American health care providers broken down by ethnicity, sex, country of birth, location, specialty, number of Asian Pacific American patients, and languages spoken. Once such data are amassed it will be possible to study whether the supply and distribution of Asian Pacific American health care providers are sufficient to meet the health needs of Asian Pacific American populations.

Notes

1. Most relevant sources of data fail to distinguish between Asians and Pacific Islanders. Instead, they refer to "Asian/Pacific Islanders." The term *Asian Pacific* refers to people in the United States whose ethnicity is Asian or Pacific Islander. Because the term does not distinguish nationality, there is some unavoidable ambiguity when discussing data based on this classification. Nevertheless, the term *Asian Pacific American* will be used in this chapter for the sake of continuity in this volume and with the source material. When possible, information will be provided on separate Asian Pacific ethnic groups even when there are no comparable data available on the range of Asian Pacific American ethnic groups.

2. There is evidence that some Asian Americans seek Western health care and some seek Eastern health care (Hessler, Nolan, Ogbrue, & New, 1975; Loo & Yu, 1984). However, when I refer to *health care professionals*, my focus is primarily on physicians, because more data are available on physicians than on any other health professionals.

References

Anderson, J. N. (1983). Health and illness in Pilipino immigrants. *Western Journal of Medicine, 139,* 811-819.

Asian and Pacific Islander American Health Forum. (1986). *Proceedings of the First Asian and Pacific Islander American Health Forum, New York City, August 22-23, 1986.* San Francisco: Author.

Association of American Medical Colleges. (1989a). *Facts: Applicants, matriculants and graduates 1983 to 1989.* Washington, DC: Author.

Association of American Medical Colleges. (1989b). *Minority students in medical education: Facts and figures* (Vol. 5). Washington, DC: Author.

Association of American Medical Colleges. (1990). *Facts: Applicants, matriculants and graduates 1984 to 1990.* Washington, DC: Author.

Babbott, D., Baldwin, D. C., Killian, C. D., & O'Leary-Weaver, S. (1989). Racial-ethnic background and specialty choice: A study of U.S. medical school graduates in 1987. *Academic Medicine, 64,* 595-599.

Bureau of Health Professions. (1984). *An in-depth examination of the 1980 decennial census employment data for health occupations: Comprehensive report* (ODAM Report No. 16-84). Rockville, MD: Author.

California Office of Statewide Health Planning and Development. (1981). *California health manpower plan: Biennial update.* Sacramento: Author.

Carr, S. (1989). Congress challenges medical schools on progress in minority representation. *Academic Medicine, 64,* 81.

Cuca, J. M. (1980). 1978 U.S. medical school graduates: Career plans by racial/ethnic identity. *Journal of Medical Education, 55,* 721-724.

Egawa, J., & Tashima, N. (1982). *Indigenous healers in Southeast Asian refugee communities.* San Francisco: Pacific Asian Mental Health Research Project.

Gaw, A. (1975). An integrated approach in the delivery of health care to a Chinese community in America: The Boston experience. In A. Kleinman, P. Kunstadter, E. R. Alexander, & J. L. Gale (Eds.), *Medicine in Chinese cultures: Comparative studies of health care in China and other societies* (pp. 327-349). Washington, DC: Government Printing Office.

Goodman, L. J., & Wunderman, L. E. (1981). Foreign medical graduates and graduate medical education. *Journal of the American Medical Association, 246,* 854-858.

Gould-Martin, K., & Ning, C. (1981). Chinese Americans. In A. Harwood (Ed.), *Ethnicity and medical care* (pp. 130-171). Cambridge, MA: Harvard University Press.

Grizzel, S., Savale, J., Scott, P., & Detroit, N. T. (1980). Refugee report: Indochinese refugees have vastly different views and use of medical care system. *Michigan Medicine, 79,* 624-628.

Hessler, R. M., Nolan, M. F., Ogbrue, B., & New, P. K. (1975). Intraethnic diversity: Health care of Chinese Americans. *Human Organization, 34,* 253-262.

Ito, K., & So, A. (1982a). *Asian American field survey: Re-analysis of health data* (Health Care Alternatives of Asian American Women Research Project, Working Paper No. 1). Los Angeles: University of California, Asian American Studies Center.

Ito, K., & So, A. (1982b). *Whom do they serve? A profile of Asian American physicians and their practices in Los Angeles, California* (Health Care Alternatives of AA Women Research Project, Working Paper No. 9). Los Angeles: University of California, Asian American Studies Center.

Kim, I. (1981). *New urban immigrants: The Korean community in New York.* Princeton, NJ: Princeton University Press.

Kitano, H., & Daniels, R. (1988). *Asian Americans: Emerging minorities.* Englewood Cliffs, NJ: Prentice Hall.

Loo, C. M., & Yu, C. Y. (1984). Pulse on San Francisco's Chinatown: Health service utilization and health status. *Amerasia Journal, 11,* 55-73.

Matsunaga-Nishi, S., & Wang, C. (1985). The status of Asian Americans in the health care delivery system in New York. *New York State Journal of Medicine, 85,* 153-156.

Muecke, M. A. (1983a). Caring for Southeast Asian refugee patients in the USA. *American Journal of Public Health, 73,* 431-438.

Muecke, M. A. (1983b). In search of healers: Southeast Asian refugees in the American health system. *Western Journal of Medicine, 139,* 835-840.

National Heart, Lung and Blood Institute. (1989). *NHLBI guidance for minority activities.* Bethesda, MD: Author.

National Institutes of Health. (1989). Initiatives for underrepresented minorities in biomedical research. *NIH Guide for Grants and Contracts, 18,* 1-7.

Olness, K. (1979). Indo-Chinese refugees: Cultural aspects in working with Lao refugees. *Minnesota Medicine, 62,* 871-874.

Peng, S. S. (1988, May 5-6). *Attainment status of Asian Americans in higher education.* Paper prepared for the Cornell Symposium on Asian Americans: Asian Americans and Higher Education, Cornell University.

Robinson, G. H., & Schriver, J. (1989). Immigration issues in hiring alien physicians as teachers. *Academic Medicine, 64,* 357-362.

Rosario, J. B. (1980). Health problems and the inadequate access to health care services for Pacific Islanders in California. In U.S. Commission on Civil Rights (Ed.), *Civil rights issues of Asian and Pacific Americans: Myths and realities* (pp. 326-329). Washington, DC: Government Printing Office.

Silverman, M. L. (1979, October 24-25). *Vietnamese in Denver: Cultural conflicts in health care.* Paper presented at the First Annual Conference on Indochinese Refugees, George Mason University.

Sue, S., & McKinney, H. (1975). Asian Americans in the community mental health system. *American Journal of Orthopsychiatry, 45*, 111-118.

Thien, T. (1990). Health issues affecting Asian Pacific American women. In U.S. Commission on Civil Rights (Ed.), *Civil rights issues of Asian and Pacific Americans: Myths and realities* (pp. 118-124). Washington, DC: Government Printing Office.

True, R. H. (1985). *Health care services delivery in Asian American communities* (Report of the Secretary's Task Force on Black and Minority Health, Vol. 2). Washington, DC: U.S. Department of Health and Human Services.

Tung, T. M. (1980). The Indochinese refugees as patients. *Journal of Refugee Resettlement, 1,* 53-60.

U.S. Department of Health and Human Services. (1990). *Guidelines for supplements for underrepresented minorities in biomedical and behavioral research supported by ADAMHA.* Washington, DC: Government Printing Office.

U.S. Department of Health and Human Services, Health Resources and Services Administration. (1987). *Minorities and women in the health fields.* Washington, DC: Government Printing Office.

U.S. General Accounting Office. (1990). *Asian Americans: A status report.* Washington, DC: Government Printing Office.

UCLA Health Team. (1975). *Asian Americans and health care in Los Angeles County.* Los Angeles: University of California, School of Public Health.

Yeatman, G. C., Shaw, M., & Barlow, G. (1976). Pseudobattery in Vietnamese children. *Pediatrics, 58,* 616-618.

15

Health Policy Framework

NINEZ PONCE

TESSIE GUILLERMO

The purpose of this chapter is to provide a framework for understanding the formulation of health policy for Asian Pacific Americans in the United States. We define *health policy formulation* as the
translation of health issues into concrete policy interventions.
Policy interventions can originate in Congress through laws or
initiatives or come from the executive branch through the U.S.
Department of Health and Human Services, which may change,
repeal, or launch health programs. Interventions through policies
can also be regulatory (e.g., restricting the supply of physicians)
or evaluative (e.g., assessing the impact of community health
centers). This chapter is written for health professionals and researchers who may be experts regarding the problems faced by the
Asian Pacific American community, yet who may be unfamiliar
with the national policy-making process. Policy makers can gain
insight into the Asian Pacific American community from the discussion of examples, considerations, and recommendations concerning health policy offered here.

The making of policy is prompted by the demand for a change in
a system in order to solve a problem, such as making the health care
delivery system accessible to limited-English-proficiency populations, or to reach a desirable objective, such as mandating the
immunization of children against measles. The successful formulation

of policy is a result of relevant and compelling information, distilled and communicated to the appropriate policy players and their staffs in a timely manner. Put simply, it is a matter of informing the right people at the right time and at the right place, with the help of good research, media promotion, and public advocacy.

Although the elements necessary for policy making will be discussed here, we do not prescribe any one set formula for the successful transformation of issues into policies. The magnitude and intensity of the various elements may differ depending on the issue (HIV prevention versus health care reform), the authorizing environment (Democratic or Republican administration), the scope of the problem (short or long term), the proposed solution (budgetary or institutional change, national or local impact), and many more conditions, circumstances, and constraints. In order to help the reader gain an understanding of the processes and analytic techniques of policy formulation, we simplify the subject by restricting the discussion to the federal government policy-making arena and by giving examples of recent policies and programs that have had impact on, or in some cases may have failed to have impact on, Asian Pacific Americans.

Our discussion involves a somewhat generic description of the federal health policy-making process, to provide a framework for discussing the particular problems, programs, and policies that are consequential to the Asian Pacific American community. We conclude with specific recommendations for the provider/ advocate, the researcher, and the policy maker to assist them in their efforts to improve Asian Pacific American health.

Who Are the Policy Actors?

There are three major actors in health policy making: the constituency, the policy maker, and the researcher. Public interest groups and their lobbyists as well as the media greatly influence policy agendas, but these will not be discussed here. The constituents in health policy among the Asian Pacific American population are similar in composition to the constituents of other groups. They are health professionals (providers, managers, academics), employers, researchers in biomedical and behavioral sciences, and users or underserved, nonusers of health services.

The Constituent Community

The first step in health policy formulation is to establish the criteria for prioritizing concerns that can be raised as issues and that can feasibly be addressed by generating alternative solutions. The community, through its leaders and health professionals, is the best detector of what has gone wrong or what could be better. Community networks, social service organizations, schools, community health centers, and ethnic media organizations have frontline mechanisms to detect not just the news of illnesses, disabilities, or deaths, but also the social and cultural contexts of these adverse health outcomes. The sequence of questions a community member may ask that could lead him or her to seek policy intervention concerning health is as follows:

- What kinds of illnesses, disabilities, genetic predispositions (such as beta-thalassemia), and behavioral risk factors (e.g., late prenatal care), have been observed or heard of that have occurred in a number of people?
- Can I discern if these occurrences have some sort of a pattern? For instance, can the incidents be grouped by ethnicity (e.g., Korean), employment, income, age, sex, nativity, refugee or immigrant status, or rural or urban geographic location?
- Why does this pattern (i.e., disparity in health) exist? Are there perceived or actual barriers to health services, laws, research, or information that have resulted in, or contributed to, these disparities?
- Can I identify among the problems/issues any that are more pressing than others and/or that have a larger impact on the community?
- Does the problem/issue need resources and/or solutions that the government must provide?
- What is at stake if this problem goes unattended?
- Who would be the best public officials to approach, and how could I best alert them to this problem?

For example, the Vietnamese community in San Jose, California, which makes up 5.3% of the total population (Asian Pacific Islander Data Consortium-ACCIS, 1992, Tables CA-T3, CA-F4) and 27.0% of the Asian Pacific American population in San Jose, may assess that smoking among men is the foremost problem requiring intervention. Because of the high proportion of Vietnamese in San Jose, the strengths of well-established community organizations, and the

funding opportunities to design and implement antitobacco programs through California's cigarette tax initiative revenues, policies
that establish tobacco education programs targeting Vietnamese
men in San Jose are politically viable and, in fact, already have been
developed (such as Proposition 99, and subsequently Assembly Bill
75, which created the Anti-Tobacco Programs in Media, Education
and Community Interventions in 1989).

The National Policy Maker

At the national level, the Vietnamese community's numerical
significance diminishes from 5.3% of the total population in San
Jose to 0.2% in the United States as a whole, and from 27% of the
San Jose city's Asian Pacific population to 8.4% of the total U.S.
Asian and Pacific Islander population (Asian Pacific Islander Data
Consortium-ACCIS, 1992, Figures US-T1, US-F2). Moving from the
local-level issue—San Jose Vietnamese men and smoking—and
generalizing this issue to all the Vietnamese men in the United
States may be valid, based on the Vietnamese community's knowledge of widespread smoking among immigrant Vietnamese men.
However, this cultural common knowledge among Vietnamese may
not be evident to policy makers, who may question the external
validity, or generalizability, of San Jose's city issue and may require
some sort of measure of the dimension of the problem at a national
level to facilitate comparisons with other groups (e.g., Hispanics,
African Americans, whites, or other Asian Pacific American ethnic
groups).

Generally, the national health policy maker's criteria have five
dimensions (Altman, 1986):

- *Cost:* What will the proposed new, or change to existing, program
  cost?
- *Access:* Will people get the health services they need?
- *Health status:* Will changes in health status occur?
- *Administrative feasibility:* Can this be done given the existing bureau-
  cratic structure and existing regulatory environment?
- *Political viability:* Will this be supported by Congress and the public?

The national policy maker, confronted by myriad issues and
trade-offs, wants to maximize the benefits in health but is faced

with constraints, and must make decisions based on competing appeals from other constituent groups. Asian Pacific American advocates may present compelling arguments based on their ability, as members of an at-risk constituent community, to articulate the community's needs, documented gaps, and desire for change. However, the attendant policy recommendations most often come in the form of wish lists rather than as concrete options with insight and analysis of who gains and who loses, by how much, and for how long.

On the other hand, particularly with regard to prioritizing the health concerns of at-risk communities of color, the national policy maker's perspective in the past has been a function of Washington's view of racial issues as having predominantly black and white dimensions. The population of Washington, DC, is 1.8% Asian Pacific American, much less than the national representation of 2.9% and certainly much less than California's 9.6% Asian Pacific American representation and Hawaii's 61.8% proportion (U.S. Bureau of the Census, 1990). The *Washington Post*, which contributes to spinning the direction of most policy agendas, has had fewer than 20 mentions of Asian Pacific Americans over the past 2 years. Hence, unless the Asian Pacific American constituency can present persuasive quantitative as well as qualitative arguments and options, the black/ white dimension will continue to dominate policy makers' attitudes and decision making. Asian Pacific American advocates must also point out that it behooves the policy maker to listen to community representatives outside of Washington, DC, who have a better grasp of service gaps, health status trends, and disease prevention priorities for Asian Pacific American communities so that their policy-making efforts can be effective throughout the nation, with all of its varied constituencies.

The Researcher

In the policy-making process, the researcher serves as a bridge between the constituent community and the policy maker. Community advocates do not always need hard data and good research to make convincing arguments to push their agendas; however, hard data are crucial for educating policy makers unfamiliar with Asian Pacific American constituencies and their needs. Empirical validation of the arguments of community advocates provides them with added legitimacy, because the use of research signals to decision makers an objective, value-free, and nonself-serving view of the problem. Policy makers rely heavily on research studies and data analysis when they attempt to assess problems normatively, weigh the alternatives, and attach value to predicted outcomes.

To illustrate, hepatitis B infection, which is correlated with the incidence of liver cancer, is prevalent among Asia-born women. Given that the prevalence of hepatitis B in the U.S. population is under 1%, it is unlikely that a policy maker would consider universal vaccination to prevent hepatitis B, because of its low prevalence in the general population and the high cost attached to that intervention. Researchers, in studying the prevalence of hepatitis B among Asian Pacific Americans, have collected data that document the prevalence rate of hepatitis B among Asian Pacific American women at 10% to 14% and have also documented that the most common mode of transmission of the virus is from mother to child at birth. The researcher can assist the community in using these empirical data to present convincing arguments for viable alternatives (perinatal screening of hepatitis B infection versus universal vaccination) that consider costs and benefits in decreasing the rate of hepatitis B among Asian Pacific Americans.

The researcher's primary role in health policy formulation is to advance the understanding of a particular biomedical, psychological, social, or economic problem with regard to Asian Pacific American health through empirical investigation. The biomedical field in health is still nascent in its understanding of Asian Pacific Americans, owing to the exclusion of Asian Pacific Americans from most pharmaceutical and clinical trials. Physical health research is at the heels of mental health research in exploring the epidemiology of disease in Asian Pacific Americans and the cultural aspects of help-seeking behavior and outcomes. Asian Pacific American mental health research has a more solid empirical base, owing in part to the research incentives provided by the National Institute of Mental Health dating back to the 1970s that supported the establishment of the Pacific Asian Mental Health Resource Center at the University of Illinois, Chicago, and subsequently the National Research Center on Asian American Mental Health at the University of California, Los Angeles.

In 1992 the federal Agency for Health Care Policy and Research funded two developmental research centers, located at UCLA and at the Pacific Research Institute in Hawaii, to conduct studies of Asian Pacific Americans on medical treatment effectiveness, otherwise known as "outcomes research." Further, given that research that examines existing data hinges on the usability of those data (e.g., secondary analysis of the National Health and Nutrition Examination Survey will not yield any dietary habit information on Asian Indians), the National Center for Health Statistics awarded cooperative agreements for fiscal years 1991 and 1992 to the Asian and Pacific Islander American Health Forum in San Francisco to investigate data issues in sampling, classification, and health indicator development.

The role of the researcher in the policy-making process as the bridge between the constituent community and the policy maker has to be underscored. As a bridge, the researcher should not see the effective dissemination of findings to the community as a departure from, or as being outside of, her or his investigative role. Most important, the researcher has to exercise responsibility in the conduct of primary research. Without conscientious planning with the community of concern on the intent of the research, the community being "researched" may justifiably believe that it is advancing an investigator's career without seeing any health benefits. Furthermore, if the researcher fails to integrate the targeted community fully in all aspects of the research, he or she may embark on a course of study that is not relevant with regard to the Asian Pacific American constituency and its health policy-making needs.

Key to health research is the dissemination of information to health professionals and community service providers in order to assure the Asian Pacific American community that efforts are under way to improve health status, healthy behaviors, and health care access, as well as to afford the opportunity to operationalize or reinforce research findings by the network of health care practitioners. A standard procedure for submission of research findings should be to write articles for Asian Pacific ethnic print media throughout the country, including *Asian Week*, the *World Journal*, or the *Philippine News*, or through national organization and Asian Pacific professional association newsletters. Other ways of informing the public, health professionals, and policy makers include actively disseminating research findings through ethnic television, radio, and local community meetings, and at national Asian Pacific American organization conventions. This effective conduct and dissemination of research, coupled with active advocacy, can result in productive health policy formation for the Asian Pacific American community.

Once the community advocate, researcher, or service provider has shaped a workable idea into a potential policy, she or he has to be familiar with the federal policy and budgetary process. We discuss this process in the next section.

The Federal Policy Process

Executive Branch

The president sets the policy agenda by presenting his budget in January of each year. Throughout the course of the year, Congress works on the president's proposal by retooling, adding, deleting, or changing budget items, levels, and allocations. Hence, although Congress may completely transform the president's budget before the start of the federal government's new fiscal year in October, the president, informed by his cabinet members, staff, and the Office of Management and Budget (OMB), is still the key policy figure who sets the agenda (Davis, 1986).

What the president announces in January is a product of the budgetary process that began in June of the previous year, when the secretary of health and human services and other cabinet members considered proposals for their respective departments. Given this schedule, the best time to approach the executive branch with issues is between mid-March and June, when the agency directors in the Department of Health and Human Services prepare for the recommendation of proposals and budget levels to present to the OMB in September. Subsequently, the OMB makes a budget recommendation to the president between September and January (Wildavsky, 1992).

Policy making as a remedy for improving health disparities should begin at the executive branch or administrative level, where resources are distributed and legislative mandates are interpreted, then transformed into regulatory requirements. Legislative remedies to problems usually involve a prolonged, complicated process and should come as a last resort, if constituents are convinced that existing laws have not been applied or interpreted appropriately by the executive branch. Therefore, the constituent community should begin the policy formation process by becoming familiar with the structure of the Department of Health and Human Services (DHHS) and all of its agencies. The organizational chart of the DHHS is shown in Figure 15.1.

Establishing communication with DHHS agency directors and their appropriate staffs should be ongoing throughout the year. The

Office of Minority Health, created in 1990 under Title XVII of the Public Health Service Act, is an important milestone for Asian Pacific American health, in that its existence institutionalizes an administrative mandate to attend to the needs of racial and ethnic populations. Most federal health agencies within the Public Health Service, and many states, have established mechanisms to focus on minority health needs, following the example of the federal Office of Minority Health.

Community policy advocates should also be familiar with the *Federal Register*, which is published daily and provides information about administrative policy initiatives, regulations changes, and funding opportunities. Although it may not be worthwhile to purchase a subscription to the *Federal Register*, as most of its announcements do not pertain directly to Asian Pacific Americans, it is worthwhile to review it regularly at libraries or through electronic databases for occasional announcements relevant to Asian Pacific American concerns.

A very important "policy vehicle" is the appointment of Asian Pacific Americans to executive branch positions as well as to advisory committees such as the National Committee on Vital and Health Statistics (which only recently appointed an Asian American member), the Institutes of Medicine, and the various study sections that review grant proposals and set forth priorities in the National Institutes of Health, the Centers for Disease Control, and the Agency for Health Care Policy and Research.

The information lag between Washington, DC, and everywhere else invokes the need for a regular Asian Pacific American presence within the Washington beltway. Although organizations may be closer to the detection of the needs of the communities they represent in states such as Washington, Hawaii, or Ohio, the policy windows of opportunity may open and shut spontaneously and quickly, and geographical remoteness from Washington, DC, can become a critical liability.

Legislative Branch

The federal fiscal year is from October to September. Between January and May, Congress works on the president's budget, passing a budget resolution usually by May. This budget resolution puts a cap on the entire U.S. budget. If specific proposals of researchers, providers, or community advocates are included in that budget, then the months between January and May are a crucial period in

406

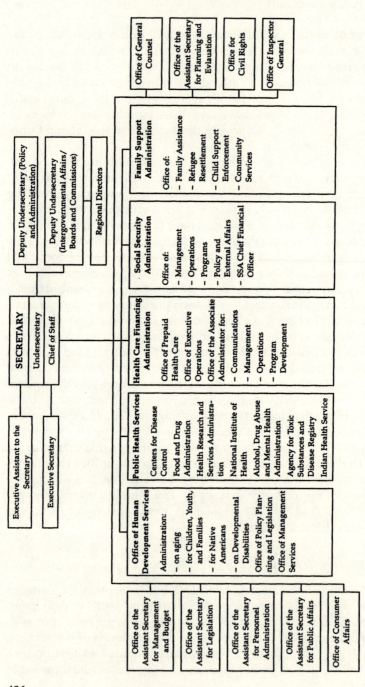

Figure 15.1. Organization of the U.S. Department of Health and Human Services

SOURCE: U.S. Department of Health and Human Services (1992).

which to approach members of Congress and their key health staff to ensure the authorization and appropriation of the programs of interest. The best time to present information and issues to legislative staff is during October through December, after members of Congress and their staffs have returned from the congressional recess in August and September and are ready to consider new ideas and proposals (Davis, 1986). These proposals can be legislated into the budget presented by the president during the congressional approval process.

Any major health legislative proposal must pass through as many as 10 committees and subcommittees in the House of Representatives and the Senate before reaching a final vote in Congress. Each committee has a function: approving the intent of a proposal, authorizing the dollar amounts, or setting the appropriation levels.

It is easy to get confused over dollar amounts. The public law may authorize funding for programs that differs widely from what is actually appropriated. For instance, the Disadvantaged Minority Health Improvement Act of 1990, P.L. 101-527, authorized a total of $12.5 million to improve the quality of health statistics for fiscal years (FY) 1991 and 1992. However, for FY 1991 and FY 1992, only $2 million was appropriated. The House and Senate Appropriation Committees decide on how much money will actually be given. Any differences in the versions of a bill passed by the House and Senate are resolved in a joint conference committee of Congress. The following is a list of the key congressional committees and subcommittees that work on health legislation:

- Senate
    Finance Subcommittee on Health for Families and the Uninsured
    Finance Subcommittee on Medicare and Long-Term Care
    Labor and Human Resources Committee
    Appropriations Subcommittee on Labor, Health and Human Services, and Education
- House of Representatives
    Ways and Means Subcommittee on Health
    Energy and Commerce Subcommittee on Health and the Environment
    Appropriations Subcommittee on Labor, Health and Human Services, and Education

Policies that affect Asian Pacific Americans and their participation in the U.S. health system are not limited to these committees. Other congressional committees, as well as the Supreme Court, have jurisdiction over related health and welfare issues such as civil rights (e.g., anti-Asian violence and "social morbidities" such as homicide and substance abuse) (Shortell & Reinhart, 1992), immigration (e.g., quotas that limit or encourage professional immigration from Asia affect the availability of Asian American health care workers such as nurses and doctors), and education (e.g., bilingual education programs to improve English proficiency, which may enhance the proclivity to access health care).

Congressional representation is a critical factor in the oversight of the Public Health Service agencies' commitment to minority health. The extensive ethnic identifiers available for Hispanics in the National Health Interview Survey, an annual survey of approximately 50,000 randomly sampled households nationwide that provides the bulk of information on the health of the nation, are the result of legislation enacted in 1976 requiring all federal agencies to collect data on Hispanics. The Hispanic Health and Nutrition Examination Survey was conducted, against the recommendation of the National Center for Health Statistics and the Office of Management and Budget, because of pressure from the congressional Hispanic Caucus and White House support. Oversampling of the black population was instituted in 1985 as a result of pressure from the congressional African American Caucus for better information on the African American population. Congressman Norman Mineta was critical in developing legislation that favored Asian Pacific American health data and bilingual service needs in 1990, with the passage of the Disadvantaged Minority Health Improvement Act. Senator Daniel Inouye was instrumental in ensuring that language noting the unique needs of underserved, indigent Asian Pacific Americans was contained in legislation authorizing the federal community health center (CHC) program.

The Use of Data for Policy Analysis

Policy makers make decisions based on current regulations or demonstrated need. Identified needs are assessed relative to the competing needs of other population groups or other issues. A case in point is provided by the current community health center program, which was established by the federal government to provide primary health care services to indigent populations in the United States. Our example centers on an appeal to increase the number of CHCs serving Asian Pacific Americans, which in turn prompted the need for a justification for increasing the number of CHCs. The current criterion that establishes a legitimate basis for a CHC is location in a designated MUA, or medically underserved area, a geographic clustering of census tracts where, among other indicators, the physician-to-population ratio falls below a standard that ensures access to a primary health care provider. A policy maker uninformed about the sociodemographics of the Asian Pacific American population may feel that there is not sufficient justification to consider the appeal or may point to data that show Asian Pacific Americans either do not live in MUAs or live in MUAs where there are CHCs already in existence.

Although geography is the primary criterion that makes a health center eligible for government subsidies, data that document the considerations of language and culture have come into play as distinctive elements by which community health providers define a "population" versus an "area" to be considered as "medically underserved." Recent attempts in Santa Clara County, California, illustrate this issue. Santa Clara County has a population of 261,466 Asian Pacific Americans, 17.5% of the total county population (U.S. Bureau of the Census, 1990). An application to establish a new CHC in Santa Clara County for Asian Pacific Americans runs up against two problems in existing policy. First, targeting all Asian Pacific Americans in Santa Clara County would require proposing a geographic service area that would not qualify as an MUA. However, the Asian Pacific American population in the county is dominated by Vietnamese, a group that has experienced phenomenal growth since 1980, clustering around the San Jose metropolitan area and constituting 5.3% of that area's population (Asian and Pacific Islander American Health Forum , 1990). The 1980 census data indicate that Vietnamese income is among the lowest of all Asian Pacific American populations, and that poverty (defined as having an annual income below $12,575 for a family with two parents and two children) is high (27.2%) within this community as well, qualifying many for subsidized care at an existing CHC in the San Jose metropolitan area (U.S. Bureau of the Census, 1980). The existing CHC, already operating at capacity and providing services to other indigent segments of the community, has no provisions to serve this mainly non-English-speaking population (88.6%) of Vietnamese (Asian American Health Forum, 1990), creating barriers to care for the indigent Asian Pacific Americans in its jurisdiction and leaving the Asian Pacific American community unserved. In the meantime, a proposal from a local, community-based provider organization that would have specifically targeted this community as a medically underserved population was not considered for review by the federal agency responsible for funding CHCs because of existing policy that disallows any geographic overlap in service area, regardless of data indicating an underserved population.

The Association of Asian Pacific Community Health Organizations (AAPCHO) has been waging an aggressive policy battle to address this unfortunate dilemma for indigent Asian Pacific American communities in need of health care. All of the above data documenting the special needs of this community have been instrumental in the consideration of changes in the regulations governing the establishment of community health centers.

Another example of the need for data in policy analysis concerns funding for prevention programs. In order to increase funding for programs that prevent and reduce deaths from homicide and suicide for Asian Pacific youth, for example, one would have to convince policy makers or their staffs that there is a relatively high proportion of homicide and suicide within these communities. The problem with this on a national level is that, given aggregate statistics at the national level, such as from the annual publication *Health, United States*, Asian Pacific Americans do not have high homicide or suicide rates compared with other populations. In 1988, homicide and legal intervention was ranked as the eighth (221 deaths) leading cause of death among Asian Pacific American males and eleventh (109 deaths) among Asian Pacific American females (U.S. Department of Health and Human Services, 1991). *Health, United States* has a standard report card function for health policy circles in Washington, D.C., and hence inclusion or exclusion of disease areas of concern or of population groups in this publication is critical in drawing the attention of policy makers. Only as recently as 1990 have Asian Pacific Americans been included in the presentation of the data.

However, in analyzing California mortality data for the age group 15 to 24, we can see empirically what we have heard of in local newspaper headlines, and community discussions, of the high homicide rates among Samoans and Cambodians. Table 15.1 and Figure 15.2 illustrate that when the data are disaggregated by ethnic group,

Table 15.1 Homicide Rates in California, by Race/Ethnicity and Gender

Race/Ethnicity	Total	Females	Males
African American	103.32	34.35	165.79
Samoan	50.87	10.31	90.39
Other Pacific Islander	28.29	0.00	58.48
Hispanic	20.56	3.97	33.76
Other Asian	15.61	9.51	21.00
Vietnamese	10.15	2.52	16.35
European American	8.72	5.72	11.51
A/PI	6.36	2.91	9.59
Filipino	5.32	3.95	6.66
Hawaiian	4.96	0.00	9.53
Chinese	4.82	1.88	7.56
Korean	4.44	1.51	7.24
Japanese	3.43	3.46	3.40
Asian Indian	2.75	2.88	2.62

SOURCE: Asian and Pacific Islander American Health Forum (1992, p. 22).

Samoans and Cambodians rank second and third to blacks in homicide deaths for both male and female groups. Although California data cannot be assumed to represent the Asian Pacific population throughout the United States, it should be noted that 39.1% of the total Asian Pacific population in the United States resided in California as of the 1990 census (see Table 15.2), as did the majority of Samoans and Cambodians in the United States. Therefore the data are significant and have relevance for national policy formation.

For both examples, the Asian Pacific American community is in a catch-22 when it comes to measures of health needs. As another example of the deficient state of health data for Asian Pacific Americans, the most adversely affected groups from the measles epidemic last year were Hmong, Laotian, and Cambodian children in California's Central Valley and Samoan children in Los Angeles. Yet *Health, United States* publishes data on measles and other disease vaccinations of children 1 to 4 years of age with only "white" and "all other" racial classifications (U.S. Department of Health and Human Services, 1990).

Under a provision of the Disadvantaged Minority Health Improvement Act of 1990, Congress authorized the National Center for Health Statistics to invest up to $22.5 million over a 3-year period to fill the information gaps in data on the health of racial and ethnic populations or subpopulations. Whereas some aspects

Table 15.2   States With the Largest 1990 Asian Pacific Populations

Rank	State	Number of Asian and Pacific Islanders	% of State Population	A/PI 1980-1990 % Increase	% of U.S. Asian and Pacific Islander Population	Cumu-lative Total
1	California	2,845,659	9.6	116.7	39.1	39.1
2	New York	693,760	3.9	109.6	9.5	48.7
3	Hawaii	685,236	61.8	16.0	9.4	58.1
4	Texas	319,459	1.9	137.6	4.4	62.5
5	Illinois	285,311	2.5	65.7	3.9	66.4
6	New Jersey	272,521	3.5	149.1	3.7	70.1
7	Washington	210,958	4.3	89.0	2.9	73.0
8	Virginia	159,053	2.6	125.4	2.2	75.2
9	Florida	154,302	1.2	246.8	2.1	77.4
10	Massachusetts	143,392	2.4	172.5	2.0	79.3
Total		5,769,651		95.7	79.3	79.3

SOURCE: Asian Pacific Islander Data Consortium-ACCIS (1992), from data in U.S. Bureau of the Census (1980, 1990).

of this provision extend broadly to omissions in data collection and research methods for all minority populations, as a subgroup, Asian Pacific Americans lag the furthest behind all other groups in the collection, analysis, interpretation, and publication of health data. P.L. 101-527 provides an opportunity to initiate deliberate efforts in the statistical coverage of small groups that have historically been left out of government surveillance systems.

Some progress has already been made in *Health, United States, 1990,* in that the publication presents tables, charts, and narratives on the Asian Pacific American population and on Japanese, Chinese, and Filipinos for natality and infant mortality, death rates, and cancer incidence and survival rates. Given that the national vital statistics system allows for encoding of Native Hawaiians and that the Surveillance Epidemiology and End Results (SEER) program registries of the National Cancer Institute encode for many Asian Pacific ethnic groups, *Health, United States* could present more detailed information. Unlike the African American and Hispanic population, Asian Pacific Americans and Native Americans are missing from charts on diabetes, hypertension, high serum cholesterol, and cocaine episodes that were derived from the National

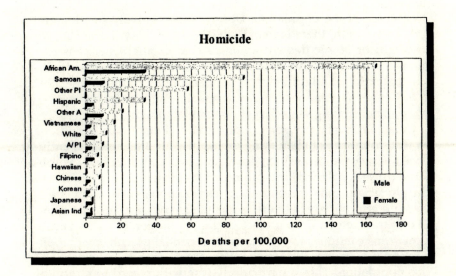

Figure 15.2. Homicide Rates in California, by Race/Ethnicity and Gender
SOURCE: Asian and Pacific Islander American Health Forum (1992, p. 22).

Health and Nutrition and Examination Survey (NHANES) and the Hispanic Health and Nutrition Examination Survey (HHANES).

Policy Themes

Although national health policy formulation concerning the Asian Pacific American community could be viewed as dealing with issues familiar to the rest of the nation (e.g., health access, health promotion/disease prevention, data quality and research), there are unique dimensions to these issues relative to the Asian Pacific American population and worthy of fresh pursuit. These dimensions, or themes, provide a framework around which Asian Pacific American health policy issues can be shaped.

Cultural Competence

As documented by the 1990 decennial census, Asian Pacific Americans represent a constituency base of more than 7 million, with a

2.9% share of the population. Despite this relatively small aggregate population, there is remarkable heterogeneity in the country of origin or ethnic descent among Asian Pacific Americans that manifests as distinctive characteristics in culture, language, political context of immigration, and socioeconomic status. In the 1990 U.S. Census tabulations, 28 Asian and 19 Pacific Islander groups were sizable enough to warrant distinct tabulations.

Culture affects perception of physical and emotional conditions as well as means of alleviating illness. Cultural factors may influence the way individuals (a) define and evaluate their health problems, (b) seek help for their problems, (c) present their problems to the physician, and (d) respond to treatment plans. Therefore effective and appropriate delivery of health care requires incorporation of cultural factors. If, as projected, the population of Asian Pacific Americans continues to experience exponential growth, health policies and programs will have to reflect more accurately the needs of this population. This is particularly true with regard to reform of the current health care system. The nonfinancial barriers faced by culturally distinct and limited-English-proficient populations will not be removed by dealing only with financing reform.

Although specific data are not yet available on language, 1980 census data indicate that an average of 85% of Asian Pacific Americans speak a language other than English at home. According to the 1990 census, Asian Pacific Americans have the highest percentage of all persons aged 5 years and over who are characterized as *linguistically isolated*, which is defined as not having any member of the household over age 14 who is bilingual in English and the primary language spoken at home. The 1990 census data indicate that in California, 32.8% of all Asian Pacific American households in which an Asian or Pacific Islander language is spoken are linguistically isolated, compared with 27.8% of Spanish-speaking households and 14.9% of households speaking "other" languages (Asian/Pacific Islander Data Consortium-ACCIS, 1992). For populations of linguistically isolated elderly, who constitute a disproportionally large proportion of the Asian Pacific population, the issue of cultural competence is more acute because they have fewer health care options to pursue compared with other segments of the population.

Population characteristics, such as diversity in ethnic origin and linguistic isolation, indicate culture and language needs that require "cultural competence" in health services delivery. Cultural competence is the key factor when dealing with health access policy and barriers to care for Asian Pacific American populations. One of the factors behind seemingly low utilization of mainstream health care system is lack of appropriate care. A culturally competent delivery system has been defined as a system that "acknowledges and incorporates—at all levels—the importance of culture, the assessment of cross-cultural relations, vigilance towards the dynamics that result from cultural differences, the expansion of cultural knowledge, and the adaptation of services to meet culturally-particular needs" (Cross, Bazron, Dennis, & Isaacs, 1989).

Each of the 28 Asian and 19 Pacific Islander groups' separately listed ethnicity connotes distinctions in language, practices, and beliefs that must be taken into consideration in the organization and structure of health services, particularly when coupled with information indicating that the overwhelming majority, 58.6%, of Asian Pacific Americans are foreign-born (Asian & Pacific Islander American Health Forum, 1990) and that this proportion will continue up to the year 2020 (LEAP Public Policy Institute, 1990).

The availability of health care services to culturally and linguistically diverse populations presents special challenges to service delivery (Asian and Pacific Islander American Health Forum, 1991) and is a major factor influencing access to care. This includes the availability of a range of culturally and linguistically appropriate care: adequately trained translators at all points of patient contact, bilingual providers and support personnel, culturally sensitive methods of care (e.g., understanding native patterns of help-seeking behavior, incorporating folk remedies with Western treatments), and the ability to obtain care within a reasonable time frame in an appropriate setting. According to data from AAPCHO, only 8 of more than 400 federally funded community health centers exist to provide comprehensive, primary care to the low-income, limited-English-speaking Asian Pacific population in the United States. These 8 centers provide care to more than 60% of the estimated Asian Pacific population eligible to receive subsidized care; the remaining 40% receive care from one of 86 centers nationwide (L. Mayeno, personal communication, September 1992).

In a recent needs assessment conducted by the Association of State and Territorial Health Officials (1992) in the United States on state-sponsored bilingual health services, only 26% of the states responding indicated that linguistically appropriate service delivery is a high priority; 54% rated it an average priority and 20% rated it a below-average or low priority. The same report indicates that bilingual/bicultural services are not offered uniformly across all service programs. Overall, the number of bilingual services offered across all state health programs ranges between 3 and 49, with STD/HIV/AIDS programs having the highest percentage of some type of bilingual/bicultural services available (Association of State and Territorial Health Officials, 1992). Immunization/tuberculosis and maternal and child health programs ranked second and third after STD/HIV/AIDS programs for bilingual/bicultural services. For distribution of educational/information services, 70% of respondent states have material in Vietnamese, 52% in Cambodian, and 21% in Chinese languages. The most utilized method of delivery for written or oral translation is to contract with individuals as needed by the different programs. Although this indicates some availability of bilingual health education, it does not guarantee that culturally competent services exist within the health care system.

Emerging Communities of Color

According to an Asian & Pacific Islander American Health Forum analysis of 1980 and 1990 census data, this population group experienced the highest decennial growth rate (95%) compared with all other population groups. This statistic gains greater significance when looked at from a state level, where increases in Asian Pacific American populations since 1980 ranged from 149% in New Jersey to 16% in Hawaii. Looking at growth by ethnic group, the Cambodian population increased at a phenomenal rate of 818%, whereas Japanese grew by only 18.3% nationally (see Figure 15.3).

Although the Office of Management and Budget accords Asian Pacific Americans a race category along with white, black, Hispanic, and Native American, most key policy documents put Asian Pacific Americans in the residual categories of "etc." and "other." The importance of Asian Pacific Americans as emerging communities of color must be brought home to national policy makers, whose decisions often affect these communities at both state and local levels. In areas where Asian Pacific Americans make up an increasingly large proportion of the total population, grouping them as "other" impedes the ability of service providers to identify and address the unique health care needs of specific ethnic groups of Asian Pacific populations most at risk. This is especially true for regions where specific ethnic groups are clustered but make up only a small portion of the general population. The increasing size

Percent Ethnicity Increase: 1980 to 1990

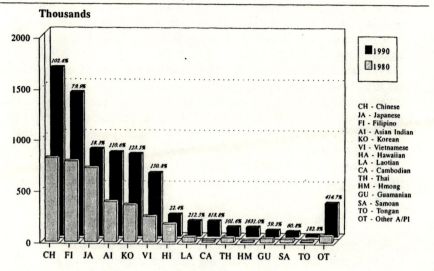

Thousands

CH - Chinese
JA - Japanese
FI - Filipino
AI - Asian Indian
KO - Korean
VI - Vietnamese
HA - Hawaiian
LA - Laotian
CA - Cambodian
TH - Thai
HM - Hmong
GU - Guamanian
SA - Samoan
TO - Tongan
OT - Other A/PI

Figure 15.3. U.S. Asian Pacific Population: Percentage Ethnicity Increase, 1980-1990

SOURCE: Asian Pacific Islander Data Consortium-ACCIS (1992), from data in U.S. Bureau of the Census (1980, 1990).

of the Asian Pacific American population has to be recognized as a specific group, not as a residual one.

Even if the Asian Pacific American population is recognized as a distinct group, this is no guarantee that the needs of individuals in that group will be addressed. In some categorization schemes, Asian Pacific Americans fall under the rubric of "special populations." *Healthy People 2000*, the "blueprint" that establishes health promotion/ disease prevention objectives for the nation, describes special populations as "population groups that now experience above average incidence of death, disease, and disability. These population groups include people with low incomes, people who are members of some racial and ethnic minority groups, and people with disabilities." The benefit of being in this rubric is that Asian Pacific Americans will be included in all initiatives that focus on or serve special populations. The drawback is that being a part of the several types of groups considered to have high risks for adverse health outcomes can dilute the amount of resources directed toward

Asian Pacific Americans. Although the special population designation is a bona fide classification for program planning and policy, it is questionable whether issues specific to the Asian Pacific American population will be addressed as such.

Whether in the context of "communities of color" or "special populations," Asian Pacific Americans in the United States are not members of the majority, and thus they have a legitimate basis to isolate policy considerations based on their distinctness from the majority. In addition to considerations based on color or other population characteristics, Asian Pacific Americans, like other minority groups, often possess additional characteristics or needs that place them at a disadvantage with regard to other populations.

Disadvantaged, Underserved, Underrepresented

With scarce resources, targeting of funds for minority populations has resulted in differentiating between minorities and "disadvantaged" minorities. The *disadvantaged* qualifier has two purposes: First, it tempers a misperception that resources are being taken away from indigent whites to go to ethnic and racial minorities who may not be disadvantaged; second, it aims to target resources not along racial lines but along socioeconomic and health status lines within races. This reasoning may ignore the physical and psychological effect of being part of a cultural, political, and linguistic minority, regardless of socioeconomic status. Furthermore, although commonly "disadvantaged" because of color, each minority group has disadvantages or needs that are particular to that group. The key to alleviating these needs lies in targeting specific populations without stigmatizing them. For example, many Asian Pacific ethnic groups suffer disproportionally from tuberculosis and hepatitis B compared with other minority groups. This disparity in health status can be defined as a disadvantage specific to Asian Pacific groups and would require policy and programs explicitly targeting those segments of the Asian Pacific population and not other segments, or other minorities that do not have a similar disparity. The understanding of needs or "disadvantage" and appropriate remedies cannot be achieved for any group if "disadvantage" is seen as identical for every group.

For Asian Pacific Americans, compared with other minorities, the term *disadvantaged* may be applied inconsistently, regardless of varying socioeconomic statuses or health needs. To elucidate this, we will examine the most prominent example of the use of the term *disadvantaged*. The Disadvantaged Minority Health Improvement Act of 1990 is a milestone health policy directive for communities of color, following the 1985 publication of the U.S. Department of Health and Human Services report on black and minority health. The provisions of the act range from establishment of an entity dedicated to minority health within DHHS to building programs targeted at specific populations and incentives to enter the health professions.

The Disadvantaged Minority Health Improvement Act includes the following provisions:

- Creation of the Office of Minority Health
- Health services for residents of public housing
- Centers of Excellence in health professions education
- Federal capital contribution to student loans
- Assistance programs for disadvantaged students in the health professions
- Loan repayment program regarding service on faculties of certain health professions schools
- Extension of the program for the National Center for Health Statistics
- Demonstration grants to states for community scholarship programs
- Bilingual assistance for primary health care providers
- Grants for health services for Pacific Islanders

Although it is clear that the intent of the legislation is to benefit disadvantaged minorities, the language is ambiguous. The specific language in the law connotes a wider beneficiary pool than racial/ethnic minorities. For example, in describing the beneficiaries, the legislative language consistently refers to "individuals from disadvantaged backgrounds, including racial and ethnic minorities." Much further into the legislation, in the section on federal capital contributions to student loans, the law states, "The term 'disadvantaged,' with respect to an individual shall be defined by the Secretary," indicating an interpretation left to the discretion of an individual public official (H.R. 5702 RDS, 101st Congress, second session). Racial and ethnic minority status is part of being disadvantaged but is not the sole criterion. Presumably, other criteria include economic disadvantage.

The ambiguity is also evident in the lack of definition of *disadvantaged minorities* at the very outset of the legislation. In the beginning of the act, there is a section enumerating the percentages of the population who are blacks, Hispanics, and Native Americans, implying that these are the only disadvantaged minority groups. Asian Pacific Americans are not mentioned until much later, in the "Bilingual Assistance Regarding Health Care" provision under the jurisdiction of the Office of Minority Health, and the "Annual Collection of Data," by the National Center for Health Statistics. Therefore, the act could be interpreted to imply that all blacks, Hispanics, and Natives Americans are disadvantaged, whereas Asian Pacific Americans are not, except in terms of language and health information gaps.

The above two provisions and the final provision that allocates grants for Pacific Islanders (the residents of the Territory of American Samoa, the Commonwealth of Northern Mariana Islands, the Territory of Guam, the Republic of the Marshall Islands, the Republic of Palau, and the Federated States of Micronesia) explicitly target Asian Pacifics. However, the needs of Asian Pacific Americans are not addressed in other provisions. The provisions for Centers of Excellence, which promote minority health professionals, have been limited to addressing gaps in African American, Hispanic, and Native American populations. Although certain Asian Pacific American populations are overrepresented in the health professions, many Asian Pacific American populations are not. Although the American Association of Medical Colleges classifies Asian Americans as overrepresented in terms of medical enrollment, the federal government includes Asian Pacific Americans as a disadvantaged group in "health manpower" (Asian & Pacific Islander American Health Forum , 1990). According to the U.S. Commission on Civil Rights (1979), from the perspective of the health manpower opportunities for Asian Americans, the majority of Asian Pacific American health care workers are second- and third-generation Asian Americans, specifically of Japanese and Chinese descent. The health manpower shortages are most pronounced in Pacific Trust Territories. A report by the University of Hawaii states that "no single jurisdiction comes close to a marginally adequate level of . . . its requirement for health manpower" (U.S. Department of Health and Human Services, 1989). For example, in the Republic of the Marshall Islands, the minimum required number of physicians is 40, but only 14 are available (U.S. Department of Health and Human Services, 1989).

Asian Americans tend to be pulled out of the disadvantaged and/or underrepresented minority group classification, most notably in policies promoting the development of minority health professions. Thresholds for affirmative action selection to health professional schools, fellowships, and training programs have largely been based on a population-parity formula. A common policy hypothesis heard in health manpower and scientific education circles is that if Asian Americans made up less than 2% of the 1980 population, but made up more than 10% of scientists and engineers in 1980, then they are no longer underrepresented. Therefore, training programs, fellowships, and admissions policies do not regard them as underrepresented minorities. A major contributor to this problem is that the National Institutes of Health, the biggest funder of health professions training programs, does not differentiate between biomedical and behavioral research. Whereas there is indeed adequate representation among many Asian American groups in biomedical research, there is a shortfall of Asian Pacific Americans in the various fields of behavioral sciences.

Moreover, there are few initiatives or grant opportunities that encourage research on Asian Pacific American health issues such as thalassemia or AIDS, hence these research topics are not addressed. Therefore the lack of incentives in health services and epidemiological research on Asian Pacific American populations contributes to the absence of a fully developed theoretical and empirical framework for strategic health policy formulation.

A key to framing coherent health policy for Asian Pacific Americans, as well as other "disadvantaged" groups, is to understand that there are problems specific to each population. Only then will policy be formulated and implemented to be population and need specific and thus be effective in improving the health of Asian Pacific Americans. But first, Asian Pacific groups must be recognized and respected as communities distinct, though not separate, from the majority and other minorities. Without this recognition, there is no basis for a consistent framework.

Summary

In this chapter we have attempted to provide a policy overview for those concerned with improving the health of Asian Pacific Americans in the United States. For Asian Pacific American health advocates, the most important thing to keep in mind is the ever-growing need for policy intervention that explicitly and effectively deals with the Asian Pacific American community as a legitimate and distinctive constituent group. Although Asian Pacific American health policy concerns often mirror those that exist in more established and visible populations, many of those involved in the policy-making process may tend to consider these issues "solved" or "addressed" using interventions designed for the other populations. It is important for the Asian Pacific health professional to be assertive about the character of Asian Pacific American communities, utilizing the above policy issues to reframe an existing, or well-worn, issue. The themes may change with changes in demographics, political administrations, and other global economic and environmental factors, but the goals of policy formulation are by definition strategic goals. Success in attaining short-term funding of a project will be short-lived if institutional or attitudinal change does not occur. Keeping this in mind, the institutional framework and the integration of approaches in the detection and the communication of the problem and its transformation into a policy should be regarded as a standard process that can be followed regardless of the issue, whether it is for today or for the year 2000.

Guidelines

For the Service Provider/Advocate

- Familiarize yourself with the policy-making process. Develop a set of principles or criteria to determine which issues need to be on the policy agenda. Develop plans and alternatives to these plans that will best address the problems of the population you serve.
- Establish the parameters of the policy problem. How many people are affected? What is the geographic area of concern? What specific risk factors are relevant?
- Define the standards for health care for your client population. Develop standards for health service translation or interpretation through a certification procedure to legitimate them. Explore all reimbursement mechanisms tied to the delivery of certified translation services.
- Determine models of service that work and don't work. Formalize your observations by collecting, recording information, and assessing impacts and outcomes.
- Challenge yourself to generate several policy alternatives. Always have a fallback position in order to negotiate successfully.

- Do your homework on policy makers: what they have or haven't done relative to your issue or target population, how much knowledge they have, and what their priorities are. Doing your homework allows you to carry on informed, fruitful discussion and to hold the policy maker accountable to her or his past decisions and future actions.
- Relate your policy issue to other existing policies. For example, language rights legislation has passed in education, employment, and voting. A connection may be made between these laws and bilingual health services.
- Seek partnerships with researchers. By exposing researchers to current concerns in the community and applied methods of program implementation and service delivery, you can keep their research better informed. They can also advise you on how to collect and utilize data for planning, evaluation, analysis, and policy formulation.

For the Policy Maker

- Congress and the administration should prioritize the integration of culturally competent and linguistically appropriate health care services delivery in all proposals for health care reform.
- Reinforce current national and state data collection and reporting systems to codify Asian Pacific populations and, where appropriate, break down morbidity, mortality, health care use, and expenditures data by specific ethnic groups.
- Public Health Service agencies should create financial and other incentives for providing community-sensitive health services and conducting outcomes research on Asian Pacific Americans.
- Public Health Service agencies should expand and fund health promotion/disease prevention programs targeted toward limited-English-proficiency populations and newcomer communities that are community based and population specific.
- As needed, increase the number of community-based primary care facilities targeted to Asian Pacific communities.
- Training institutions should modify minority education and training program eligibility to include Asian Pacific American health professionals from ethnic communities that are at risk, underserved, and underrepresented.
- Create financial and other incentives to encourage the development of more primary care providers available to serve the Asian Pacific community, and motivate a redistribution of providers to match the population demographics and geography more accurately.

For the Researcher

- Seek community participation in formulating, conducting, and drawing conclusions in your research to conduct investigations that are needed by the population.
- Collect, analyze, and report on demographic and socioeconomic variables that have explanatory power for Asian Pacific Americans. These variables are ethnicity, nativity, age at immigration or proportion of life in the United States, primary language spoken at home, and per capita income versus family/household income.
- Conduct primary research sampling from the 1990 census-designated "linguistically isolated" households. A larger empirical base would bolster appeals to policy makers for bilingual/bicultural services and programs.
- Use data sets that have extensive ethnic identifiers of Asian Pacifics, such as vital statistics registries, the SEER database, and the National Health Interview Survey.
- If you are a biomedical scientist, conduct investigations on the disease areas described in this book, with particular attention to the gaps in our understanding of Asian Pacific health and different subgroups.
- Augment rigorous techniques with second-best "policy-usable" measures. For example, although regional Asian Pacific data may not be representative of all Asian Pacific Americans, they may be used with other data or anecdotal reports.
- Include broad dissemination of findings, beyond publication in scientific and academic journals, as your responsibility. Publicize your research using Asian Pacific media and community provider networks.

References

Altman, D. E. (1986). Two views of a changing health care system. In L. H. Aiken & D. Mechanic (Eds.), *Applications of social science to clinical medicine and health policy* (pp. 100-112). New Brunswick, NJ: Rutgers University Press.

Asian & Pacific Islander American Health Forum. (1990). The development of Asian/Pacific Islander health professionals: The myth of overrepresentation. In *Dispelling the myth of a healthy minority: The Third Biennial Forum of the Asian and Pacific Islander American Health Forum* . San Francisco: Author.

Asian & Pacific Islander American Health Forum. (1991). *Nationwide survey of health promotion/disease prevention programs for Asian Pacifics* (Asian and Pacific Islander American Health Forum Strategic Health Development Program). Unpublished manuscript.

Asian & Pacific Islander American Health Forum, Survey and Research Program. (1992). *Teen and young adult mortality in California: Analysis of state of California mortality data 1986-1988*. San Francisco: Author.

Asian Pacific Islander Data Consortium-ACCIS. (1992). *Our ten years of growth: A demographic analysis on Asian Pacific Americans*. San Francisco: Author.

Association of State and Territorial Health Officials. (1992). *State health agency strategies to develop linguistically relevant public health systems: Report and recommendations*. Washington, DC: ASTHO Bilingual Health Initiative.

Cross, T. L., Bazron, B. J., Dennis, K. W., & Isaacs, M. R. (1989). *Towards a culturally competent system of care: A monograph on effective services for minority children who are severely emotionally disturbed*. Washington, DC: Georgetown University Child Development Center/CASSP Technical Assistance Center.

Davis, K. (1986). Research and policy formulation. In L. H. Aiken & D. Mechanic (Eds.), *Applications of social science to clinical medicine and health policy* (pp. 113-125). New Brunswick, NJ: Rutgers University Press.

LEAP Public Policy Institute. (1990). *Population projection project*. Los Angeles: Author.

Shortell, S. M., & Reinhart, U. E. (1992). Creating and executing health policy in the 1990s. In S. M. Shortell & U. E. Reinhart (Eds.), *Improving health policy and management* (p. 3-36). Ann Arbor, MI: Foundation for Health Services Research, Health Administration Press.

U.S. Bureau of the Census. (1990). *Census of the population 1990* (CD-ROM Series, Summary Tape File 1A). Washington, DC: Government Printing Office.

U.S Bureau of the Census. (1980). *Asian Pacific populations in the United States: 1980* (Publication No. PC 80-2-1E). Washington, DC: Government Printing Office.

U.S. Commission on Civil Rights. (1979). *Civil rights issues of Asian and Pacific Americans: Myths and realities*. Washington, DC: Government Printing Office.

U.S. Department of Health and Human Services. (1989). *A reevaluation of health services in United States associated Pacific Island jurisdictions*. Honolulu: University of Hawaii, School of Public Health.

U.S. Department of Health and Human Services. (1991). *Health, United States, 1990* (DHHS Publication No. PHS 91-1232). Washington, DC: Government Printing Office.

U.S. Department of Health and Human Services. (1992). *National health directory*. Gaithersburg, MD: Aspen.

Wildavsky, A. (1992). *The new politics of the budgetary process* (2nd ed.). New York: HarperCollins.

Index

About the Contributors

Shirley Cachola is a native Californian of Filipino descent. She received her B.A. and M.P.H. from the University of California, Berkeley, and her M.D. degree from the University of California, San Francisco. She has served as Administrative and Medical Director of the South of Market Health Center, a community-based clinic in San Francisco, and as Co-Chairperson of the State Task Force on Hypertension in Asian/Pacific Islanders in California. Currently she is on the clinical faculty at UCSF Department of Family and Community Medicine and a staff physician at Kaiser Permanente Medical Group.

Douglas E. Crews, Ph.D. (Pennsylvania State University, 1985), is Assistant Professor of Anthropology and of Preventive Medicine at The Ohio State University, Columbus. His major research interests include human biological variation, adaptability, human population biology, and Asian Pacific Americans. His research has appeared in the *American Journal of Public Health, Epidemiology, Human Biology, American Journal of Human Biology, Ethnicity & Disease,* and *Social Science and Medicine.* His current research is directed toward documenting ethnic variability in lifestyle, physiology, and genetic markers for aging, diabetes, and coronary heart disease risk factors in Samoan, Asian, and African American samples. He is a previous Associate Editor and currently serves on the Editorial Board of *Ethnicity & Disease*. He is also currently Chair of the Publications Committee of the Human Biology Council and Editor of the *Association for Anthropology and Gerontology (AAGE) Newsletter*. He is coeditor, with Ralph M. Garruto, Ph.D., of *Biological Anthropology and Aging: Perspectives on Human Variation Over the Life Span* (Oxford University Press, 1993) and he has just completed a review manuscript for the *Annual Review of Anthropology* titled "Biological Anthropology and Human Aging: Some Current Directions in Aging Research."

Robert Gardner holds a Ph.D. in demography from the University of California at Berkeley, where he did his dissertation on mortality patterns and determinants in Japan. For 21 years he lived in Hawaii, where he was a Research Associate and Assistant Director at the Population Institute of the East-West Center. His early work there focused on the demography of Hawaii; more recently he has concentrated on immigration to the United States from Asia and on the demography of Asian Americans. In addition, he regularly taught courses in the Population Studies Program at the University of Hawaii and has taught and done research in several Asian countries. He is coeditor of *Migration Decision Making*, coauthor of the recent census monograph *Asians and Pacific Islanders in the United States*, and author of numerous journal articles and papers. In 1985-1986 he was the Sloan Visiting Fellow at the Population Reference Bureau in Washington. In 1992, he moved to Brunswick, Maine, where his wife teaches at Bowdoin College and he does demographic consulting.

Terry S. Gock, Ph.D., M.P.A., is a clinical and forensic psychologist in private practice in Alhambra, California. He is also the Associate Director of the Pacific Clinics Asian Pacific Family Center in Rosemead, California. In addition, he is an organizational trainer and consultant for a variety of private nonprofit and government entities. He received his doctorate in clinical psychology from Washington University, St. Louis, Missouri, and his postdoctoral training in forensic psychology at the Institute of Psychiatry, Law, and Behavioral Sciences, University of Southern California School of Medicine. He also received his master's degree in public administration from the University of Southern California. He has extensive clinical, community organizing, policy development, and advocacy experience on HIV/AIDS-related concerns. He was the founding chair of the HIV/AIDS Committee of the Asian Pacific Planning Council in Los Angeles, and he is currently a senior faculty member of the HOPE Program, a training program on HIV/AIDS-related psychosocial issues of the American Psychological Association funded by the National Institute of Mental Health. He has also served on the HIV/AIDS advisory committees of a number of community organizations, including United Way and California Community Foundation.

Tessie Guillermo is Executive Director of the Asian American Health Forum, a nonprofit health advocacy organization based in San Francisco that provides policy analysis, information dissemination, and technical assistance on a broad range of health care concerns for Asians and Pacific Islanders in the United States. Prior to her work at the AAHF, she worked for 8 years in community health as an administrator at a community health center in Oakland, California, serving indigent, monolingual Asians and Pacific Islanders in Alameda County. In addition to her work at the AAHF, she has cofounded a number of organizations serving the Asian and Pacific Islander community, including the Filipino Task Force on AIDS, the Asian Pacific Data Consortium, the California Asian and Pacific Islander Health and Human Services Network, and the Coalition of Asian Pacific Americans for Fair Reapportionment. She serves as a board and advisory member on several organizations and committees, including the California Prevention 2000 Advisory Committee, the California Managed Care Council, and the Association of State and Territorial Health Organizations' Bilingual Health Subcommittee.

Hie-Won Lee Hann, M.D., graduated from Seoul National University College of Medicine and received residency and oncology fellowship training for 7 years at Harvard Medical School. In 1971 she went to Fox Chase Cancer Center, where she joined the research group headed by Dr. Baruch S. Blumberg (1976 Nobel Laureate for the discovery of the hepatitis B virus). For the next 17 years she studied the relation of hepatitis B virus and primary liver cancer as well as the effect of iron on cancer. During this period she held an academic appointment at the University of Pennsylvania School of

Medicine. In 1988 she became Professor of Medicine and Director of the Liver Disease Prevention Center at Jefferson Medical College's Thomas Jefferson University Hospital. She has authored or coauthored more than 140 scientific papers and abstracts. Since 1983, along with her husband, Dr. Richard S. Hann, she has been actively engaged in the campaign for the prevention of hepatitis B and the primary liver cancer that are common diseases among Asian Americans. They have screened more than 15,000 Korean Americans for hepatitis B infection by making visits to East Coast Korean churches. She received the 1990 Outstanding Service Award of the Pan-Asian Association of Greater Philadelphia and recently the 1993 Philip Jaisohn Award, both of which acknowledged her efforts to combat hepatitis B.

Richard S. Hann, M.D., is an allergist and immunologist with extensive interests in infectious diseases. He received his M.D. degree from the Seoul National University Medical School. He received all his postgraduate medical training at Harvard Medical School-affiliated hospitals, from internship and residency training in pediatrics to fellowship in infectious diseases at the Children's Hospital Medical Center in Boston. In 1971, he joined the Temple University School of Medicine in Philadelphia with an Immunology Fellowship at St. Christopher's Hospital for Children as an NIH Immunology/Cancer Fellow. Afterward he was appointed Director of Pediatric Immunology at Hahneman University Medical College, where he served for more than 5 years. At present he is back at Temple University School of Medicine at St. Christopher's Hospital for Children as a Senior Immunologist. He has published a number of articles in the areas of infectious diseases and immunology.

Sherry M. Hirota is Executive Director of Asian Health Services, Inc., in Oakland, California. She has worked in Asian American community organizations for more than 25 years and has been in health care for the past 17 years. Under her direction, Asian Health Services has become a model for multilingual, multicultural health care services targeting Asian immigrants and refugees. Her particular interest is in health advocacy and language access for underserved Asian and Pacific Islander populations. She helped found, and serves on the executive committees of, the Asian & Pacific Islander American Health Forum and the Association of Asian

Pacific Community Health Organizations. Her leadership in the public policy arena, such as serving as Cochair of Lieutenant Governor Leo T. McCarthy's Asian Pacific Islander Health Hearings, has helped attract local, state, and national attention to the myriad health access issues (language, cultural, financial, availability) and health status problems of the country's fastest-growing minority group. She currently serves on the Cultural Competency Task Force, Institute for the Study of Social Change, UC Berkeley; the Health and Human Services Commission for the City of Oakland; and the Managed Care Council for Alameda County. She has testified in Congress and consults regularly on issues of language and cultural access for the underserved, particularly in the context of managed care and health care reform.

Christopher N. H. Jenkins, M.A., M.P.H., is the Project Director of *Suc Khoe La Vang!* the Vietnamese Community Health Promotion Project in the Division of General Internal Medicine at the University of California, San Francisco, which develops and evaluates health promotion projects in the areas of smoking prevention and cessation, diet and nutrition, and cancer prevention among Vietnamese Americans in California. He serves as a member of the Executive Committee of the Board of Directors of the Asian & Pacific Islander American Health Forum and is a member of the National Research Advisory Council on Asian and Pacific Islander Health. In addition, he is a member of the Public Education Workgroup of the State of California Breast and Cervical Cancer Detection Program. He is the author of numerous research articles and abstracts in the areas of cancer prevention and cancer epidemiology among Asian Pacific Americans.

Marjorie Kagawa-Singer, R.N., M.N., Ph.D., is a nurse-anthropologist and Associate Researcher at the National Research Center on Asian American Mental Health. She received her master's degree in nursing from the UCLA School of Nursing and her master's and doctorate in anthropology also from UCLA. She is a Fellow of the American Anthropological Association and has been a Lecturer on the faculty of the School of Nursing at UCLA. Her clinical area for the past 25 years has been oncology, and her research focuses on the influence of culture on the emotional and physical adaptation to chronic, life-threatening illnesses such as cancer. She is currently a member of the American Cancer Society, California Division, Committee for the Underserved, and Chairperson on the Los Angeles, Coastal Cities Unit Multicultural Subcommittee. She has published in various journals on a variety of issues in cross-cultural health care and has lectured extensively on the influence of culture on patient and family responses to chronic diseases as well as the dynamics involved in multicultural staff interactions. She is working on defining and developing standards of cultural competence in clinical practice and serves as consultant to community groups to develop demonstration projects to reach underserved populations with cancer education and services.

Jeannie Huh Kim, M.A., is a doctoral student in the Counseling/Clinical/School Psychology Program at the University of California, Santa Barbara. She received her bachelor's degree in psychology at the University of California, Irvine, and her master's degree in counseling/clinical/school psychology at the University of California, Santa Barbara. She has taught in the Asian American Studies Program, emphasizing Asian American history. Her current research interests include evaluation of health risk behaviors among Asian Americans, substance abuse patterns in Asian communities, acculturation, and psychotherapy with ethnic minority clients.

William T. Liu, Ph.D., is Professor Emeritus of Sociology, Psychiatry and Public Health at the University of Illinois of Chicago, and Professor of Sociology at Hong Kong University of Science and Technology. He was Director of the Pacific/Asian American Mental Health Research Center at the University of Illinois from 1976 through 1989. His fields of interest include comparative family systems, mental health, and aging. He is currently conducting research, with a binational team, on the elderly in Shanghai and in Hong Kong. He has authored and edited books on Chinese society, on family and fertility in the Philippines, on Vietnamese refugees in America, and, more recently, on economic development in Southeast Asia and China. He has contributed more than 100 papers and chapters to journals and books in sociology, anthropology, and psychiatry.

Laurin Mayeno is Executive Director of the Association of Asian Pacific Community Health Organizations, a network of community health centers dedicated to the promotion of comprehensive community-based primary care services for Asian Pacific Americans. She serves as an advocate for increased efforts to develop culturally and linguistically appropriate primary care services. In this capacity, she has presented at numerous conferences and served on several statewide and national task forces and advisory groups. She also works to develop educational, research, and clinical programs to enhance the quality and accessibility of primary care services geared toward these populations. She has more than a decade of experience working on local, statewide, and national health projects, with a focus on developing and advocating for bilingual or bicultural programs.

Ninez Ponce is currently an Agency for Health Care Policy and Research Fellow at the RAND Corporation in Santa Monica, California. She served as Deputy Director and Manager for the Survey and Research Program at the Asian & Pacific Islander American Health Forum in San Francisco for 4 years. She received her master's degree in public policy from the John F. Kennedy School of Government at Harvard University and an undergraduate degree in nutrition and food sciences at the University of California at Berkeley. Prior to joining the Asian & Pacific Islander American Health Forum, she worked for Catholic Relief Services in Bangkok, Thailand, as a project manager for a health and development project in Northeast Bangkok. She has also worked as a policy consultant for the World Bank in Washington, D.C., and for the West Bay Health Systems Agency in San Francisco. She has written extensively on the issues of health data collection, analysis, and reporting for Asians and Pacific Islanders in the United States.

Stanley Sue is Professor of Psychology at the University of California, Los Angeles, and Director of the National Research Center on Asian American Mental Health, an NIMH-funded research center. His B.S. is from the University of Oregon and his Ph.D. is from UCLA. Prior to his faculty appointment at UCLA, where he has also served as Associate Dean of the Graduate Division, he served for 10 years on the psychology faculty at the University of Washington. His research has been devoted to the study of the adjustment of, and delivery of mental health services to, culturally diverse groups. In recognition of his work in this area, he has been the recipient of many honors, including the 1989 Award for Distinguished Contributions to Clinical Psychology from the Los Angeles County Society of Clinical Psychologists, the 1990 Distinguished Contributions Award from the Asian American Psychological Association, and the

1993 Janet E. Helms Award for Mentoring and Scholarship from Columbia University Teacher's College. He has served as Chair of the APA Board of Convention Affairs and is cofounder of the Asian American Psychological Association. He is Past President of the Division of Clinical and Community Psychology for the International Association of Applied Psychology and Past President of the Society for the Psychological Study of Social Issues (APA Division 9). For 5 years, he regularly taught in Mainland China and is Visiting Professor of Psychology at South China Normal University in Guangzhou.

David T. Takeuchi, Ph.D., is a sociologist and Associate Director of the National Research Center on Asian American Mental Health at UCLA. He received his doctorate from the University of Hawaii and spent 2 years at Yale University on a postdoctoral fellowship. His areas of expertise center on the social factors that predict psychological distress, help seeking, and service utilization. He has conducted one of the nation's first studies of Asian American children receiving mental health services. Currently, he is principal investigator of the first major epidemiological study on mental health disorders of Chinese Americans funded by the National Institute of Mental Health. He has written widely on issues pertinent to Asian Americans and other minority groups and his work has been published in some of the top journals in the country, including *Journal of Health and Social Behavior, Journal of Marriage and the Family, American Journal of Community Psychology, Journal of Consulting and Clinical Psychology, Social Forces, Sociology of Education*, and *Archives of General Psychiatry*. He serves on the Initial Review Group, Social and Group Processes, for the National Institute of Mental Health. In addition to his scholarly work, he has assisted numerous community groups in conducting needs assessment and evaluation studies. He has written technical reports for community and state agencies on issues related to homelessness, discrimination confronting Hmong refugees and Filipino immigrants, multicultural education, Native Hawaiian health and mental health needs, and youth correctional programs.

Ayala Tamir, M.Sc., is a Research Associate in the Survey and Research Program at the Asian & Pacific Islander American Health Forum in San Francisco. She received her master's in exercise physiology at the Tel Aviv University School of Medicine, Israel.

Her areas of expertise are cardiac rehabilitation and prevention programs, and she has had extensive experience in analyzing data related to cardiovascular risk factors and rehabilitation techniques. Currently, she is directing a project for the Asian & Pacific Islander American Health Forum, funded by the National Center for Health Statistics/Centers for Disease Control, focusing on defining the health status of rare Asian and Pacific Islander populations and developing racial classification methods. She has also performed a wide range of secondary data analysis on health, demographic, and socioeconomic information and has used this information for program planning and policy development. Her areas of interest include the relationship between socioeconomic and demographic status to health status and its impact on access to and utilization of health services among Asian and Pacific Islander populations in the United States. She has participated in review groups of the Office of Minority Health emphasizing Asian and Pacific Islander American needs and has also served in work groups of the California Health Information and Policy Project, advocating for the urgent need for health information on Asian Pacific Americans.

Laura Uba received her B.A. in psychology and sociology from UCLA and her Ph.D. in psychology from the University of Colorado, Boulder. Subsequently she had two postdoctoral fellowships dealing with issues in Asian American communities. She is now a part-time Lecturer in the Asian American Studies Department at California State University, Northridge. Her recent article "Cultural Barriers to Health Care for Southeast Asian Refugees" appeared in *Public Health Reports* (1992), and she has written a forthcoming book on Asian American personality patterns and mental health.

Kathleen N. J. Young, M.A., is a graduate student in the Clinical Psychology Program at the University of California, Los Angeles. She received her bachelor's degree in philosophy and political science at the University of Hawaii and her master's degree in clinical psychology at the University of California, Los Angeles. She is currently conducting research at the National Research Center on Asian American Mental Health. Her research interests include the acculturation of Asian Americans, psychotherapy with culturally diverse populations, Asian and Pacific Islander mental health, and the relationship between the conceptualization of mental health problems and help-seeking strategies. She has received a National

Science Foundation Minority Graduate Fellowship and is currently a recipient of a Ford Foundation Predoctoral Fellowship.

Elena S. H. Yu, Ph.D., M.P.H., is Professor of Epidemiology in the Division of Epidemiology and Biostatistics in the Graduate School of Public Health at San Diego State University, San Diego, California. Raised in a Filipino family environment, she speaks Filipino and Chinese languages, besides formal English and Spanish. Her areas of interest include minority health, aging and dementias in the aged, caregiving and the burdens of caregivers, and women's health. She has published several book chapters on these topics and numerous original research articles in the *American Journal of Public Health, American Journal of Epidemiology, Journal of Clinical Epidemiology, International Journal of Epidemiology, Neurology, Annals of Neurology, Survey Methodology,* and *International Migration Review,* among other journals.

Nolan W. S. Zane, Ph.D., is Associate Professor in the Counseling/ Clinical/School Psychology Program and Asian American Studies Program at the University of California, Santa Barbara. He received his doctorate in clinical psychology at the University of Washington. He has been the Associate Director of the National Research Center on Asian American Mental Health and currently serves as the leader of the center's research program on treatment process and outcomes. His research interests include the development and evaluation of culturally responsive treatments for Asian and other ethnic minority clients, change mechanisms in psychotherapy, program evaluation of substance abuse and mental health programs, and the cultural and physiological determinants of addictive behaviors among Asians. He has authored numerous articles on Asian American mental health treatment and services, cultural differences in assertion, and substance abuse patterns in Asian communities. Currently, he is completing studies on ethnic differences in the role of loss of face in interpersonal relationships. He has served as a consultant on research strategies for culturally diverse populations for the National Institute on Drug Abuse, the National Institute of Mental Health, and the Center for Substance Abuse Prevention. At present, he is a member of the Initial Review Group, Medical Treatment Effectiveness Program, for the Agency for Health Care Policy and Research. He has been a member of the Board of Directors of the Asian American Psychological Association and has

served as President (1991-1993) of this association. In 1992 he was
the recipient of the Emerging Young Professional Research Award
of Division 45 of the American Psychological Association.